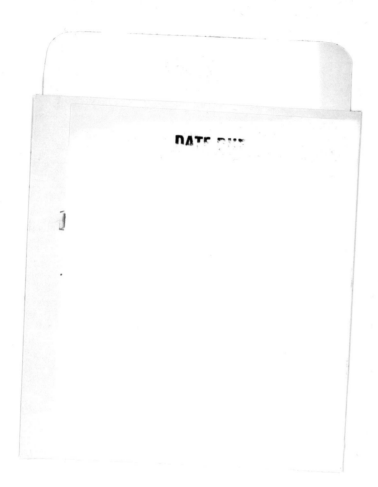

DATE DUE

INSTRUMENTAL INSEMINATION

CLINICS IN ANDROLOGY 8

E.S.E. HAFEZ, *series editor*

1. J.C. Emperaire, A. Audebert, E.S.E. Hafez, eds., Homologous artificial insemination, 1980. ISBN 90-247-2269-1.
2. L.I. Lipshultz, J.N. Corriere Jr., E.S.E. Hafez, eds., Surgery of the male reproductive tract, 1980. ISBN 90-247-2315-9.
3. E.S.E. Hafez, ed., Descended and cryptorchid testis, 1980. ISBN 90-247-2299-3.
4. J. Bain, E.S.E. Hafez, eds., Diagnosis in andrology, 1980. ISBN 90-247-2365-5.
5. G.R. Cunningham, W.-B. Schill, E.S.E. Hafez, eds., Regulation of male fertility, 1980, ISBN 90-247-2373-9.
6. E.S.E. Hafez, E. Spring-Mills, eds., Prostatic carcinoma: biology and diagnosis, 1980. ISBN 90-247-2379-5.
7. S.J. Kogan, E.S.E. Hafez, eds., Pediatric andrology, 1981. ISBN 90-247-2407-7.

Series ISBN: 90-247-2333-7.

INSTRUMENTAL INSEMINATION

edited by

E.S.E. HAFEZ
Detroit, Michigan, USA

and

K. SEMM
Kiel, FRG

1982

MARTINUS NIJHOFF PUBLISHERS
THE HAGUE / BOSTON / LONDON

Distributors:

for the United States and Canada

Kluwer Boston, Inc.
190 Old Derby Street
Hingham, MA 02043
USA

for al other countries

Kluwer Academic Publishers Group
Distribution Center.
P.O. Box 322
3300 AH Dordrecht
The Netherlands

Library of Congress Cataloging in Publication Data   CIP

Main entry under title:

Instrumental insemination.

(Clinics in andrology ; v. 8)
  Proceedings of the World Conference on Embryo Transfer, In Vitro Fertilization, and Instrumental Insemination,
held Sept. 24-27, 1980, in Kiel, West Germany.
  Includes index.
  1. Artificial insemination, Human – Congresses. 2. Semen – Congresses. I. Hafez, E.S.E., 1922-
II. Semm, K.   III. World Conference on Embryo Transfer, In Vitro Fertilization, and Instrumental Insemination
(1980 : Kiel, Germany)   IV. Series.
[DNLM: 1. Insemination, Artificial – Congresses. 2. Fertilization in vitro – Congresses. 3. Embryo transfer – Congresses.
WJ 700 C641 1980 v. 8]
RG134.I56   618.1'78   81-18910
                        AACR2

ISBN 90-247-2530-5 (this volume)
ISBN 90-247-2333-7 (series)

PRINTED IN THE NETHERLANDS

TABLE OF CONTENTS

II. TECHNOLOGY OF INSEMINATION

III. ETHICAL AND THEOLOGICAL ASPECTS

CONTRIBUTORS

ANGERER, B.: Puppenweg 42, 8000 Munich 83, FRG

BALERNA, M.: Servizio di Endocrinologia Ginecologia, Ospedale Distrettuale 'La Carita', 6600 Locarno, Switzerland

BARKAY, J.: Fertility Clinic, Department of Gynecology & Obstetrics, Central Lemek Hospital, Afula, Israel

BERGQUIST, C.A.: Division of Reproductive endocrinology, Department of Gynecology/Obstetrics, The Johns Hopkins Hospital, Baltimore, MD 21205, USA

BLAQUIER, J.A.: Institute de Biologia y Medicina Experimental Obligado 2490, 1428 Buenos Aires, Argentina

BROOM, T.J.: Department of Obstetrics/Gynaecology, The University of Adelaide, The Queen Elizabeth Hospital, Woodville, South Australia 5011, Australia

BULLIMORE, N.J.: Department of Obstetrics/Gynaecology, University of Nottingham, Hucknall Road, Nottingham, UK

CAMPANA, A.: Servizio di Endocrinologia Ginecologica, Ospedale Distrettuale 'La Carita', 6600 Locarna, Switzerland

CAPPIELLO, W.: Department of Obstetrics/Gynecology, Division of Reproductive Endocrinology, Mount Sinai Hospital, 500 Blue Hills Avenue, Hartford, CT 06112, USA

CHECK, J.H.: Department of Obstetrics/Gynecology, Division of Gynecologic Endocrinology, Thomas Jefferson University Hospital and Medical School, Philadelphia, PA 19107, USA

CHONG, A.P.: Department of Obstetrics and Cynecology, Division of Reproductive Endocrinology, Mount Sinai Hospital, 500 Blue Hills Avenue Hartford, CT 06112, USA

COHEN, J.: Department of Endocrinology, Growth and Reproduction, Erasmus University, Rotterdam, The Netherlands

COX, L.W.: Department of Obstetrics and Gynaecology, The University of Adelaide, The Queen Elizabeth Hospital, Woodville, South Australia 5011, Australia

CRICH, J.P.: Department of Pathology, University of Nottingham, Hucknall Road, Nottingham, UK

DELECOUR, M.: Department of Gynecology/Obstetrics, C.H.R. Lille, Maternité H. Salengro, 14, rue Malpart 59045, Lille Cedex, France

DELGADO, N.M.: Seccion de Enzimologia, Division de Bioquimica, Unidad de Investigacion Biomedica, CMN: Apartado postal 73-231, Mexico 73, Mexico

EPPENBERGER, U.: Hormonlabor, Universitäts-Frauenklinik, Basel, Switzerland

FABBRO, D.: Hormonlabor, Universitäts-Frauenklinik, Basel, Switzerland

FRENSILLI, F.: 5530 Wisconsin Avenue, Chevy Chase, MD 20015, USA

GASNAULT, J.P.: Department of Gynecology/Obstetrics, C.H.R. Lille, Maternité H. Salengro, 14, rue Malpart 59045, Lille Cedex, France

GAVIN, M.S.: Laboratoire d'Histologie et Cytogénétique, Faculte de Médecine, 38700 La Tronche, France

GIGON, U.: Kantonales Frauenspital Schanzeneckstr. 1, 3012 Berne, Switzerland

GOEUSSE, P.: Department of Gynecology/Obstetrics, C.H.R. Lille, Maternité H. Salengro, 14, rue Malpart, 59045 Lille Cedex, France

GROSSGEBAUER, K.: Department of Cryosperm Research, Klinikum Steglitz, Institute for Medical Microbiology, Free University of Berlin, Berlin, FRG

HAFEZ, E.S.E.: Department of Gynecology and Obstetrics, C.S. Mott Center for Human Growth and Development, Wayne State University School of Medicine, Detroit, MI 48201, USA

HARRISON, R.: Department of Obstetrics/Gynaecology, University of Dublin, Trinity College Unit, Rotunda Hospital, Dublin, Ireland

HERMANNS, U.: Staedtisch Frauenklinik Osnabrück, Osnabrück, FRG

HERNÁNDEZ,O.: Seccion de Enzimologia, Division de Bioquimica, Unidad de Investigacion Biomedica, CMN, Apartado postal 73-231, Mexico 73, Mexico

HINRICHSEN, M.J.: I. Frauenklinik und Hebammenschule der Universität München, Maistrasse II, 8000 Munich 2, FRG

HUACUJA, L.: Seccion de Enzimologia, Division de Bioquimica, Unidad de Investigacion Biomedica, CMN, Apartado postal 73-231, Mexico 73, Mexico

JEQUIER, A.M.: Department of Obstetrics/Gynaecology, University of Nottingham, Hucknall Road, Nottingham, UK

JONES, G.S.: Department of Obstetrics/Gynecology, Eastern Virginia Medical School, 603 Medical Tower, Norfolk, VA 23507, USA

KADEN, R.: Department of Cryosperm Research, Klinikum Steglitz, Institute for Medical Microbiology, Free University of Berlin, Berlin, FRG

KATZORKE, T.: Fertility Institute Essen, Cryo Center Nordshine, Kettwiger Strasse 2-10, 4300 Essen 1, FRG

KERIN, J.E.: Department of Obstetrics and Gynaecology, The University of Adelaide, The Queen Elizabeth Hospital, Woodville, South Australia 5011, Australia

KREMER, J.: Department of Obstetrics/Gynecology, University Hospital, Utrecht, The Netherlands

KREYSEL, H.W.: Department of Dermatology, University of Bonn and Department of Andrology, University of Hamburg, FRG

LAURITZEN, C.: Department of Obstetrics/Cynecology, University of Ulm, Prittwitzstrasse 43, 7900 Ulm/Donau, FRG

LETO, S.: Washington Fertility Study Center, 2600 Virginia Avenue, Washington, DC 20037, USA

LITSCHGI, M.: Universitäts-Frauenklinik, Schanzenstr 46, 4004 Basel, Switzerland

LYNCH, A.: Department of Philosophy, University of Toronto, Toronto, Canada

MAIRE, F.: Kantonsspital, 4410 Liestal, Switzerland

MALEIKA, F.:Department of Obstetrics/Gynecology, University of Ulm, Prittwitzstrasse 43, 7900 Ulm/Donau, FRG

MATTHEWS, C.D.: Department of Obstetrics and Gynaecology, The University of Adelaide, The Queen Elizabeth Hospital, Woodville, South Australia 5011, Australia

MOOYAART, M.: Department of Automatic Signal Processing, Erasmus University, Rotterdam, The Netherlands

MÜLLER, B.: Department of Biology and Zoology, Phillipps-Universität, Marburg, P.O. Box 1929, 3550 Marburg, FRG

NISSEN, H.P.: Department of Dermatology, University of Bonn and Department of Andrology, University of Hamburg, Hamburg, FRG

PAULSON, J.D.: 4801 Kenmore Avenue, Alexandria, VA 22304, USA

POTIER, A.: Department of Gynecology/Obstetrics, C.H.R. Lille, Maternité H. Salengro, 14, rue Malpart 59045, Lille Cedex, France

ROCK, J.A.: Division of Reproductive Endocrinology, Department of Gynecology/Obstetrics, The Johns Hopkins Hospital, Baltimore, MD 21205, USA

ROSADO, A.: Universidad Autonoma Metropolitana, Unidad lztapalapa Apartado postal 73-231, Mexico 73, Mexico

SAINT-POL, P.: Laboratory of Histology, Faculty of Medicine, Place de Verdun 59045 Lille Cedex, France

SCHILL, W.B.: Dermatologische Klinik u. Poliklinik d. Universität, Frauenlobstrasse 9, 8 Munich 2, FRG

SCHIRREN, C.: Department of Dermatology, University of Bonn and Department of Andrology, University of Hamburg, Hamburg, FRG

SCHÜTTE, B.: Abteilung für Andrologie der Universität Hamburg, Martinistr. 52, D-2000 Hamburg, 20, FRG

SOMFAI, B.: Regis College, Toronto School of Theology, Toronto, Canada

SPERLING, K.: Institut für Hamangenetik, Herbnerweg 6, D-1000, Berlin 19, FRG

STAHL, N.L.: Department of Obstetrics and Gynecology, University of Tennessee, Center for the Health Sciences, Clinical Education Center, Chattanooga, TN 37403, USA

USTAY, K.: Department of Obstetrics/Gynecology, Hacettepe School of Medicine, Ankara, Turkey

VREEBURG, J.T.M.: Department of Endocrinology, Growth and Reproduction, Erasmus University Rotterdam, The Netherlands

WEINRIEB, S.: Department of Obstetrics and Gynecology, Division of Reproductive Endocrinology, Mount Sinai Hospital 500 Blue Hills Avenue, Hartford, CT 06112, USA

YANAGIMACHI, R.: Department of Anatomy and Reproductive Biology, University of Hawaii, School of Medicine, Honolulu, HI, USA

ZEILMAKER, G.H.: Department of Endocrinology, Growth and Reproduction, Erasmus University, Rotterdam, The Netherlands

ZEINDL, E.: Institut für Hamangenetik, Heubnerweg 6, D-1000, Berlin 19, FRG

FOREWORD

This volume represents the Proceedings of the World Conference on Embryo Transfer, In Vitro Fertilization and Instrumental Insemination held on September 24–27, 1980 in Kiel, West Germany. Professor Dr. L. Mettler and Dr. H.H. Riedel of Frauenklinik der Universität in Kiel were the local co-chairpersons, who contributed very richly to the program.

Basic research, clinical trials, preparation of manuscripts, editorial assistance and presentation of results were generously supported by the following institutions and organizations:
Kulturministerium des Landes Schleswig-Holstein
Medizinische Fakultät der Christian-Albrechts-Universität, Kiel
Wayne State University School of Medicine; Detroit, Michigan, USA
C.S. Mott Center for Human Growth and Development; Detroit, Michigan, USA
Universitäts-Frauenklinik und Hebammenlehranstalt; Kiel, West Germany
Serono GmbH; Freiburg, West Germany
Hutzel Hospital; Detroit Medical Center; Detroit, Michigan, USA
Deutsche Gesellschaft für Gynaekologie und Geburtshilfe; West Germany
Deutsche Gessellschaft zum Studium der Fertilität und Sterilität; Sektion Andrologie

Thanks are also due to Aponti GmbH (5000 Köln 21), Bayropharm GmbH (5000 Köln 80), Deutsche Lufthansa (5000 Köln), Organon GmbH (8024 Oberschleissheim), Winthrop GmbH (6080 New Isenburg), and Wisap GmbH (8029 Sauerlach), for financial assistance.

Sincere appreciation and gratitude are due to the contributors who meticulously prepared their chapters; to Ms Jackie Mucci for editorial skills and assistance, and Ms. Jackie Smieska for editorial help. Thanks are also due to Dr. H.D. Brackebusch for his assistance during the conference; to Ms. E. Seiss for her secretarial assistance; and to Mr. Jeffrey Smith and the editorial staff of Martinus Nijhoff Publishers for their continued cooperation during the publication of this volume.

E.S.E. HAFEZ
Detroit, USA

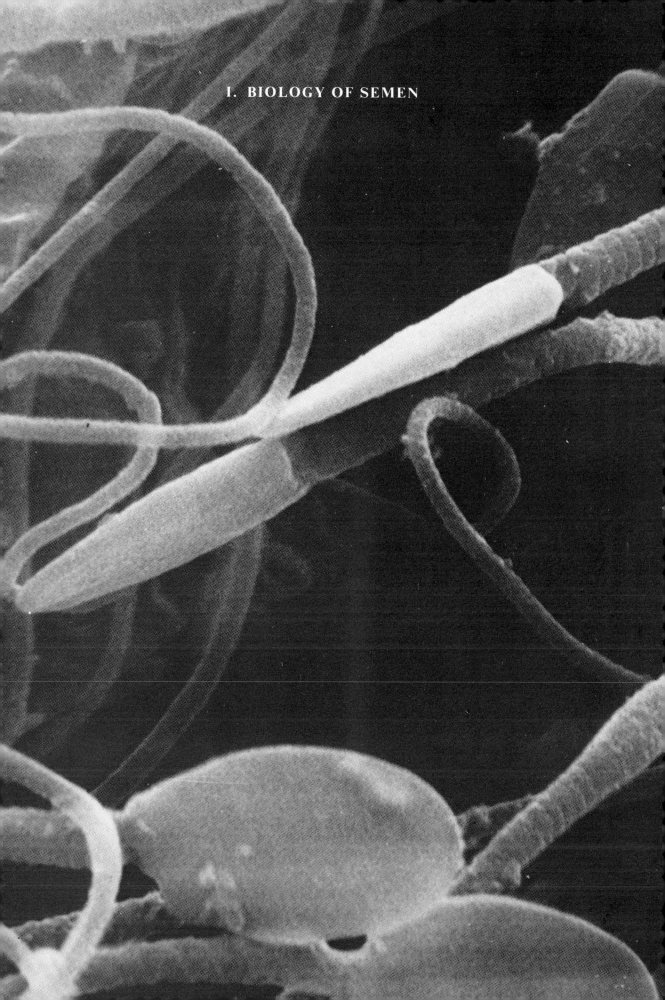

1. BIOLOGY OF HUMAN INSEMINATION

E.S.E. HAFEZ

This chapter deals with some physiological and biochemical parameters of human semen including clinical, endocrine and other methods used for the evaluation of the donor and the couple before insemination; advances in insemination technology; donor artificial insemination (AID); semen cryobanking; and conception and pregnancy following insemination (AID and AIH).

1. BIOLOGY OF SEMEN

Several physiological, biochemical, and microbiological parameters have been utilized to evaluate the whole and split ejaculate, e.g., fructose, citrate, acid phosphatase, glutamic acid, and free carnitine. The clinical significance of some of these analyses is still in doubt. The determination of concentration of enzymatic/nonenzymatic components of the seminal plasma does not contribute to the proper evaluation of semen for insemination. However, there seems to be a relationship between semen of low fertility and a decrease in total acrosin, and proacrosin in spermatozoa. Spermatozoa are equipped with two different pools of enzymes, one of which is activated and utilized to effect the acrosome reaction, while exposing a second pool to be activated at a subsequent stage for the penetration of zona pellucida by the fertilizing spermatozoon.

Some of the basic seminal plasma proteins and proteinases are similar to those in uterine secretions both electrophoretically and isoelectrophoretically. Attempts have been made to apply high resolution techniques to obtain specific patterns of seminal plasma and discrete sperm fractions from normal and infertile men. This approach may have some diagnostic value at a molecular level in certain pathological conditions.

The microbiological quantitative analysis of semen from infertile men failed to show any correlation between microorganisms and infections and/or between microorganisms and poor quality semen. The mechanism of action of decreased motility of spermatozoa due to trichinosis is secondary to the need of spermatozoa of fructose for their metabolism.

2. INSEMINATION TECHNOLOGY

2.1. Medical evaluation before insemination

Various direct and indirect methods have been employed to monitor follicular growth, e.g. BBT, daily measurement of estrogen level, improvement in cervical mucus quality, and ultrasonic scanning. The LH preovulatory surge which follows the sensitization of anterior pituitary gonadotrophes to appropriate levels of follicular estrogens may be measured in the blood or urine by RIA. The rapid RIA for serum LH, with a 3 h incubation period can be used routinely to detect the time of ovulation. There is no evidence suggesting a mid-cycle surge of GnRH which can be detected in peripheral plasma.

Ultrasonography has been applied to evaluate Graafian follicle growth in spontaneous and induced ovulatory menstrual cycles (Hackloer et al., 1978). A correlation exists between incremental follicular growth and increasing estrogen levels in peripheral venous blood. This method has been applied to measure the daily follicular growth in the ovaries of women undergoing AID with cryopreserved semen. Thus, insemination can be timed to the day before and the day of rupture of the eminent Graafian follicle with considerable precision. It is rather difficult to evaluate the efficacy of

Hafez ESE & Semm K (Eds) Instrumental insemination.
© *1982 Martinus Nijhoff Publishers, The Hague/Boston/London. ISBN 90-247-2530-5. Printed in the Netherlands.*

specific pharmacological agents for the regulation of ovulation because spontaneous ovulation may also occur without these drugs. A high ovulation and pregnancy rate can be achieved, however, by midcycle administration of LH-RH and its analogues. A step-by-step method for the selection and assessment of donors and recipients for AID has been standardized.

The decision for ovulation timing in a given patient should be individualized based on various parameters such as case history, psychological character of the patient and her response to AID treatment. Since spontaneous ovulations may always occur, one must avoid inducing an alteration of the menstrual cycle which otherwise would have been spontaneously normal.

Initial luteinization of the unruptured follicle is reflected biochemically by a rise in the secretion of progesterone or its metabolite pregnanediol. This is accompanied by a rise in 17β-hydroxyprogesterone (Dodson et al., 1975), testosterone, dihydrotestosterone and androstenedione (Vermeulen and Verdonck, 1976). The measurement of these steroids however, has no advantage over the simpler and more rapid estimations of LH for ovulation detection. While a well sustained rise in BBT may be reasonable evidence of ovulation, the thermal nadir (if any) and subsequent BBT rise correlate poorly with LH peak and ovulation.

2.2. Insemination techniques

Several techniques have been used for AIH and AID; a) intrauterine, b) intravaginal, c) intracervical, and d) the use of insemination cap.

Evidence that antibody-affected spermatozoa may fertilize if they reach the egg offers an indication for intrauterine insemination in couples with a poor cervical mucus penetration test and autoantibodies in serum and seminal plasma of the male. There is no indication that intrauterine insemination induces immune responses to spermatozoa or seminal plasma (Hansen and Hjort, 1980). The split ejaculate technique has been used when relatively high semen volume is associated with a low sperm count. The semen qualities of the first fraction is superior to the whole semen.

AIH is usually performed for six cycles. If conception does not occur, the patients are reevaluated

according to the following schedule: a) re-examination of the utero-tubal conditions, b) management of luteal insufficiency, c) investigation of insemination method, and d) improvement of semen qualities.

2.3. Behavioral aspects

The decision to accept AIH and AID may be an approach behavior (leading to surplus satisfaction in a relatively positive psychological situation, or an avoidance behavior leading to ceasing of an adverse situation). The behavior depends on different person-specific variables and on characteristic emotional changes. It would appear that there is an increasing emotional stress induced by consecutive inseminations, expressed as an influence of the female hormonal cycle. An attempt should be made to avoid irregularity of ovulation, perhaps by the early application of ovulation timing agents.

There are factors common to all women undergoing AID or AIH: the obligation to follow a basal body temperature chart, to see one's doctor at precise dates and to delay work without giving an explanation since the infertility of the husband is kept as a secret (Cabau, 1980).

3. DONOR ARTIFICIAL INSEMINATION

In artificial insemination by donor (AID), the natural (social) father is replaced by a biological (genetic) father to satisfy the parental needs of an infertile couple. AID has become popular in recent years for several reasons: a) the decline in availability of children for adoption, b) the increase in availability of semen banks and AID clinics using frozen semen from large numbers of donors, and c) dramatic changes in the patterns of human reproduction as accepted by the community (Hafez, 1977; Emperiare et al., 1980; Wood, 1980; David and Price, 1980; Richardson et al., 1980).

The recent development of AID in the USA and Europe has been faster than in other countries due to the availability of frozen semen banks (Table 1). Being a relatively new technique, AID is surrounded by social uncertainty, and there is comparatively little research or follow-up studies on the social

Table 1. Application of instrumental insemination (AIH and AID) and organization and management of semen cryobanks in some countries (data from David and Lansac, 1980; David and Price, 1980; Sherman, 1977, 1980).

Country	Application of instrumental insemination
Belgium	AID on a very small scale was first performed in the mid 1940s or early 1950s; there are no published data since the cases were very few. Up to the mid 1950s, roughly 100 pregnancies resulted from AID. In 1956 AID has been widely applied.
Canada	The first artificial insemination was performed in 1968; at least over last decade, 1500 births resulted from insemination. Currently, about 15 nonprofit University affiliated fertility centers practice artificial insemination.
Denmark	In 1967 first semen cryobank was established at Frederiksberg Hospital in Copenhagen. A few years later, other banks were established in connection with other gynecological departments. A semen bank established in Copenhagen delivers semen to clinics all over the country; in 1980, over 1000 babies were born from AID in Denmark (population 5.1 million)
France	In 1973, the first two sperm banks were established and AID was accepted as a service of the public hospitals (Necker and Bicetre) in Paris. Prof. G. David formulated three principles for the semen banks (Centres d'Etudes et de Conservation du Sperm: CECOS); a) all sperm donations must be given voluntarily without payment, like organ donations; b) semen donation must come from a couple with at least one child, and the donor's wife must give her consent. At present, there are 15 sperm banks, 14 of which make up the Centers for the Study and Preservation of Semen (CECOS) and 1 of which is independent — the Center of Human Functional Exploration (Cefer) in Marseilles. CECOS centers, located in University-Hospital centers are managed by an Administrative Board including representatives of Ministry of Health, hospital administration, Social Security and other medical disciplines, e.g. gynecology, pediatrics, genetics, virology and endocrinology. Statistical evaluation includes donor recruitment, semen preparation, recording AID requests, verifying indications for semen preservation and AID, selection and provision of semen for insemination, collection of data, and the use of findings to improve the efficacy of procedures. Based on current demand, there is a need for one sperm bank per 2 to 4 million inhabitants.
Japan	In 1948 AIH was performed in Tokyo; in 1951 the first baby born from AID was reported. Freeze preservation of spermatozoa for insemination was performed in a specific preservative (K-S medium).
Italy	In 1776, Lazzaro Spallanzani was the first to succeed in preserving human semen by means of freezing. In 1943 Prof. G. Traina reported the success of a few cases of AID; this caused severe criticism and disagreement. In 1974, during the 3rd Updating Course on Sterility in Married Couples which was held in Palermo, it was possible to report the results achieved from 1949 and after.
Spain	In 1978, Marina established a private human semen bank in Barcelona.
Switzerland	In 1970, the first semen bank for AID using liquid nitrogen as a freezing agent and glycerol as a protective medium was established at St. Gallen. In 1977, the Swiss Work Group for Artificial Insemination coordinated the activities of the centers, standardizing working methods and carrying out scientific programs on a joint basis. As of 1980, there are 5 AID centers in Switzerland.
United Kingdom	In 1973, the British Medical Association Panel on AID recommended the establishment of AID centers. At present, there is no national coordinated system of AID centers, but there are at least 24 centers which provide AID. Some 1000 to 1200 marriages out of the 400 000 marriages annually will be possible candidates for AID.
United States	AID is performed in most states and in 1980 AID was performed to single women and surrogates in California and Michigan. Eleven semen cryobanks are recognized as active centers for use of frozen semen. In 1976, seven of the fifty states had definite statuses dealing with AID.

implications. AID is the appropriate treatment for an infertile couple when the wife is normal and the husband is azoospermic or has pathological semen characteristics. Except in azoospermic men, male infertility should be considered in relationship to unsuspected female infertility. Men with relatively low sperm counts may appear to be infertile with one partner and fertile with another. Thus, accurate evaluation of the wife, infertile with an oligozoospermic husband, is as important to AID as if her husband has a normal sperm count. AID is also indicated for men who have received heavy testicular irradiation or chemotherapeutic treatment which may be associated with a high risk of new mutation. AID should not be considered for couples who have children with the relatively common birth defects such as neural tube defects, renal agenesis, cleft lip and palate.

The physical and mental characteristics and ethnic origin of the semen donor are matched with those of the recipient. The characteristics of ABO and Rh bloodtypes are also considered whenever possible except where AID is used to overcome Rh incompatability. Men afflicted by dominantly inherited genetic diseases should not be used as donors in AID.

There are no standardized procedures for the medical evaluation of a couple for AID. The medical investigations of the couple may follow one or more interviews by a trained team specializing in the social, psychological and logistic aspects of AID.

It is necessary to make a rigorous selection among women requesting AID, considering age, personal medical history, hysterogram and laparo-scopy. It may be possible to predict cases with little hope of success, e.g. obstruction of Fallopian tube, ovulatory dysfunction, anovulation, abnormal cervical mucus, chromosomal abnormalities or psychological problems.

Intercourse should be avoided close to the time of AID to avoid any possible immunological interaction between donor's semen and the husband's ejaculate. This practice has not been totally advocated by others however (Quinlivan and Sullivan, 1977).

The possible psychological risks to AID children are the main disadvantages of AID.

There are several advantages to the use of frozen semen for AID.

1. Immediate and convenient access to semen from a diverse group of carefully screened donors of known genetic constitution. This eliminates the inconvenience of last minute calls to donors and the attendant difficulties of proper coordination with the patient's ovulatory cycle.
2. Multiple inseminations in a given ovulatory cycle

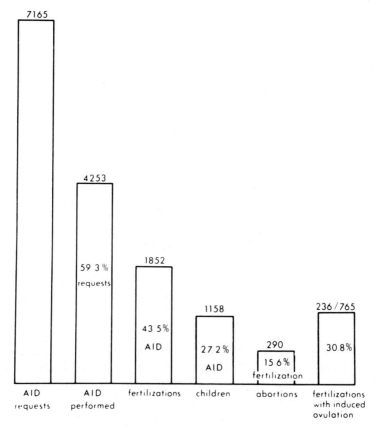

Figure 1. Results collected from all French AID centers from their opening up until 1978 (Bremond et al., 1980).

may be done, enhancing the probability of conception.

3. Access to comprehensive and detailed information with regard to each semen specimen you use: race and ethnic background, blood group and Rh type, height, weight, eye and hair color, education, religion and special talents. A semen analysis, including post-thaw motility, also accompanies each donor sample.

4. Tests of the donor's blood and semen for venereal disease and gonococcus cultures are performed on all specimens, increasing the safety to the patient.

5. The same donor may be used for subsequent pregnancies for full siblings, if donor semen is reserved in advanced.

4. SEMEN CRYOBANKING

In Italy over some 200 years ago, Spallanzani first reported his observations on the effects of low temperatures on human spermatozoa. The concept of semen cryobanking was then utilized in the USA in the mid-1950s. Recently, there has been a remarkable increase in the number of births resulting from frozen-thawed semen (Richardson et al., 1980).

Spermatozoa can be frozen with relative ease,

due to their lower water content (about 50%) as compared to other mammalian cells (80–90%). This low water content seems to reduce the lethal risk of intracellular ice formation during freezing or thawing. However, cold shock or rapid initial cooling exert adverse effects on sperm survival and some biochemical parameters, e.g. lipid fractions, cell membrane recovery and microfilaments important for sperm motility. In general, freezing damage causes reduction in the number of surviving spermatozoa, as well as failure of the normal acrosome reaction to occur in the vicinity of the ovum, or loss of acrosomal enzymes. Only semen samples of high characteristics should be used for freezing. The spermatozoal structures most frequently affected by freezing in cryoprotector medium are, in decreasing order: the acrosome coarse fibers, fibrous sheath, mitochondria and axoneme (Escalier and Bisson, 1980) (Table 2). Research on ultrastructure of spermatozoa during freezing and thawing should provide a basis for: a) structural and functional alterations in sperm, b) cryoinjury at the site and character of ice formation, c) rates of freezing as it relates to the nature of ice formation, and d) effect of cryoprotectants on cryoinjury and ice formation.

Several procedures have been adopted for the freezing of semen such as the use of the deep-freeze units with liquid nitrogen, or controlled freezing

Table 2. Various parameters for semen cryobanking.

Parameters	Description
Freezing techniques	a) Semen and glycerol are mixed in the proportion of 10 to 1; freezing is performed in vapors of liquid nitrogen b) Semen is mixed in the proportion 1 to 1 with a glycerol–egg yolk–citrate buffer then frozen in liquid nitrogen
Containers for handling and storage	French straws, glass of plastic ampules, glass vials, pellets.
Cryopreservatives	Glycerol, buffered glycerol (5–10%) Buffered glycerol with egg yolk
Indications and application of semen cryobanking	a) Timed multiple inseminations for AIH and AID b) Storage, pooling, concentration for AIH c) Failure of AIH d) Storage after in vitro improvements for AID e) Retention of fertilizing capacity in absence, death or hazard exposure of husband or donor, which may cause male infertility f) After accidents causing paraplegia associated with decreased fertility g) On demand AID, with wide selection traits h) Pre-vasectomy and pre-prostatectomy storage i) Pre-radiation storage in cases of malignancy

chambers — all followed by immediate immersion in liquid nitrogen. The cooling and freezing of semen are accomplished in liquid nitrogen vapor or cooled air (freezer). Packaged semen is placed on a horizontal tray in the cooled air, or liquid nitrogen vapor at a certain height above the surface of liquid nitrogen, or in a freezing unit. Automatic controlled freezing units can be programmed to give a very accurate controlled rate of cooling, with improved repeatability of freezing and more predictable success in terms of conception rate. Longevity and motility of sperm after cryopreservation and thawing seem to be improved by glass wool column filtration and the addition of α-amylase.

Table 3. Some ultrastructural changes in human spermatozoa after cryopreservation (data from Escalier and Bisson, 1980; Hafez et al., 1981).

Anatomical regions		*Ultrastructural changes*
Head	Plasmalemma	Absent, discontinuous, vesicular, granular, wavy, swollen
	Acrosome	Asymmetrical, destroyed, vesiculated not parallel to nucleus, enlarged, thinned, High or low or hetergeneous density, Absent, granular, discontinuous, vesicular or wavy internal or external membrane
	Postacrosomal cap	Absent, abnormal, discontinuous or detached
	Nucleus	Deformed, abnormal condensation, several large vacuoles Indistinct, absent, discontinuous or swollen nuclear membrane
	Posterior nuclear space	Absent, enlarged, open, heterogenous Swollen, thinned or granular wall
Middle piece	Cytoplasmic excess Implantation plate	Absent, large, small, vacuoles, granular or lipid droplets Contour indistinct, discontinuous, not parallel to nucleus Abnormal diameter, dissociated
	Centriole	Abnormal, indistinct contour
	Mitochondria	Dispersed, high or low number, discontinuous external membrane, indistinct architecture Heterogeneous or darkly stained contents Rounded, dilated or flattened form Cristae peripherally placed, dilated, narrowed or of variable thickness Membrane space enlarged, narrowed or of variable width High or granular cristae density Low or granular matrix density
	Axoneme	Abnormal, deformed, disorganized, indistinct contour, dense matrix, peritubular densification, tubules less or more than 9 Absent, excess or reduced number, doubled, decreased density or separated from tubules
	Annulus	Indistinct or absent
Principle piece	Plasmalemma	Absent, irregular, swollen, granular or discontinuous
	Axoneme	Absent, deformed, indistinct contour Indistinct radial spokes Dense, granular or enlarged matrix Peritubular densification
	Course fibers	Absent, indistinct contour, abnormal disposition, fibers separated from tubules Number is less or more than 9 Low or heterogeneous density
	Fibrous sheath	Indistinct contour, discontinuous Circumferential strands massed or dissociated Increased, reduced or variable thickness Low or heterogeneous density
	Longitudinal columns	Absent, indistinct, increased volume or indistinct contour

Frozen semen is packaged as frozen pellets or in glass and plastic ampules or vials with 0.5 ml straws in a wide range of colors (Table 3). Straws are preferred to ampules in terms of semen fertility, ease of handling, identification, storage, transport, and ease of insemination. Frozen pellets are formed by pipetting drops of semen directly into small wells made in dry ice. The frozen pellets are then either kept in direct contact with liquid nitrogen or packaged and stored. This method has several disadvantages in storage, identification, contamination, ease of thawing, and insemination.

The storage of frozen semen is usually on a short term basis to overcome difficulties in obtaining fresh semen at the time that it is required for insemination. However, long term storage of frozen semen acts as an insurance against complete loss of reproductive capability, which is practiced by men undergoing vasectomy and those whose work is unduly hazardous to life. Semen obtained from donors selected for supposedly favorable genetic characteristics might be stored in view of controlling production of children with these desired characteristics at some later time.

The andrologist has to rely on the donor remaining free of infection throughout the period of semen collection. In the case of frozen semen, the culture results are available before insemination and all specimens are cultured prior to cryopreservation. The pathogenicity of the gonococcus organism may be retained after freezing and thawing of semen. The American Association of Tissue Banks (AATB) has initiated close working relations among its members for the exchange of information in research and development for sperm and embryo banks. The AATB has also initiated proposals for standards on cryobanking of human semen that satisfy criteria for processing long-term maintenance of a biological product that is both clinically safe and effective.

5. CONCEPTION AND PREGNANCY AFTER INSEMINATION

The levels of sperm count, motility and morphology which are compatible with normal fertility, are lower than originally reported. High indices of semen characteristics are not necessarily associated with extra fertility, whereas semen with lower indices do not necessarily have a lesser fertility potential. Little is known about the minimal number of spermatozoa necessary for conception. Whereas conception may be achieved using low sperm numbers, larger numbers of motile sperm appear necessary for AID. At least two insemina-

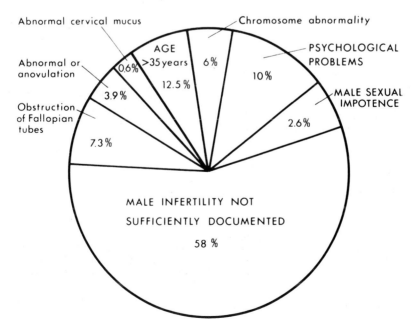

Figure 2. Study of 150 medical records of couples not accepted for French AID (CECOS of Grenoble, Lille, Lyon, Nancy, Rennes, Toulouse and Tours) (Bremond et al., 1980).

tions per cycle are recommended but more than two inseminations per cycle do not seem to improve the conception rate. Under ideal conditions of normal intercourse, the exposure of 100 ova to fertile spermatozoa is followed by the birth of 31 live children. Even among the clinics with the highest conception rates, human fertility following AID is reduced by 50% of Leridon's model. In women with correctable inovulation or normal reproductive organs, AID causes a conception rate of 40–70%. The conception rate declines in women with disorders such as endometriosis, tubal disease, pelvic adhesions and uterine abnormalities.

Even with a history of regular ovulatory cycles, some 30% of women start to ovulate irregularly or infrequently when they undergo instrumental insemination. Physical parameters and endocrine profiles for ovulation detection are time-consuming and occasionally impracticable, particularly when the patient lives away from the insemination center. Thus, it is important not only to detect, but to predict the time of ovulation so that a single properly timed insemination can result in a pregnancy.

Conception rate after AID is determined primarily by the fertility potential of the recipient provided that all other parameters (quality of semen, insemination technique, timing, etc.) are adequate.

In large random groups of women with normal ovulatory functions, the time required to establish pregnancy after instrumental insemination is longer with the use of frozen semen than with fresh semen. However, in cases of ovulatory, tubal, uterine or cervical dysfunction in the recipient, the use of frozen semen delays the occurrence of conception but is also associated with a lowered conception rate (Bremond et al., 1980). There is physiological interaction between the fertility potentials of each partner which influences the overall fertility potential of the couple as a unit. If the fertility potential of both partners is high, conception rate is high and pregnancy occurs promptly. However in the case of a female infertility or male infertility, conception is delayed. If both male and female factors are present, conception is delayed and pregnancy rate is decreased (Steinberger et al., 1980).

In order to improve AID pregnancy rate, future research is needed to improve semen cryopreservation and ovulation detection. Improved cryopreservation techniques will reduce the presently inevitable drop in post-thaw motility of spermatozoa. A reliable, non-invasive and inexpensive method is needed to predict and detect the fertile preovulatory period in the women. Several factors will determine future standards for AID, adequate documentation of insemination procedures and follow-up as to the immediate and long-term outcome for the patients and AID children. To review AID programs, complete and accurate records are kept for the ongoing retrieval and analysis of donor data. In several AID clinics, a punch-card system is used for computer storage and retrieval for this data. Future research is needed to evaluate the possible effects of AID on family structure and human culture.

Unexplained AID failure may be due to failure to detect the accurate time of ovulation or to unsuspected anovulation, frequently without disturbance of menstrual rhythm. AID failure may also result from loss of fertilizability of semen with motile spermatozoa.

REFERENCES

Bremond A, Cottinet D, Lansac J (1980) Evaluation of female fertility before AID. In: David G, Price WS, eds. Human artificial insemination and semen preservation. New York: Plenum.

Cabau A (1980) Modifications of female fertility in AID due to psychological factors. In David G, Price WS, eds. Human artificial insemination and semen preservation. New York: Plenum.

David G, Lansac J (1980) The organization of the study and preservation of semen in France. In: David G, Price W.S., eds. Human artificial insemination and semen preservation. New York: Plenum.

David G, W.S. Price, eds. (1980) Human artificial insemination and semen preservation, pp 625. New York: Plenum.

Dodson KS, Macnaughton MC, Coutts JRT (1975) Infertility in women with apparently ovulatory cycles. Brit J Obstet Gynec 82:615.

Emperaire JC, Audebert A, Hafez ESE, eds. (1980) Homologous artificial insemination (AIH). The Hague: Martinus Nijhoff.

Escalier D, Bisson JP (1980) Quantitative ultrastructural modifications in human spermatozoa after freezing. In David G, Price WS, eds. Human artificial insemination and semen preservation. New York: Plenum.

Hackloer BJ, Fleming R, Robinson HP, Adam AH, Coutts JRT (1978) Ultrasound assessment of follicular growth: a new technique for observation of ovarian development. Int symp on the functional morphology of the human ovary, Glasgow, Scotland.

Hafez ESE, ed. (1977) Techniques of human andrology. Amsterdam: Elsevier/North Holland.

Hansen KB, Hjort T (1980) Intrauterine insemination as a treatment of immunological infertility in the male. In David G, Price WS, eds. Human artificial insemination and semen preservation. New York: Plenum.

Quinlivan WLG, Sullivan H (1977) Spermatozoal antibodies in guman seminal plasma as a cause of failed artificial donor insemination. Fertil Steril 28: 1082.

Richardson DW, Joyce D, Symonds EM, eds. (1980) Frozen human semen. The Hague: Martinus Nijhoff.

Sherman JK (1977) Clinical results and proposed standards in cryobanking of human semen. In Sell KW, Perry VP, Vincent MM, eds. Proceedings of the 1977 annual meeting, American Association of Tissue Banks, AATB, pp 139–40.

Sherman JK (1980) Historical synopsis of human semen cryobanking. In David G, Price WS, eds. Human artificial insemination and semen preservation. New York: Plenum.

Steinberger E, Rodriguez-Rigau LJ, Smith KD (1980) Comparison of results of AID with fresh and frozen semen. In David G, Price WS, eds. Human artificial insemination and semen preservation. New York: Plenum.

Vermeulen A, Verdonck A (1976) Plasma androgens during the menstrual cycle. Am J Obstet Gynec 125: 491.

Wood C, ed (1980) Artificial insemination by donor AID. Melbourne, Australia: Brown Prior Anderson.

Author's address:
Dr E.S.E. Hafez
Department of Gynecology and Obstetrics
C.S. Mott Center for Human Growth and Development
Wayne State University
School of Medicine
Detroit, MI 48201, USA

APPENDIX I

AID SEMEN REQUEST FORM

Doctor _____

Address _____

_____

_____

Phone # _____

Number of insemination units: _____

Number of disposable inseminators _____

Date required _____

HUSBAND		WIFE
_____	EYES	_____
_____	HAIR	_____
_____	COMPLEXION	_____
_____	HEIGHT	_____
_____	WEIGHT	_____
_____	BLOOD TYPE	_____
_____	RH	_____
_____	NATIONALITY/ ETHNIC BACKGROUND	_____
_____	EDUCATION	_____

OTHER IMPORTANT CHARACTERISTICS DESIRED:

_____

_____

LAB USE ONLY: Donor Recommended _____

(From IDANT Laboratories, 645 Madison Avenue, New York, NY 10022)

APPENDIX II

INSEMINATION WITH FROZEN SEMEN

I. PREPARATION

SEMEN SHOULD BE USED WITHIN TWO OR THREE MINUTES AFTER ITS REMOVAL FROM THE TANK OF LIQUID NITROGEN. THEREFORE THE PATIENT SHOULD BE PREPARED FOR INSEMINATION BEFORE THE FROZEN SEMEN IS WITHDRAWN.

1. Remove the top from the tank and locate the proper can which contains the required insemination units.
2. Check donor to verify identification.
3. Lift the cane to the mouth of the tank and remove one straw (insemination unit) of semen. The straw may be removed from the can with tweezers or directly with the fingers.
4. It is not necessary for the semen to thaw prior to loading the inseminator.

II. LOADING THE INSEMINATOR

1. Unpack the inseminator and remove the metal plunger from the inseminator.
2. Hold the straw level — horizontal — and cut the seal off each end of the straw. Do not hold the straw vertically or the semen may run out.
3. Holding the inseminator level — horizontal — slide the straw — white plug end _last_ — into the inseminator (the end with the large rubber ring).
4. Using the metal plunger, push the straw — _by the straw edge, not the plug_ — down into the inseminator. The straw must slip over the cone end in the inseminator tip.
5. Still pressing the straw edge — _not the plug_ — tap the straw several times to firmly seat the straw over the cone tip. If the straw is not tightly seated, the semen will leak out.
6. Now slide the plunger past the straw end to the white plug. The inseminator is now ready for use.

III. INSEMINATION PROCEDURE RECOMMENDATIONS

1. Remove excess cervical mucus, if present, leaving a small amount in the cervical os.
2. Insert inseminator about 1 cm into the cervical canal and slowly instill the semen into the cervical canal.
3. Inseminate the woman daily commencing two days prior to the anticipated date of ovulation, stopping on the way of ovulation.
4. Check cervical and vaginal mucus pH.

(From IDANT Laboratories)

2. CARBOHYDRATES OF GLYCOPROTEINS OF HUMAN SEMINAL PLASMA

H.P. Nissen, H.W. Kreysel and C. Schirren

Although the physiological importance of sugar units in complex carbohydrates was long ignored, there has been an increase in the study of glycoproteins in recent years (Gottschalk, 1972; Heide and Schwick, 1973). Sugar units play an active role in a variety of cellular phenomence which include cellular adhesion, cellular recognition and density dependent inhibition of growth. The possibility that complex carbohydrates like nucleic acids and proteins might serve as an informational molecule has created intensive interest and research on the structure, metabolism and function of glycoconjugates. The present investigation was undertaken to determine the sugar components of glycoproteins of human seminal plasma and to correlate the chemical analyses with the clinical diagnosis.

acetates were used, because they have an advantage over other derivates resulting in single peaks for each saccharide (Lehnhardt and Winzler, 1968).

Table 1. Size of groups.

Diagnoses	Number of patients
Asthenozoospermia	18
Oligozoospermia	20
Azoospermia	15
Teratozoospermia	17
Total	70

The results of the different diagnoses were statistically analysed by using the U-Test from Mann and Whitney (Van der Waerden, 1957).

1. METHODOLOGY

Human semen was obtained by masturbation from 70 andrological patients. The size of the individual groups was arranged according to clinical diagnoses (Table 1). The analysis of the neutral sugars was carried by gas-liquid chromatography. The alditol

2. GLYCOPROTEINS IN SEMINAL PLASMA

The concentration of neutral sugars of glycoproteins in human seminal plasma is given in Table 2. A comparison between the neutral sugar content of the different clinical diagnoses shows that the concentration of fucose and galactose was significantly

Table 2. Carbohydrate concentration of glycoproteins from human seminal plasma.*

Carbohydrate	Asthenozoospermia	Oligozoospermia	Diagnostic azoospermia	Teratozoospermia
D-galactose	9.23 ± 2.57	9.62 ± 2.25	24.9 ± 7.82	12.00 ± 3.42
D-mannose	3.98 ± 1.08	7.37 ± 3.71	17.1 ± 12.60	13.00 ± 6.40
D-glucose	1.02 ± 0.28	6.12 ± 4.76	2.44 ± 0.61	1.12 ± 2.20
L-fucose	4.85 ± 1.68	15.70 ± 5.84	25.4 ± 7.16	8.01 ± 1.55
D-xylose**	0.10 ± 0.06	3.75 ± 3.31	2.94 ± 2.26	0.22 ± 0.13
L-arabinose**	0.40 ± 0.35	2.66 ± 2.31	4.65 ± 2.72	1.29 ± 0.87
D-rhamnose**	0.02 ± 0.02	4.61 ± 3.72	0.69 ± 0.40	0.42 ± 0.42
D-ribose**	1.75 ± 0.69	5.63 ± 3.17	7.91 ± 3.37	4.65 ± 1.71

* Values are mean concentrations of carbohydrates (mg/ml ejaculate) $\pm$ S.E. $\times 10^{-2}$.
** Carbohydrate could be identified only in some ejaculates.

Hafez ESE & Semm K (Eds) Instrumental insemination.
© *1982 Martinus Nijhoff Publishers, The Hague/Boston/London. ISBN 90-247-2530-5. Printed in the Netherlands.*

larger in the group with azoospermia than in the other three groups.

The significance of the high fucose and galactose concentration in azoospermia is presently difficult to assess. There may be a correlation between glycoproteins and the density of spermatozoa must be taken into account. For further investigations, glycoproteins were isolated from pooled human semen (diagnosis: normazoospermia and oligozoospermia) by gel-chromatography on Bio-Gel A 0.5 m. The two glycoproteins of different molecular weight were analysed for carbohydrate and amino acid content (Tables 3, 4 and 5). In order to elucidate the chemical structure of the glycopeptide

Table 3. Carbohydrate composition of glycoproteins from human seminal plasma.*

Parameters	^{GP}I Normo	^{GP}I Oligo	^{GP}II Normo	^{GP}II Oligo
Neutral sugar	4.6	4.0	2.7	2.5
Hexosamine	2.3	2.2	2.0	1.8
Sialic acid	2.0	1.7	0.7	0.3
Total	8.9	7.9	5.4	4.6
Molar ratio:				
N-acetylglucosamine N-acetylgalactosamine	0.78	0.84	3.1	7.75

* Expressed as a percentage of the total glycoprotein.

Table 4. Neutral sugar composition.*

Parameters	^{GP}I Normo	^{GP}I Oligo	^{GP}II Normo	^{GP}II Oligo
Fucose	34.0	27.7	10.7	3.7
Xylose	0.7	1.0	2.3	1.0
Galactose	60.7	63.1	19.8	26.1
Mannose	3.5	6.4	30.6	33.5
Glucose	1.0	1.2	36.5	35.7

* Expressed as a percentage of the total neutral sugar.

Table 5. Amino acid and amino sugar composition of glycoproteins of human seminal plasma (moles per 100 moles amino acid).

Amino acids	^{GP}I Normo-	^{GP}I Oligo-	^{GP}II Normo-	^{GP}II Oligo-
Asp	6.07	11.15	11.59	12.03
Thr	9.11	8.99	7.89	7.33
Ser	8.29	11.42	13.31	9.25
Glu	8.06	8.53	8.15	7.29
Pro	6.19	4.88	2.69	6.41
Gly	5.02	8.82	9.16	9.66
Ala	4.44	4.33	4.06	5.50
Cys	1.40	0.33	0.90	2.24
Val	2.80	2.94	5.27	4.76
Met	1.29	—	0.41	—
GlcN	8.29	4.88	0.95	7.36
GalN	10.63	5.81	0.30	0.95
Ileu	1.87	1.24	4.90	2.02
Leu	5.26	3.80	9.24	4.79
Tyr	0.58	0.86	4.58	0.87
Phe	2.10	0.99	3.14	0.62
Orn	1.99	—	—	—
Lys	3.62	7.67	1.87	5.95
His	3.62	8.62	7.29	9.72
Arg	9.34	4.66	4.32	3.25

bonds, glycopeptide fractions were prepared from the glycoproteins by digestion with pronase.

The resulting glycopeptides were purified by gel filtration on Bio-Gel P-6. The polypeptides of the glycoproteins with the lower molecular weight did not undergo alkaline-elimination. The attachment of the oligosaccharide chains to the polypeptide is an N-glycosidic bond between C_1 of N-acetyl-glucosamine and asparagine. The bond of the other glycoprotein is under investigation. Studies of the sequence of the sugars in the carbohydrate unit with

glycosidases are difficult because the isolated glyco-proteins are heterogeneous. There are still dif-ferences in the carbohydrate and amino acid com-position of the two andrological conditions. If the molecules show a high degree of heterogeneity and if pooled samples are used, it may be possible to give average values for the composition.

Further investigations on single ejaculates with a refined technique are necessary to elucidate the function of glycoproteins, and especially of their carbohydrate unit, in reproduction.

REFERENCES

Gottschalk A (1972) Glycoproteins, their composition, structure and function. Zweite Aufl BBA library, Bd. 5. Amsterdam: Elsevier.

Heide K, Schwick HG (1973) Chemie und Bedeutung des Kohlenhydrat-Anteils menschlicher Serum-Glykoproteine. Angew Chem 85: 803.

Lehnhardt WF, Winzler RJ, (1968) Determination of neutral sugars in glycoproteins by gas-liquid-chromatography. J Chromatogr 34: 471.

Van der Waerden B (1975) Mathematische Statistik. Berlin: Springer.

Author's address:
Dr H.P. Nissen
Univ. Klinik für Hautkrankheiten
Abtg. für experimentelle Dermatologie
Venusberg, 5300 Bonn 1, FRG

3. HIGH-RESOLUTION SEMINAL PLASMA PROTEIN PATTERNS IN NORMAL AND INFERTILE MEN

M. Balerna, A. Campana, D Fabbro and U. Eppenberger

Seminal plasma has been the subject of studies dealing with its composition, homeostatic regulation and interaction with spermatozoa in men, and especially in non-human primates, for a long time (cf. Mann, 1975, 1977). Even today, however, there does not exist a unitary concept about its role(s). The older view (i.e. of seminal plasma as a transport and possible buffering fluid) is rapidly changing as our physiological and biochemical knowledge evolves. The investigations on split-ejaculates as well as the numerous analytical studies made in recent years have in fact revealed several metabolic, enzymologic, immunologic and sperm protecting functions (Mann, 1977; Tauber et al., 1975, 1976; Lindholmer et al., 1974; Umapathy et al., 1980; Chang et al., 1977; Oliphant, 1976). Clinical evidence also begins to suggest that the ejaculate in its integrity (and not only the spermatozoon) is of importance for the achievement of high pregnancy rates in artificial insemination (J. Kremer, personal communication).

Because of our interest in normal and infertile human sperm, we recently started an analytical and possibly systematical study on the protein composition of the seminal plasma (SP) derived from the semen of both patients and donors visiting our clinic. This paper focuses on the methodological approaches we developed for proper analysis of SP proteins by isoelectrofocusing and high-resolution eletrophoresis techniques as well as on the evaluation of some of the results so far obtained.

1. THE SEPARATION OF SP PROTEINS BY ISOELECTROFOCUSING (PAGIEF)

1.1. Methodology

Urea and non-ionic detergents as well as SDS are today widely used in combination with PAGE or PAGIEF, to break molecular aggregates and to improve the resolution of complex protein mixtures such as those found in body fluids. The same approach is extensively applied also in view of bi-dimensional separations (the interested reader is referred to "Electrophoresis '79" (Radola, 1980) for an updated methodological overall review). We also tried to use these agents (such as Nonidet P-40 and Triton X-100, as well as urea) in various combinations and proportions during sample preparation and gel run but, at least in our hands, superior quality separations of SP-proteins have been obtained without these agents. The gel formula finally adopted for routine analysis of SP samples is given in the Appendix, and was derived from current formulations used in PAGIEF routine (Winter et al., 1977).

SP was obtained from centrifugation at room temperature (2000 g/20 min) of fresh or frozen-thawed sperm and was diluted 1/3 (v/v) with de-ionized water.

The gels (250 × 100 × 1.5 mm) were always prepared the day before use and left overnight at room temperature. About 30–60 min before the run, the gels were cooled to $+4°$ C, mounted on a Multiphor LKB-apparatus (LKB, Sweden) and provided with the electrode filter strips (1 M NaOH, 1 M $H_3 PO_4$). The samples (usually 5–10 μl of diluted SP, i.e. about 80–160 μg of proteins) were deposed on small rectangular filter papers (Pharmacia) and the gel run first at constant current, then at constant power (for a 250 × 110 × 1.5 mm gel: 30 mA ($\sim 90 \rightarrow \sim 520$ V), 9 W). The gel was cooled with running tap water (12–13° C) and the run terminated after 130 min (reproducibly optimal running time using LKB ampholines) by immediate fixation with the trichloroacetic–sulfosalicylic acid mixture followed by staining and destaining as recommended (Winter et al., 1977).

Hafez ESE & Semm K (Eds) Instrumental insemination.

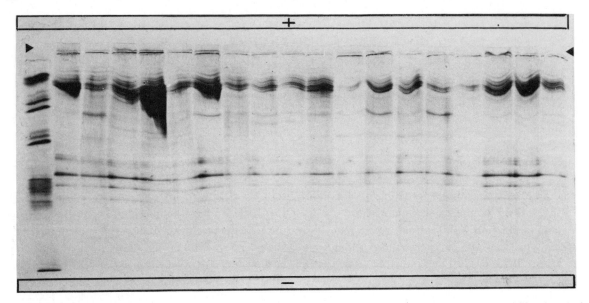

Figure 1. Comparative PAGIEF run of the SP proteins derived from 18 different sperm samples. Ten microliters of diluted seminal plasma (1/3 with water) were focussed on a 250 × 110 × 1.5 mm gel (5% T, 5.4% C see Appendix) for 130 min at 12–13° C. The samples were applied anodically (arrow on the top). Left: pI-markers. Please note the 'constitutive' proteins (present in every lane) as well as the pattern variability.

1.2. Routine screening

An example of the separation of SP proteins by the described PAGIEF is shown in Fig. 1. The analytical parameters finally chosen, the large capacity of the PAGIEF-system (up to 30 samples) and the reproducibility of the patterns obtained by strict standardization of the procedure allow for a rapid and efficient screening of the proteins. Up to 30 different protein and peptide bands are detectable by Coomassie coloration and the bands are found to by smoothly distributed on about 90% of the gel surface, many (but not all) of these bands are present in every lane. The overal impression one gets from patterns like those given in Fig. 1 is that the protein and peptide distribution is fairly constant in all samples and that most of them have a neutral–acidic pI. The bands seen in Fig. 1 are not only single proteins but also protein complexes (bi- or multi-component aggregates, see section IV).

The analysis performed on over 200 "normal" and "abnormal" sperm samples revealed, however, that this pattern constancy has at least two important exceptions:

1) a remarkable richness in neutral–basic proteins (pI 7 to 8.4) has been found in some SP obtained from normal wealthy sperm donors (see Figs. 2b and 2c) as well as in some pathological cases (Fig. 3);

2) in some of these pathological sperms one finds an almost quantitative lack of the "acidic complex" (around pI 4, Fig. 3).

The patterns of Fig. 2 offer two other important pieces of information:

1) the protein pattern does not change when the centrifugation conditions are changed (here from 1650 to 100000 *g*, Fig. 2a);

2) the SP protein composition in the same individual seems to be time variant (Figs. 2b and 2c). Variability exists in the composition of seminal plasma constituents in individuals belonging to the same species (Mann, 1975; see also Fig. 1). Figure 2c shows that a (cyclic?) variability, at least in the protein contents and types, seems to be present for this individual as a function of time. The fact that the basic bands and not the acidic region seem to be involved in this phenomenon, as well as its physiological and clinical implications, are not understood at the moment.

1.3. Other studies

The same analytical procedure can also be applied to all sort of studies centered on SP proteins. As an example, the result of an autoproteolysis study is shown in Fig. 4. PAGIEF reveals that proteolysis hardly operates in this as well as in other samples

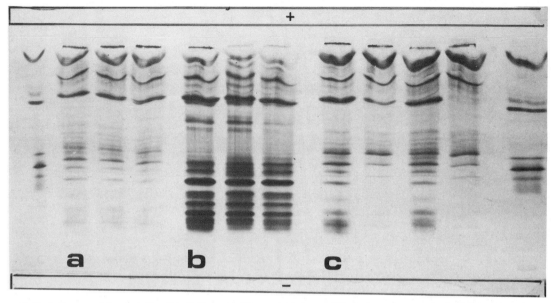

Figure 2. *2a*: Influence of the centrifugation field on the SP protein pattern. 500 μl of a sperm sample were diluted with 1000 μl of NaCl 0.9% (154 mM). After gently mixing, the sperm was sequentially centrifuged for 20 min at 1650, 12000 and 100000 g (from left to right). A 10 μl aliquot was withdrawn after each step and applied on small filter papers on the gel. *b and c:* Sp protein patterns of normal sperm donors as a function of time: *2b:* sperm obtained at days 1, 13 and 15; *2c:* sperm obtained at days 1, 18, 24 and 28. Liquefied sperms were frozen at $-25°$ C, then thawed, centrifuged (see text) and the SP diluted and processed on PAGIEF. Left and right: pI markers. Run conditions as in Fig. 1.

we analyzed, at least during the first 6–8 h at 37° C. Longer incubation times (24 and 36 h at 37° C, last two bands on the right in Fig. 4) show limited, but easily detectable, changes in the protein pattern.

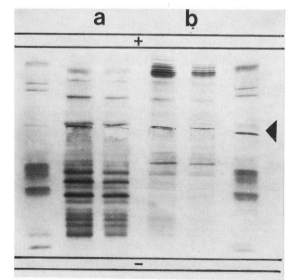

Figure 3. PAGIEF of SP. *3a:* SP proteins of AT-patient (astheno-teratozoospermia). *3b:* SP proteins from a patient with normal sperm parameters. Two aliquots (10 and 5 μl, about 160 and 80 μg protein) of the 1/3 diluted SPs were applied on the center of a $125 \times 110 \times 1.5$ mm gel (arrow) and run at 15 mA/5 W. The other experimental conditions are as in the legend of Fig. 1 (left and right: pI markers).

These results support those recently published by other authors (Thangnipon and Chulavatnatol, 1979) but do not explain the sudden rise of free amino acid content in SP after its liquefaction reported originally by Jacobsson (1950).

1.4. Limitations of PAGIEF

Despite their good quality, the patterns obtained by PAGIEF cannot give the full protein analytical detail of SP. This can easily be demonstrated by performing a 2d-electrophoretic run with the same samples: the number of peptides and proteins detected in this case is at least twice as high (see section IV). A major drawback encountered in the use of PAGIEF with SP proteins has been the impossibility (under our experimental conditions) to use this method for a comparative study of blood plasma proteins and SP proteins coming from the same individual. The fairly strong complexes formed by blood plasma proteins call for the use of a high urea concentration in both sample and gel to obtain high-resolution separations (Atland and Hackler, 1980). This was expressly avoided in the present work; one of the aims of this study was in fact to obtain SP proteins for future (e.g. immuno-

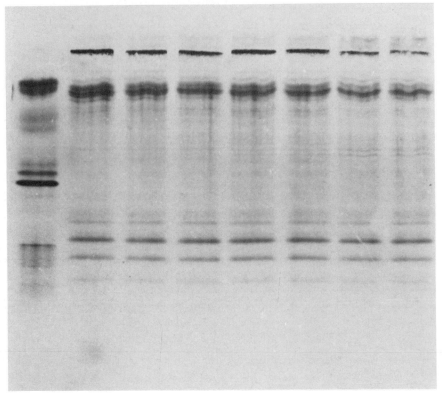

Figure 4. Autoproteolysis in SP. A sperm sample was left to liquefy over 40 min at 37°C (t = 0). At t = 0, 2, 4, 6, 8, 24 and 32 h (37°C). An aliquot of 100 μl was withdrawn, centrifuged (2000/20 min) and the supernatant immediately frozen (−25°C). For analysis, the aliquots were thawed, diluted and processed by PAGIEF as described (see Appendix and Fig. 1). Note that minor shifts in the protein pattern can be observed only at the longest incubation times. Left: pI markers.

chemical, enzymologic) work in their native state. The usefulness of PAGIEF for comparative purposes, however, has not been matched by other electroanalytical procedures used in this study.

2. THE SEPARATION OF SP PROTEINS BY SDS-POLYACRYLAMIDE GEL ECTROPHORESIS (SDS-PAGE)

By this powerful electrophoretic method (probably the most widely used in biochemical research today) only limited information could be obtained when comparing "normal" and "abnormal" SP proteins patterns. The resolution can be made nearly optimal (Fig. 5), but in all cases tested most of the bands gather together near the front (the 10 to 20 kilodalton region) despite the use of acrylamide gradients (5–15 or 10–20%) and of a discontinuous system (Laemmli, 1970). Under the strongly denaturing conditions used for the preparation of the samples (1% SDS, 5% β-mercaptoethanol, 10 min

95–100°C), no bands of $M_r \geqslant 80000$ were normally found. The major bands in the 20 to 70 kilodalton region had an M_r of 75000, 68000 (albumin), 49000 and 32000 (Fig. 5a), but represent only about 5–10% of the total Coomassie peak integral. These technical limitations make the comparison between the different samples more difficult.

3. SEPARATION OF SP PROTEINS BY NORMAL PAGE

The observation that SP proteins do not form strong complexes *in vivo* (see section 1 above), and the limitations for comparative studies encountered by the use of SDS-PAGE, prompted us to try the continuous Tris–glycine PAGE system devised and successfully applied to blood plasma proteins by Hoffmeister and co-workers (Abraham et al., 1970). Figure 6a shows an example of the results obtained.

The following comments can be made:
1) The resolution obtained with blood plasma-

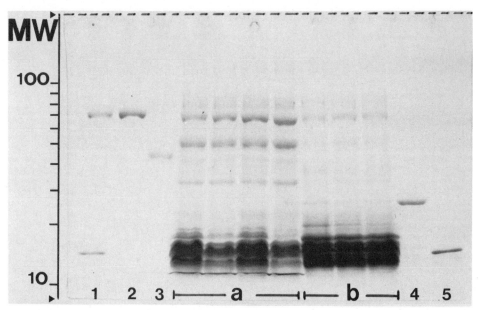

Figure 5. 5a: Polyacrylamide-gel ectrophoresis of SP proteins in the presence of sodium dodecylsulfate (SDS-PAGE, Laemmli). Lanes (from left to right): 1: lysozyme and BSA; 2: BSA (68000 daltons) 3: ovalbumin (45000 daltons); a: the four SP samples (donor sperm) given in Fig. 2c; b: the three SP samples (donor sperm) given in Fig. 2b; 4: chymotrypsinogen (25500 daltons; 5: lysozyme (14400 daltons). The broken line on the top indicates the top of the separation gel. Gel dimensions (sep.gel): 115 × 150 × 2 mm. Run conditions: RT, 90–200 V, 5 h. Staining–destaining with Coomassie Brillant Blue as described by Fairbanks et al. (1970). The MW scale (log-scale) on the left is given in daltons × 10^{-3}. *5b:* SDS-PAGE of SP obtained from normal sperm. Gel thickness was in this case 0.8 mm. Other conditions as in 5a. The arrow indicates the albumin band. The resolution is better than in gel 5a, but again band comparision is problemátic.

proteins (used as an internal standard) is not obtained in the case of the SP proteins samples.

2) The bands are smoothly distributed on the whole gel surface.

3) The gel conditions are non-denaturing.

The lack of resolution (point 1) could be due to the relatively high ionic strength of the sample or to the stacking (concentrating) effect on the gel surface. It was found (by simple dilution of the samples) that the ionic strength is probably not responsible for the effect observed. The resolution could only partially be improved even by utilizing a discontinuous system (e.g. the classical Ornstein–Davis system (see Fig. 6b) which is much less sensitive to I-effects (Maurer, 1974). The SP proteins are probably present in vivo as loose complexes which are, however, sensitive to mechanical compression, amongst other things.

TWO-DEMENSIONAL ELECTROPHORESIS

Since the publication of the excellent work on 2d-electrophoresis by O'Farrel (1975), and the systematic studies undertaken by N.G. Anderson and his group on the protein composition of human body fluids (see Anderson et al., 1980 and references therein), the term "molecular anatomy" was created. The impressive resolution acieved by combining the resolving power of PAGIEF (normally in the presence of urea and/or non-ionic detergents) with that of SDS-PAGE allowed for the analysis of extremely complex protein mixtures, e.g., those of whole mouse embryos (Klose et al., 1980). We explored the possible use and applications of this technique to SP proteins by combining our slab-gel PAGIEF (without detergent or urea, see section 1) with gradient SDS-PAGE (see section 2) (Fig. 7).

In the cases analyzed, the Coomassie coloration (Racine and Langley, 1980) revealed the presence of at least 60–70 protein and peptide spots indicating that PAGIEF or SDS-PAGE alone are not sufficient to obtain the full analytical detail of the SP protein composition. The number of detectable spots varied however from sample to sample, indicating a far-reaching heterogeneity in their protein content. The neutral–basic bands (see section I and Figs. 2b, 2c and 3) were found to migrate in the 10–30 kilodaltons zone. With the intent to further improve the quality of the detection method, we

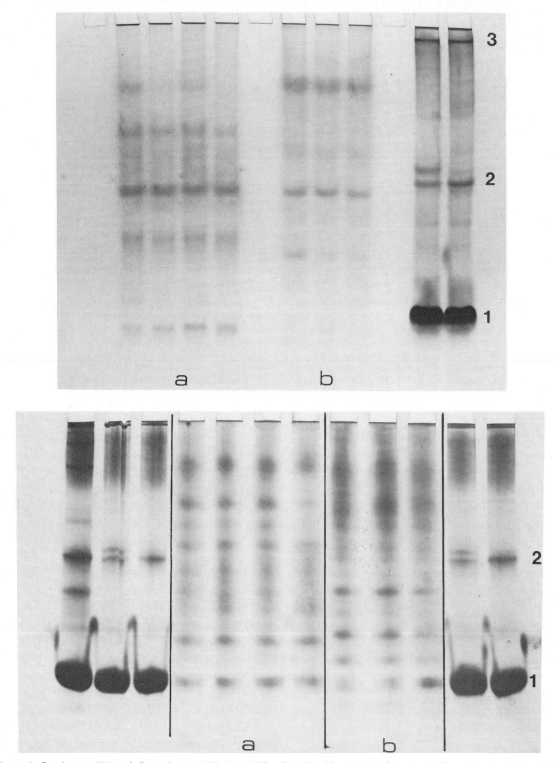

Figure 6. Continuous (6a) and discontinuous (6b) "normal" polyacrylamide-gel ectrophoresis of SP samples on slab gels. For comparative purposes, the samples used in PAGIEF (Fig. 2) and SDS-PAGE (Fig. 5) experiments are again shown here. *6a:* From left to right: SP of donor 11 (a), SP of donor 7 (b) and two blood plasma samples. Double-gel, continuous buffer and run conditions as given in Appendix. 1 = albumin, 2 = transferrin, 3 = α_2-macroglobulin. *6b:* The same samples as in 6a (with one more blood plasma sample at the extreme left). Ornstein–Davis (pH 8.9) discontinuous PAGE (see Appendix). The reader should compare Figs. 2, 5 and 6 to observe the different resolutions achieved by the different systems. Also note the differences in the number of bands between 6a and 6b and the lack of correspondence between blood and SP samples (with the exception of albumin at the bottom).

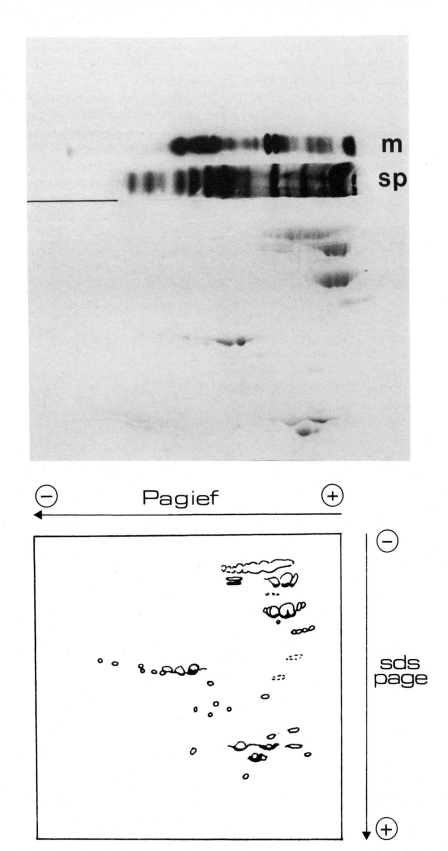

Figure 7. Two-dimensional electrophoresis of an SP sample obtained from a normal sperm. Above (from the top): PAGIEF of marker proteins, PAGIEF of SP proteins, SDS-PAGE separation gel. Experimental conditions: see Appendix. Below: drawing of the pattern shown above.

also tried to utilize the very recently published silver-stain procedure (Merril et al., 1979). The results, however, were rather disappointing (not shown) because of the amount of background coloration obtained.

CONCLUDING REMARKS

This chapter has explored the application of a certain number of high-resolution electroanalytical techniques to the study of SP proteins, obtained from normal and from infertile sperms. No pools of sperm samples were made. Each SP is, in fact, a special item and must be treated as such. The best method for SP protein analysis was found to be PAGIEF. Neither urea nor non-ionic detergents are needed to obtain patterns useful for analysis, or comparative studies. SDS-PAGE and normal PAGE (both continuous and discontinuous) were not as useful as PAGIEF for the same comparative studies, at least in their applications. 2d-electrophoresis, although extremely resolutive and powerful, remains at present a "method of the future", because of its complicated technicalities. In fact, the coloration procedure, the spots identification and cataloging, as well as the difficulties encountered when running a high number of samples under strictly identical conditions, do not yet allow for an easy and large-scale clinical application of 2d-electrophoresis to andrological diagnosis.

The present study has revealed the presence of a set of neutral–basic bands (PAGIEF) of unknown origin and role in the SPs of some normal as well as in some infertile semen. Sometimes these proteins constituted more than 50% of all protein and peptide bands detected by Coomassie staining. Futhermore, when analyzed under strong denaturing conditions, these components were found to migrate in SDS gels in the low-MW region (10–30 kdalton). There are fine variations between the patterns of the different SPs samples, and this goes for almost all individuals analyzed. These heterogeneities in protein constituents most probably reflect the quantitative and qualitative changes deriving from the individually different contributions of the accessory male glands secretions (Ahmed et al., 1979). The SP protein composition was observed to be time-dependent in the same individual.

Whether this phenomenon is a more general and genuine characteristic of SP protein composition is unclear at the moment. This phenomenon, however, deserves particular attention because of its possibly far-reaching (possibly clinical) consequences. During the development of this work the authors felt that a complex study like this needed a more profound and up-to-date knowledge about the proteins and enzymes contributed to SP by the accessory male glands (prostata, seminal vescicles, epididymis) in order to understand the features and properties of each SP better.

APPENDIX

A. Composition of PAGIEF gels (for 25 ml total volume)

1. A/B is (28.38 g/1.62 g made up to 100 ml with H_2O)   4.165 ml
2. Glycerol   1.75 ml
3. Ampholytes   pH 4–6   0.14 ml
   (Ampholines, LKB)   pH 5–7   0.14 ml
        pH 9–11   0.26 ml
        pH 3.5–10   0.84 ml
4. Persulfate $((NH_4)_2S_2O_8, 100$ mg/ml)   0.15 ml
5. H_2O (ditto)   ad 25.0 ml

The resulting gels are 5% T (= % total gel concentration) and 5.4% C (= % crosslinker). Electric conditions are given in section 1.

The pH-gradients were measured with a Micro-Combination pH probe (MI-410) from Microelectrodes Inc., Londonderry, New Hampshire (USA) directly after the run.

B. Composition of SDS-PAGE gels

As given by Laemmli and Favre (1973) with the exception of the A/Bis solution (which was the same as that used in A above). Initial setting: 80 V (200 V max). Running time: ~5 h.

C. Composition of the normal PAGE gels

1. Continuous system: as described by Abraham et al. (1970). Running conditions: 100 V (const), 5 h.
2. Discontinuous system: 7.5%, pH 8.9 gels (System Nr. 1 given in Maurer's (1971) book. Running conditions: 90–200 V, 5 h.
Staining: 1vol. of 1% Coomassie R-250 + 19 vol. of 12.5% TCA solution
Destaining: Several changes of 7% acetic acid.

D. Two-dimensional electrophoresis

1. First dimension: as described under A above. Strips of 3 mm were cut and transferred.
2. Equilibration: 5 min in the transfer solution (Solution O of O'Farrel (1975)).

3. The gels were loaded onto the second dimension slab gel as described in O'Farrel (1975).

4. Second dimension: 10–20% acrylamide gradient slab-gel. Gel composition as described under B above.

Staining and destaining was done as described in Racine and Langley (1980).

ACKNOWLEDGMENTS

The present work has been partially supported by the Swiss National Science Foundation (Grant 3.886–0.79). The authors gratefully acknowledge the assistance of Mr. F. Schloss (for carefully reading the manuscript), of Miss N. Rusconi (for work in the andrologic lab) and of Miss D. Albertoni and Mrs. R. Waters for secretarial work.

REFERENCES

Abraham K, Schütt K, Müller I, Hoffmeister H (1970) Kontinuierliche Polyacrylamid-Elektrophrese I. Untersuchungen und Normaliseren. Z Klin Chem Klin Biochem 8:92.

Ahmed K, Wilson MJ, Goueli SA, Steer RC (1979) Functional biochemistry. In Hafez ESE, Spring-Mills E eds. Accessory glands of the male reproductive tract, pp 69–108. Ann Arbor: Ann Arbor Science Publishers.

Anderson L, Anderson NG (1977) High resolution two-dimensional electrophoresis of human plasma proteins. Proc Natl Acad Sci USA 74: 5421.

Anderson NL, Edwards JJ, Giometti CS, Willard KE, Tollaksen SL, Nance SL, Hickmann BJ, Taylor JJ, Coulter B, Scandora A, Anderson AG (1980) High-resolution two-dimensional electrophoretic mapping of human proteins. In Radola BJ, ed Electrophoresis '79, pp 313–328. Berlin and New York: W de Gruyter.

Atland K, Hackler R (1980) Double one-dimensional slab-gel electrophoresis. In Radola BJ ed. Electrophoresis '79, pp 53–66. Berlin and New York: W de Gruyter.

Chang MC, Austin CR, Bedford JM, Brackett BG, Hunter RHF, Yanagimachi R (1977) Capacitation of spermatozoa and fertilization in mammals. In Greep RO, Proj. Dir. Frontiers in reproduction and fertility control pp 434–451. Cambridge: The MIT Press.

Clavert A, Montagnon D, Brun B (1980) Studies on the origin and nature of seminal proteins by cellulose acetate electrophoresis. Andrologia 12:338.

Fairbanks G, Steck Th L, Vallach DFH (1971) Electrophoretic analysis of the major polypeptides of the human erythrocyte membrane. Biochemistry 10: 2606.

Klose J, Nowak J, Kade W (1980) Two-dimensional electrophoresis: high resolution of proteins and automatic evaluation of the patterns under different methodical conditions. In Radola BJ, Electrophoresis '79 ed., pp 297–312. Berlin and New York: W de Gruyter.

Jacobsson L (1950) Free amino acids in human semen. Acta Physiol Scand 20:88.

Laemmli KK, Favre MJ (1973) Mol Biol 80:575.

Lindholmer C, Carlström A, Eliasson R (1974) Occurrence and origin of proteins in human seminal plasma with special reference to albumin. Andrologia 6:181.

Mann Th (1975) Biochemistry of semen. In Greep RO, Astwood EB, eds. Handbook of physiology, Vol 5, pp 461–471. Baltimore: Williams & Wilkins 1975.

Mann Th (1977) Semen: metabolism, antigenicity, storage and artificial insemination. In Greep, Proj. Dir. Frontiers in reproduction and fertility control, pp 427–433. Cambridge: The MIT Press.

Maurer HR ed. (1971) Disc electrophoresis and related techniques of polyacrylamide electrophoresis. Berlin and New York: W de Gruyter.

Merrill CR, Switzer RC, Van Keuren ML (1979) Trace polypeptides in cellular extracts and human body fluids detected by two-dimensional electrophoresis and a highly sensitive silver stain. Proc Natl Acad Sci USA 76: 4335.

Oliphant G (1976) Removal of sperm-bound seminal plasma components as a prerequisite to induction of the rabbit acrosome reaction. Fertil Steril 27: 28.

O'Farrel PH (1975) High resolution two-dimensional electrophoresis of proteins. J Biol Chem 250:4007.

Racine RR, Langley CH (1980) Genetic heterozygosity in a natural population of *Mus musculus* assessed using two-dimensional electrophoresis. Nature 283: 855.

Radola BJ ed. (1980) Electrophoresis '79, Advanced methods, biochemical and clinical applications. Proceedings of the 2nd int conf on electrophoresis. Berlin and New York: W de Gruyter.

Tauber PF, Zaneveld LJD, Propping D, Schumacher GFB (1975) Components of human split-ejaculates. I. Spermatozoa, fructose, immunoglobulins, albumin, lactoferrin, transferrin and other plasma proteins. J Reprod Fert 43: 249.

Tauber PF, Zaneveld LJD, Propping D, Schumacher GFB (1976) Components of human split-ejaculates. II. Enzymes and proteinase inhibitors. J Reprod Fert 46: 165.

Thangnipon W, Chulavatnatol M (1979) Autoproteolysis in human seminal plasma under acidic conditions. Int J Fertil 24:260.

Umapathy E, Manimekalai S, Govindarajulu P (1980) Lipid pattern in split-ejaculate and Klinefelter's syndrome. Fertil Steril 33:294.

White IG, Darin-Bennett A, Poulos A (1976) Lipids of human semen. In Hafez ESE ed. Human semen and fertility regulation in man, p 144. St Louis: CV Mosby.

Winter A, Ek K, Anderson UB (1977) Analytical electrofocusing in thin layers of polyacrylamide gels. Application note 250, LKB-Produkter AB, Bromma, Sweden.

Author's address:
Dr M. Balerna
Servizio di Endocrinologia Ginecologica
Ospedale Distrettuale "La Carità"
Locarno, Switzerland

4. SEMINAL PLASMA PROTEINS IDENTICAL TO UTERINE SECRETION PROTEINS

B. MÜLLER

1. INTRODUCTION

The biochemistry of semen is a relatively modern, but rapidly expanding field of reproductive physiology. Apart from the spermatozoa, the seminal plasma and its components have been the subject of many investigations. The accessory organs that secrete the seminal plasma are under hormonal control (Mann, 1974) and any changes in the hormonal level may change its composition (Eliasson, 1973; Mann, 1974). As a result, a change in their influence on the spermatozoa or the egg wil follow.

In addition to many studies of inorganic ions (Emmens, 1947; Lindholmer, 1974) and of non-protein components (Mann, 1964; Murdoch and White, 1966; Peterson and Freund, 1971) there have also been investigations of the proteins of the seminal plasma (Weil and Finkler, 1958; Lavon, 1972; Yantorno et al., 1972; Zappi et al., 1972; Kirchner and Schroer, 1976; Müller and Kirchner, 1978, Müller and Kirchner, 1980). However, in only a few cases for some animals has it been possible to assign a function to these proteins, by starting from the biological function and then trying to find out its cause: in the bovine it has been possible to find a sperm forward motility protein (Brandt et al., 1978); in man a seminal plasma proteinase has been found which accelerates migration of spermatozoa through cervical mucus in vitro (Syner and Moghissi, 1972); and a peptidase, which is involved in the ejaculate liquefaction has also been found (Koren and Lukač, 1979).

In the rabbit some functional data have indicated a sperm-coating antigen which blocks fertilization (Hunter and Nornes, 1969), an iron-binding protein (O'Rand, 1974), a reversible decapacitation factor (Eng and Oliphant, 1978), and a protein which supports spermatozoan motility (Müller and Kirchner, 1978).

Very much in contrary to the above, however, are certain cases where a characteristic protein or group of proteins is of special interest, and becomes the source of functional analysis which can be difficult and time consuming.

The present report demonstrates such a characteristic group of proteins which do occur in the rabbit seminal plasma as well as in the uterine fluid six days post coitum at the time of implantation, but not in the serum. Biochemical data are given and an attempt is made to assign a function to at least some of the proteins.

2. PROTEIN CLASSES OF SEMINAL PLASMA

The seminal plasma generally contains proteins of two different origins: the first type is derived from the serum and these proteins reach the genital tract by exudation through the lumen walls. The second type is synthesized and released by the male genital tract itself. Some proteins of the latter type also occur in the uterine fluid six days post coitum, but these are synthesized by the female genital tract (Kirchner and Schroer, 1976; Müller and Kirchner, 1980). In these types of protein it is clearly of interest to obtain more detailed information about their hormonal control and their effect on the spermatozoa and/or the egg, most particularly with regard to their possible involvement in the process of reproduction.

2.1. Disc-electrophoretical classification

In disc-electrophoresis, rabbit seminal plasma showed a very specific protein pattern which is generally not comparable to rabbit serum and rabbit uterine fluid. One of the few proteins common to all three protein sources is the band of

Hafez ESE & Semm K (Eds) Instrumental insemination.

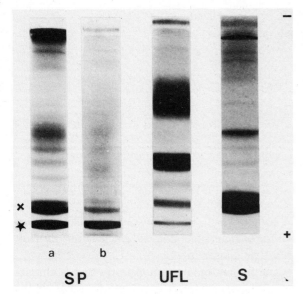

Figure 1. PAA gel electrophoresis of seminal plasma (SP), a) after protein staining and b) after carbohydrate staining in comparison to flushed uterine fluid on day six post coitum (UFL) and to serum (S). The band of albumin common to all three protein sources in indicated by × whereas 'pre-albumin' occurring in SP and UFL is marked by ★ (from Müller and Kirchner 1980).

2.2. Immunological classification

With antiserum against seminal plasma from the sheep 22 antigens were found (Table 1): antigens E, appearing only in the seminal plasma (E for ejaculate); antigens EU, appearing in the seminal plasma and the uterine fluid, for example the 'pre-albumin'; antigens ES, appearing in the seminal plasma and the serum; and finally antigens EUS, common to seminal plasma, uterine fluid and serum, for example the albumin (Fig. 2a). To find out which antigens belong to which group of proteins, the antiserum against all proteins was neutralized with uterine fluid, serum, and uterine fluid plus serum. With these partially neutralized antisera the seminal plasma, the uterine fluid, and the serum was developed after electrophoresis in agar gel. For one example, it could be shown that among the 22 seminal plasma antigens there are five antigens (EU) appearing in the seminal plasma and the uterine fluid but not in the serum (Table 1 and Fig. 2b).

albumin (Fig. 1). Another protein common to only two protein sources is the band of the so-called 'pre-albumin'. Using the PAS-carbohydrate staining (Schwick, 1965) its glycoprotein nature is obvious (Fig. 1). With these mere descriptions all possibilities of the electrophoretic method have been exhausted and a further characterization of the seminal plasma antigens can be achieved by immunological methods alone.

3. THE EU ANTIGENS

To assess further biochemical characteristics the isolation of two proteins of this antigen type was carried out. One protein was isolated by the immunoabsorption technique using Sepharose 4B to which antibodies against uteroglobin were covalently bound. When seminal plasma was coupled

Table 1. Reaction combinations between rabbit seminal plasma, rabbit uterine secretion and rabbit serum to give precipitates of the following antigen types: E, antigens specific for seminal plasma; EU, antigens present in the seminal plasma and the uterine secretion; ES, antigens present in seminal plasma and serum; EUS, antigens present in seminal plasma, uterine secretion and serum.

Antiserum ↓	Antigen →	Seminal plasma		Uterine secretion		Serum
Anti-seminal plasma		22	E (12) EU (5) ES (2) EUS (3)	8	EU EUS	5	ES EUS
Anti-seminal plasma + uterine secretion		14	E ES		—	2	ES
Anti-seminal plasma + serum		17	E EU	5	EU		—
Anti-seminal plasma + uterine secretion + serum		12	E		—		—

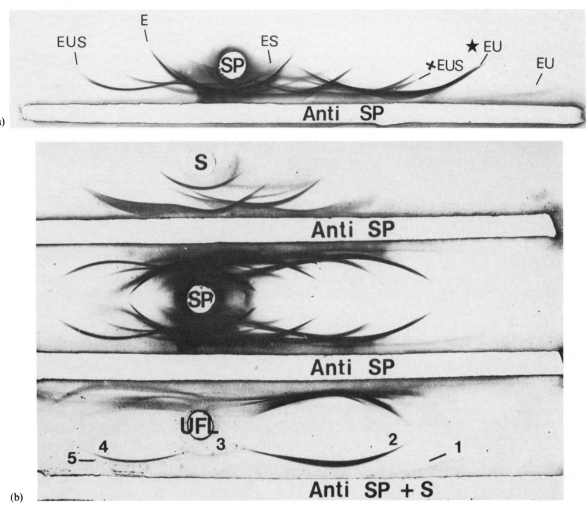

Figure 2. (a) Immuno-electrophoresis of rabbit seminal plasma (SP) in agar gel developed with antiserum against the seminal plasma (Anti SP). The precipitate of albumin is indicated by × and the precipitate of 'pre-albumin' by ★. Precipitates belonging to the different antigen types of the seminal plasma are marked by E, EU, ES and EUS as examples only (see also Table 1). *(b)* Immuno-electrophoresis of serum (S) and seminal plasma (SP) and uterine fluid (UFL) in agar gel with antiserum against the seminal plasma (Anti SP) developed. Uterine fluid was also developed with Anti SP, which was neutralized with serum (S). The precipitates (no. 1–5) document the EU antigens, among them the 'pre-albumin' (no. 2).

to the matrix the absorbed material showed, as expected, immunological identity with uteroglobin from the uterus and the lung. Moreover, all three proteins had the same isoelectric point, showed the same mobility in agar, and eluted the same level when their original protein sources were chromatographed on Sephadex G 75 SF. From these data it might be concluded that this protein is the uteroglobin, but additional data, such as exact molecular weight, protein subunits and progesterone binding studies are needed to confirm its identity (Table 2). For these tests, however, a large amount of this protein has to be isolated from the seminal plasma,

a difficult problem considering its very low level in this protein source.

The second protein, already mentioned as 'prealbumin', was isolated in three steps by gel filtration of seminal plasma on Sephadex G 75 SF, ionexchange chromatography on DEAE-Sephacel and finally, absorption chromatography on Concanavalin A – Sepharose 4 B, using its glycoprotein nature. This glycoprotein, molecular weight 24 500, has a carbohydrate content of about 40% and an isoelectric point of 4.05 (Table 3). In the female the rate of synthesis of this protein is very high at the time of implantation (Beier, 1974); moreover it is

Table 2. Biochemical characterization of uteroglobin deriving from seminal plasma (SP), uterine fluid (UFL), and from the lung (LUNG).

Source	Immunological identity	Mobility in agar	R_f in PAA 6%	IEP	Elution on G 75 SF	Molecular weight	Progesterone induced	Steroid binding
SP	+	+	?	5.6	58%	?	—	?
UFL	+	+	0.73	5.6	60%	13 000	+	+
LUNG	+	+	0.73	5.6	61%	13 000	—	+

+ = identical, — = not identical for all three protein sources.
? = not determinable.

Table 3. Biochemical characterization of the seminal plasma acid glycoprotein deriving from the seminal plasma (SP) and from the uterine fluid (UFL).

Source	Immunological identity	Mobility in agar	R_f in PAA 6%, 10%	IEP	Molecular weight	Carbohydrate content	Steroid induced	Steroid binding
SP	+	+	1.0	4.05	24 500	41%	—	—
UFL	+	+	1.0	4.05	24 500	41%	Prog.?	—

+ = identical, — = not identical for both protein sources.
Prog.? = possibly progesterone induced.

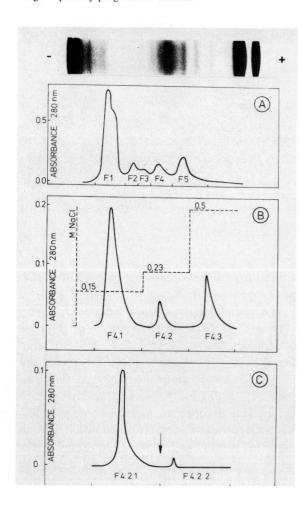

contained in the blastocyst fluid (Beier, 1968; Kirchner, 1969). Its migration in immuno-electro-phoresis as an α_1 protein leads to its α_1 acid glycoprotein character and the name 'seminal plasma acid glycoprotein' is to be preferred to 'pre-albumin'. The function of this striking protein remains unclear (Fig. 3). Attempts to assign any enzymological activity to this protein have given no result to date, nor does there appear to be any steroid-binding ability comparable to that of the similar serum-acid glycoprotein (Müller and Kirchner, 1980).

Data about the biological functions of the other three proteins belonging to the EU antigen type

Figure 3. Isolation of the seminal plasma acid glycoprotein from rabbit seminal plasma (see the disc-electrophoresis above). A. Elution profile of 100 mg seminal plasma proteins on Sephadex G 75 SF with 50 mM Tris HCl (pH 8.0). B. Elution profile of fraction F4 DEAE-Sephacel with stepwise elution by 0.15, 0.23, and 0.5 M NaCl in 50 mM Tris HCl (pH 8.0). C. Elution profile of fraction F 4.2 of the ion-exchange chromatography on Concanavalin A Sepharose 4 B. Coupling buffer was 50 mM Tris HCl (pH 8.0), containing 0.5 M NaCl and MgCl₂, CaCl₂ and MnCl₂ (each 2 mM). Seminal plasma acid glycoprotein was eluted with 20 mM borate buffer (pH 7.0), containing 0.5 M NaCl 50 mM α-methyl-D-mannoside and MgCl₂, CaCl₂ and MnCl₂ (each 2 mM) as indicated by the arrow (from Müller and Kirchner, 1980).

were obtained when the isoelectric focusing technique was combined with immunological and enzymological procedures. Isoelectric focusing of uterine fluid (pH 3.5–11) followed by a second run in agar-gel containing antiserum against the seminal plasma proteins which was neutralized with serum also produced five EU antigen precipitates (Fig. 4a). One of them is uteroglobin, IEP 5.6 (precipitate no. 3) and the other the seminal plasma acid glycoprotein, IEP 4.05 (precipitate no. 2).

Upon incubation of focused runs of uterine fluid and rabbit seminal plasma in 0.1 M diethanolamine buffer, containing 10 mM p-nitrophenol, pH 10.5, three alkaline phosphatase reactions were observed in the uterine fluid and five reactions in the seminal plasma. For both the uterine fluid and the seminal plasma there was an alkaline phosphatase reaction at IEP 7.4, and an immunological cross-reaction with the neutralized antiserum (precipitate no. 4). This indicated that one of the last three EU antigens is an alkaline phosphatase (Fig. 4b). A simple Ilford Pan F film strip was used as the substrate for proteinase activity tests. By laying the film directly onto the gel surface of focused uterine fluid and seminal plasma for a suitable incubation time (1 h, 37° C), proteinase activities were obvious by a lysis of the gelatine on the film right at the site of their isoelectric points. From the total number of seven proteinases found in the uterine fluid and of eight in the seminal plasma, one enzyme activity was common to uterine fluid and seminal plasma at the IEP of 10.5. This antigen showed an immunological cross reactivity with the partially neutralized antiserum too (precipitate no. 5) (Fig. 4b). The function of the final (fifth) EU antigen, IEP 3.9 (precipitate no. 1), apparent molecular weight 40 000, remains unclear.

4. CONCLUDING REMARKS

This synopsis on the five rabbit seminal plasma proteins common to uterine fluid and seminal plasma but not to serum might serve as a pilot study concerning genital tract specific proteins and their possible importance for the gametes and/or the normal development of the embryo.

Taking into account that uteroglobin in the uterus might, despite the high progesterone level during pregnancy, serve as a progesterone-neutralizing agent (Kirchner, unpublished results), it might be assumed that a uteroglobin in the rabbit seminal plasma will have another function, since it occurs at a very low level. Concerning the alkaline phosphatase, the precise role of the enzyme in deciduation and early embryonic development is unclear. The fact that the basic proteinase reaches its highest level in the uterus one day before implantation (Kirchner, 1972) suggests that it might be one of the implantation-initiating factors. Moreover, the increase of seminal plasma acid glycoprotein at the time of implantation at least suggests a particular importance for the development of the embryo. Its biological role in the seminal plasma remains unclear.

The problems concerning some of the non-serum proteins, identical to uterine fluid and seminal plasma, could only be solved if it were possible to isolate a large amount of each protein and test only its function. In this case perhaps the inactivation of these protein syntheses or function could assist in finding new ways of contraception or could help in some disorders of embryonic development.

ACKNOWLEDGMENTS

This work was supported by grant Ki 154/8 from the Deutsche Forschungsgemeinschaft.

The author is grateful to Professor Dr C. Kirchner for his encouragement in writing this paper and for use of his laboratory facilities, to Dr B. Broughton (London) for reading the manuscript and to Mrs R. Roller-Müller for her typing.

REFERENCES

Beier HM (1968) Biochemisch-entwicklungsphysiologische Untersuchungen am Proteinmilieu für die Blastocystenentwicklung des Kaninchens (Oryctolagus cuniculus). Zool Jb Anat 85: 72.
Beier HM (1974) Oviducal and uterine fluids. J Reprod Fert 37: 221.
Brandt H, Acott TS, Johnson DH, Hoskins DD (1978) Evidence for an epididymal origin of bovine sperm forward motility protein. Biol Reprod 19: 830.
Eliasson R (1973) Parameters of male fertility. In Hafez ESE Evans, eds. Human fertility, conception and contraception. Harper & Row.
Emmens CW (1947) The mobility and viability of rabbit spermatozoa at different hydrogen-ion-concentrations. Ann NY Acad Sci 121: 404.

32

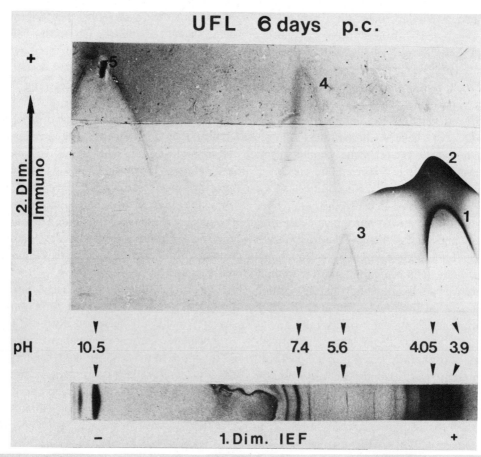

(a)

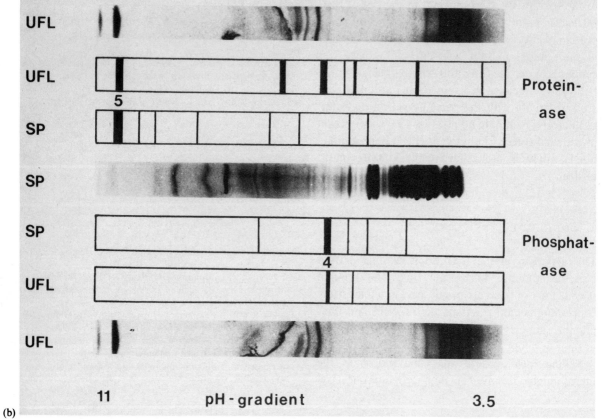

(b)

Eng LA, Oliphant G (1978) Rabbit sperm reversible decapacitation by membrane stabilization with a highly purified glycoprotein from seminal plasma. Biol Reprod 19: 1083.

Hunter IG, Nornes J (1969) Characterization and isolation of a sperm-coating antigen from rabbit seminal plasma with capacity to block fertilization. J Reprod Fert 20: 419.

Kirchner C (1969) Untersuchungen an uterusspezifischen Glykoproteinen während der frühen Gravidität des Kaninchens (Oryctolagus cuniculus). Wilhelm Roux Arch Entw Mech 164: 97.

Kirchner C (1972) Uterine protease activities and lysis of the blastocyst covering in the rabbit. J Embryol Exp Morph 28: 177.

Kirchner C, Schroer HG (1976) Uterine secretion-like protein in the seminal plasma of the rabbit. J Reprod Fert 47: 325.

Koren E, Lukac J (1979) Mechanism of liquefaction of the human ejaculate. I. Role of collagenase-like peptidase and seminal proteinase. J Reprod Fert 56: 501.

Lavon U (1970) Characterization of boar, bull, ram and rabbit seminal plasma proteins by gel disc electrophoresis and isoelectric focusing on polyacrylamide. J Reprod Fert 31: 29.

Lindholmer C (1974) Toxity of zinc ions to human spermatozoa and the influence of albumin. Andrologia 6: 181.

Mann T (1964) Biochemistry of semen and the male reproductive tract. London: Methuen.

Mann T (1974) Secretory function of the prostate, seminal vesicle and other male accessory organs of reproduction. J Reprod Fert 37: 179.

Murdoch RN, White IG (1966) Metabolism of glucose, acetate, lactate and pyruvate by ram, bull, dog and rabbit spermatozoa. J Reprod Fert 12: 271.

Müller B, Kirchner C (1978) Influence of seminal plasma proteins on motility of rabbit spermatozoa. J Reprod Fert 54: 167.

Müller B, Kirchner C (1980) Purification and properties of a carbohydrate-containing glycoprotein specific to rabbit genital tract. Biol Reprod, in press.

O'Rand MG (1974) Isolation of an iron-binding rabbit seminal plasma antigen. J Reprod Fert 39: 349.

Peterson RN, Freund M (1971) Glycolysis by human spermatozoa: levels of glycolytic intermediates. Biol Reprod 5: 221.

Schwick HG (1965) Chemisch-entwicklungsphysiologische Beziehungen von Uterus zu Blastocyste des Kaninchens. Wilhelm Roux Arch Entw Mech 156: 283.

Syner RN, Moghissi KS (1972) Purification and properties of a human seminal proteinase. Biochem J 126: 1135.

Weil AJ, Finkler AE (1958) Antigens of rabbit semen. Proc Soc Exp Med 98: 794.

Yantorno C, Vides MA, Vottero-Cima E (1972) Studies of the macromolecular and antigenic composition of rabbit seminal plasma. J Reprod Fert 29: 229.

Zappi E, Smith DJ, Shulman S (1972) Preparative separation of seminal plasma and immunochemical study of the resulting fractions. Int J Fert 17: 145.

Author's address:
Dr B. Müller
Department of Biology, Zoology
Philipps-Universität Marburg
P.O. Box 1929, 3550 Marburg, FRG

Figure 4. (a) Isoelectric focusing (pH 3.5–11) of uterine fluid (1. Dim.) followed by an immuno-electrophoresis in agar gel containing antiserum which was neutralized with serum (2. Dim.). The numbered precipitates document the EU antigens, the arrows indicate the corresponding IEPs. *(b)* Isoelectric focusing (pH 3.5–11) of uterine fluid (UFL) and seminal plasma (SP). Proteinase and alkaline phosphatase activities were indicated with small or broad black bars, depending on enzyme activity. The numbers are identical to the numbers of the EU antigens; number 4: alkaline phosphatase, number 5: proteinase.

5. ROLE OF SEMINAL PLASMA AND SPERM FERTILIZABILITY

A. Rosado, N.M. Delgado, L. Huacuja and O. Hernández

Motility of spermatozoa is one of the most important factors in evaluating the potential fertility of a given male. No consistent standards for the evaluation of this fundamental characteristic of the spermatozoa have yet been defined. While some groups use the evaluation of sperm motility in the seminal plasma as criteria, others study the rate of penetration of spermatozoa through natural cervical mucus, or artificial media.

Most of the problems of all the systems used depend on not being able to give adequate answers to one or more of the following requirements: 1) ease of performance, 2) quantitative, 3) an adequate estimation of the number of motile cells in the whole sample, 4) an adequate estimation of rate and direction of movement, 5) an estimate of the range of time the spermatozoa can preserve their motility characteristics. Although there are some methods that actually allow the adequate quantification of the parameters mentioned above (Jouannet et al., 1977), they are rather sophisticated and not useful in the common laboratory.

Good estimations of most of the required parameters can be obtained by the combined use of two recently proposed methods: 1) the stroboscopic photographic method of Makler (1978) which permits the determination of the rate and direction of movement and of the relative proportion of cells moving in a small representative sample of the specimen, and 2) the procedure of Atherton et al. (1978) which exploits the marked optical characteristics of sperm suspensions submitted to flow orientation (Walton, 1952) and thus permits the quantification of the number and rate of motility of sperm suspensions taken directly from the specimen under study. The relative facility of this procedure allows the determination of motility characteristics of the specimen at two or more intervals of time.

Spermatozoa are immotile during their stay in the epididymis. Upon ejaculation sperm cells become actively motile with a characteristic progressive motility. In spite of the transcendent significance of this change, relatively little work has been done towards understanding the mechanisms of initiation of sperm motility.

The acquisition of motility by spermatozoa may be explained by: 1) simple reduction of sperm cell to cell contact; 2) reduction of the hyperosmolality of epididymal fluid at ejaculation; 3) specific ion requirements, particularly those of calcium and potassium; 4) sudden loss or decrease in concentration of a specific inhibitor of metabolism such as zinc, carnitine, glyceryl phosphoryl choline (GPc) etc.; 5) addition of a stimulator of a pre-existing sperm system such as the adenylate cyclase system, the ion or metabolite transporting system; 6) the addition of specific motility activators such as the forward motility protein, etc.

Sperm leaving the testis are not capable of acquiring forward motility. Development of this capacity takes place during epididymal maturation. Depending on the species, sperm removed from the caput epididymis and diluted or washed may move in tight circles, twitch, or not move at all; but in no species are they capable of moving progressively forward. Sperm removed from the cauda of all species show, in contrast, vigorous forward progression on dilution or washing. This apparent hedge with regard to washing or dilution is necessary, since caudal sperm in situ are immotile and the act of dilution with fluids from other accessory glands at the time of ejaculation is an important part of the motility initiation process.

Presently, semen analysis is still primarily based on ratings pertaining fundamentally to spermatozoa. Relatively little has been done to relate the composition and biochemistry of seminal plasma to infertility problems and the few attempts made have

Hafez ESE & Semm K (Eds) Instrumental insemination.

been oriented more to the understanding of the male accessory gland function than to the importance of seminal plasma by itself. Much more could be learned about male reproductive function in fertility, infertility and family planning if seminal chemistry were studied. However, at present we are just beginning to understand the complex interaction existing between spermatozoa and seminal plasma that results in the attainment of the necessary progressive motility, the regulation of the fertility potential and the preparation for capacitation and acrosomal reaction of the spermatozoa.

This chapter deals with some recent developments over some components of seminal plasma which may play a role in the acquisition, preservation or development of the fertilizing ability of the spermatozoa.

1. PHYSICO-CHEMICAL PROPERTIES

1.1. Osmolality

Recently, renewed attention has been focused on studies of the biochemical composition of human seminal plasma under both normal and pathological conditions. Although much is known about specific components of seminal plasma and the participation of specific ionic species, particularly Na^+, K^+ and Ca^{++} (Guerin and Czyba, 1979), on the development of spermatozoa motility, such important general properties of seminal plasma as osmolality and conductivity have almost been neglected. Although none of these properties are specific for any particular component, they serve as a quantitative measure of the total concentrations of active, ionized, and unionized, particles in the studied secretions, and may therefore give some explanation of the changes in seminal plasma composition that may be present in cases of infertility.

Epididymal plasma obtained in vivo by micropuncture (Johnson and Howards, 1977) experiments is extremely hyperosmotic. The osmolality in the caput epididymal fluid is over 400 mOsm/ml and declines through the subsequent zones of the epididymis to a concentration of 340 mOsm/l in the cauda epididymis. Reduction of osmolality during ejaculation may play an important role in the development of progressive motility.

Most human spermatozoa are motile, move rapidly, and consume oxygen when they are in a medium isotonic with blood plasma. A hypotonic medium causes a reduction in percentage motility and oxygen consumption, whereas hypertonic conditions cause a reduction in mean velocity. Through microscopic observation, (Guerin and Czyba, 1977), it is clear that hypotonic conditions cause the greatest loss of motility with an apparent flagellar dysfunction.

The influence of the osmotic pressure on the percentage motility and on the average velocity of spermatozoa was studied simultaneously on ten ejaculates from different donors (Guerin and Czyba, 1979). The spermatozoa from each ejaculate were divided into three aliquots which were resuspended in hyper-, normo- or hypotonic media. Ejaculates from seven other individuals were similarly divided and used for the study of oxygen consumption. The spermatozoa performed best in isotonic medium (310 mOsmoles). The percentage motility was equally affected by a rise or fall in the osmotic pressure of the medium, whereas the mean velocity was more severely affected at higher, and the oxygen consumption at lower, osmotic pressures. The osmotic pressure of the medium was indeed an important cause of the variations and most of the variation, especially in the percentage motility, was related to the individual donor.

1.2. Osmolality and conductivity

The possible correlation between two important general properties of seminal plasma, osmolality and conductance, and the presence of some pathological conditions of human semen, asthenospermia and oligoasthenospermia, have been studied. Osmolality was measured under carefully controlled conditions by the freezing point depression method and conductance with a Wheatstone bridge. Volume, by an isotopic dilution method, and pH were also determined (Velázquez et al., 1977).

The mean semen volume of the asthenospermic group (1.76 ± 0.68 ml) was significantly lower than the semen volume of the control group (3.05 ± 0.8 ml). However, no significant difference in ejaculate volume was found between the oligo-asthenospermic group (2.63 ± 0.37 ml) and the normal group. Osmolality of normal human semen was significantly higher (366 ± 16 mOsm/kg) than the reported osmolality of human blood serum (310 ± 285 mOsm/kg) (Table 1). Seminal plasma obtained from astheno- and oligoasthenospermic subjects showed a still higher value of osmolality (428 ± 38 and 457 ± 49 mOsm/kg respectively) (Table 1). Incubation of normal seminal plasma for 24 h at room temperature produced a significant increase in osmolality (from 366 ± 16 to 430 ± 31 mOsm kg) while pathological seminal plasma failed to show any modification (Table 1).

Table 1. Osmolality of normal and abnormal human seminal plasma. Estimated by the freezing point depression method the data express the mean $\pm$ the standard deviation of number of cases indicated in parentheses and expressed as mOsm/kg.

	Incubation time ($37°C$)	
	1 h	24 h
Normospermic	366 ± 16 (29)	430 ± 31 (29)
Asthenospermic	428 ± 38 (17)	434 ± 37 (17)
Oligoasthenospermic	457 ± 49 (9)	460 ± 45 (9)

(Modified from Velázquez et al., 1977).

Specific conductance (mhos $\times 10^{-3}$) and osmolality (mOsm/kg) of normal human semen were significantly and inversely correlated with the sample volume, the former (Fig. 1) obeying the equation mhos $\times 10^{-3} = -0.61$ ml $+ 11.9$ with correlation coefficient $r = -0.45$ and the latter (Fig. 2) the equation mOsm/kg $= -16.3$ ml $+ 416.2$ with an $r = -0.65$. Both correlation coefficients had a $p < 0.05$ significance level. Concerning osmolality, in pathological semen, although significant differences with the control group were observed in mean values (Table 1; Fig. 2), neither astheno- nor oligoasthenospermic seminal plasma osmolalities showed any correlation with semen volume (Fig. 2); $r = 0.027$ and 0.042 for asthenospermic and oligoasthenospermic respectively.

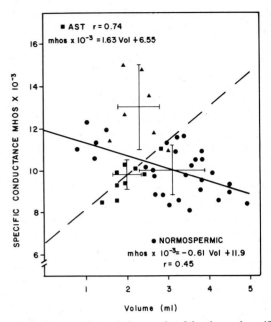

Figure 1. Scatter and correlation graphs of the observed specific conductance (Wheatstone bridge) values plotted against the ejaculated volumen in normal and abnormal human seminal plasma. The traced lines are the theoretical lines obtained from the values of normal (●) and asthenospermic men (■) by method of least squares and obey the equations indicated. The correlation coefficient found is also indicated. No correlation was observed in the oligoasthenospermic group (▲). (Modified from Velázquez et al., (1977).

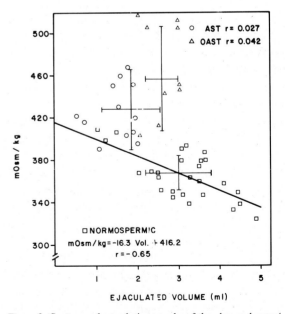

Figure 2. Scatter and correlation graphs of the observed osmolality plotted against volume values in normal (□) and abnormal seminal plasma. The line is the theoretical line found by the method of least squares and obeys the equation pointed out above. The correlation coefficients for asthenospermic (○) and oligoasthenospermic (△) subjects are also indicated. (Modified from Velázquez et al., 1977).

2. ZINC: A FUNDAMENTAL COMPONENT OF SEMINAL PLASMA

2.1. Role on metabolism and motility of spermatozoa

In comparison with those found in other body fluids and cells, seminal plasma and spermatozoa of certain mammals contain high concentrations of zinc (Rosado et al., 1977) (Table 2). Although zinc is an important cofactor in the activity of some enzymes, its role in sperm cells is important in the regulation of the metabolism of these cells (Delgado et al., 1975) rather than that of a prosthetic metal.

Table 2. Elemental composition of human seminal plasma as determined by atomic absorption spectroscopy. The data express the mean ± the standard deviation of the number of indicated in the last column.

Element	$\mu g/ml$	meq/l	No. of cases
Na^+	3804 ± 98	165.4 ± 4.3	12
K^+	1163 ± 64	29.3 ± 1.6	12
Ca^{++}	216 ± 15	10.8 ± 0.4	12
Mg^{++}	107 ± 12	8.8 ± 0.5	12
Zn^{++}	119 ± 21	3.6 ± 0.6	12

(Huacuja and Delgado, unpublished observations).

Zinc participation on the processes which are conducive to the development of adequate fertility potential by the spermatozoa is confronted with a multitude of contradictory results, from those which show that seminal zinc concentration and sperm motility (Danscher et al., 1978) or fertilizing ability (Swarup and Sekhon, 1976) are inversely correlated, to those which show that high sperm motility can be correlated to high zinc content (Stankovic and Mikac-Devic, 1976). There seems to be no correlation between zinc concentration of seminal plasma and spermatozoa motility (Frenkel-Paz et al., 1977; Janick et al., 1971).

The fundamental parameters are not the concentrations of the metal in seminal plasma, but the zinc concentration of the sperm cells and the mechanisms that regulate binding and release of this metal by the sperm cells.

Some dynamic studies should be considered of the participation of zinc in human spermatozoa metabolism and motility, which relates the spontaneous and induced release of zinc with the oxygen uptake and motility of these cells (Huacuja et al., 1973). Zinc content of human seminal plasma was 3.5 ± 1 $\mu Eq/ml$ and of spermatozoa, 2.5 ± 0.24 $\mu g/10^8$ cells. (Data represent the mean ± the standard deviation of 15 different determinations.) If we consider that in 1.0 ml packed sperm cells there are approximately 1.5×10^{11} spermatozoa (Sosa et al., 1972), we can calculate that the zinc content is 115 $\mu Eq/ml$ of packed cells; thus the concentration of zinc in the human sperm cells is almost 33 times higher than in the seminal plasma.

Incubation of washed human spermatozoa in the presence of 6 mM concentrations of EDTA, histidine and cysteine induces a release of about 75% of the zinc bound to the cells. No zinc is released by human spermatozoa when incubation is done in done in the absence of the reagents mentioned. No detectable amounts of calcium or magnesium were released by the sperm cells under any of the experimental conditions tested. Zinc release induced by the presence of EDTA, histidine and cysteine is accompanied by: 1) a significant increase in oxygen uptake, both under basal conditions and in the presence of some substrates (glucose, pyruvate and succinate), and 2) a significant increase in motility. This increase was greater with cysteine than with histidine, and greater with the latter than with EDTA. Zinc release induced by the presence of chelating agents was also accompanied by: 1) a significant increase in the utilization of exogenous ^{14}C-labeled glucose, which was reflected in an increase in the production of $^{14}CO^2$, 2) a small but significant decrease (14%) in the utilization of fructose when this sugar was added as exogenous substrate, and 3) a highly significant decrease in the endogenous sperm phospholipids ($>30\%$), an effect which was not inhibited by the addition of exogenous substrates. No preferential utilization of any phospholipid species occurred under these conditions. The amount of lipoproteins or proteolipids, which run as the first spot in chromatograms, did however show a significant decrease, indicating the deaggregation of these complexes when zinc was chelated out of the sperm cells (Delgado et al., 1976).

2.2. In accessory gland secretions

If an ejaculate is collected by the split ejaculate

technique, even though the morphology of the spermatozoa is similar in all fractions, the viability and the motility can be significantly different, being less in the final fractions. This difference is due to the presence of some factor(s) in the vesicular secretion that have a detrimental effect on sperm functions and to some factor(s) in prostatic fluid which protect the spermatozoa from the inhibitors in vesicular fluid and some other components that stimulate the motility of spermatozoa (Lindholmer, 1974).

Prostatic and vesicular fluids also have distinct effects on the uptake of zinc by the spermatozoa. Although concentration of zinc in seminal plasma is 5–10 times higher in the initial fractions of the split ejaculate, spermatozoa recovered from the last fractions have significantly higher concentrations of zinc ($p < 0.001$) (Lindholmer and Eliasson, 1972). Washed human spermatozoa incubated in prostatic and vesicular fluids take up higher amounts of zinc in the vesicular than in the prostatic fluid despite the presence of almost three times more zinc in the prostatic fluid.

In a survey of the functional properties of spermatozoa from fertile and infertile men (Lindholmer and Eliasson, 1974), the most dramatic difference found between the groups was the zinc content of the spermatozoa. In the fertile group, the mean value was 3.3 $\mu g/10^8$ spermatozoa, while in the infertile group, figures of over 6 $\mu g/10^8$ spermatozoa were frequently found, reaching values of up to 100 $\mu g/10^8$ spermatozoa in some samples with obvious deficiencies in motility.

The importance of zinc for the regulation of human sperm motility is further stressed by the selectivity of these changes. The uptake of magnesium by washed spermatozoa was the same when incubated in the "prostatic" as in the "vesicular" secretion. The higher uptake of zinc by spermatozoa in the "vesicular" secretion is probably specific for that ion and not a nonspecific uptake of divalent cations (Lindholmer and Eliasson, 1974b). Similarly, induced release of zinc by incubation in the presence of chelating agents does not produce the release of any other divalent cation (Huacuja et al., 1973; Westmoreland et al., 1967). There is an increasing uptake of zinc, but not of magnesium, by the spermatozoa during the first 24 h after the ejaculation when the spermatozoa were stored at 30° C.

Zinc content of human spermatozoa changes during the simple storage of normal ejaculates (Eliasson, 1974). During the first hour there was a significant decrease, followed by a "steady state" that lasted 2 h. During this time sperm motility was kept constant or showed a slight increase. During the following 3–5 h of storage there was a significant ($p < 0.05$) increase in the uptake of zinc by spermatozoa, and there was also an increase in the percentage of immotile or dead spermatozoa. During the entire observation period the magnesium content in the spermatozoa was unchanged (Lindholmer and Eliasson, 1972).

2.3. Role in nuclear decondensation

Condensation and stabilization of mammalian sperm chromatin, a process which gives characteristic properties to the mammalian sperm nuclei, occurs during spermatogenesis and is usually completed during the initial steps of maturation of eutherian spermatozoa in the epididymis. Chromatin condensation is due to the presence in sperm cells of specific DNA properties (Hernández et al., 1978) and to the formation of large numbers of disulfide bonds within the chromatin (Bedford and Calvin, 1974; Calvin and Bedford, 1971). This complicated process needs to be reversed after fertilization as a requirement for the transcription of the sperm genetic information.

Although nuclear decondensation has been induced in vitro by a wide variety of treatments, little is known of the mechanisms involved in sperm nuclear swelling and DNA synthesis in vivo. Acid mucopolysaccharides have been involved in the transition from the heterochromatic to the euchromatic state of somatic nuclear chromatin and they simultaneously increase the template availability of nuclear DNA. The addition of acidic polymers, heparin or polyxanthilic acid to rabbit sperm heads, previously exposed to disulfide reducing agents, releases sperm DNA template restriction.

Decondensation of human spermatozoa nuclei has been induced by exposure of intact spermatozoa to heparin, while the spermatozoa of rabbit, ram, and bull remained highly condensed under similar experimental conditions (Delgado et al., 1980). This process occurred in the complete absence of any disulfide bond cleaving reactant, stressing the importance of the participation of non-covalent interaction on the mechanisms of condensation and decondensation of human spermatozoa nuclei (Hernández et al., 1973). Swelling of human spermatozoa nuclei commenced about 30 min after the addition of heparin and depended on heparin concentration reaching 83% of swelled nuclei after 6 h of incubation with 5000 USP of heparin per ml. Addition of 10 mg/ml of trypsin soybean inhibitor did not interfere with the swelling action of heparin. Electron microscope observations of human spermatozoa nuclei treated with heparin revealed that the chromatin is organized into "hublike" nuclear bodies joined by a network of cross-linked and branched chromatin fibers ranging in thickness from 25 to 1.5 nm. The activity of heparin on the decondensation of sperm nuclei depends on the presence of specific membrane receptors for the mucopolysaccharide (unpublished results) (Fig. 3).

Seminal plasma of prostatic origin has the ability to rapidly protect ejaculated spermatozoa against

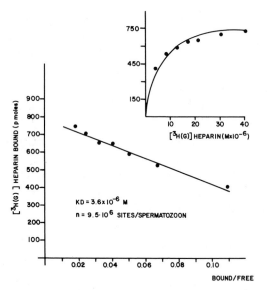

Figure 3. Inset: The interaction of heparin sodium salt ^{3}H (G) with human spermatozoa as a function of the total concentration of heparin added. The amount of heparin ^{3}H (G) bound is indicated in the ordinates. A Scatchard plot is indicated in the main figure. The concentration of free heparin was obtained by subtracting the amount of heparin initially added to the reaction mixture. KD was obtained from the slope of the Scatchard plot, calculated by the method of least squares, by evaluating the molar concentration of heparin from the total amount of ligand bound in 1.0 ml of reaction mixture. N, the number of binding sites per sperm cell, was obtained from the "y" intercept and the number of spermatozoa added to the incubation mixture. (Delgado et al., unpublished observations).

swelling in sodium dodecyl sulfate (SDS) (Kvist 1980a). A considerable increase of the spermatozoa chromatin resistance against swelling in SDS already takes place during the first 15 min after ejaculation. The prostatic origin of this component is shown by the fact that semen from donors with adequate secretory function of the prostate were more resistant to nuclear swelling than spermatozoa from men with impaired prostatic function. Spermatozoa in the first ("prostatic") portion of the ejaculate were more resistant to sodium dodecyl sulphate (SDS) than spermatozoa from the second ("vesicular") portion. Spermatozoa sensitized to SDS in this manner regained their SDS resistance upon exposure to normal prostatic fluid (Kvist 1980b).

The possible identification of this prostatic component acting as a nuclear chromatin stabilizer in seminal plasma with zinc has been proposed by Kvist (1980c) who found that spermatozoa subjected to SDS were found to undergo nuclear chromatin decondensation if previously or afterwards treated with substances known to deplete the spermatozoa of zinc (albumin and EDTA). Zn^{++}, but no other, "prostatic" cations (Ca^{++}, Mg^{++}), inhibited the experimentally induced nuclear decondensation. Zinc may have exerted its inhibitory effect by reversibly binding to intracellular thiols, which are derived from the cleavage of S–S bridges present in chromatin. Spermatozoa free ("unprotected") thiols are readily oxidized in an atmospheric milieu (Marushige and Marushige, 1975). However, thiols bound to zinc are considerably less susceptible to oxidation, and the main physiological importance of spermatozoa zinc might be to protect thiols from oxidative destruction after ejaculation (Kvist, 1980d). The spermatozoon may have an intrinsic mechanism for nuclear decondensation that is preserved by temporary zinc inhibition and may be reactivated by zinc removal within the female tract (Kvist and Eliasson, 1980).

Studies of heparin decondensing capacity of ejaculated human spermatozoa have also shown that the polysaccharide is necessary to produce this phenomenon. However, previous release of sperm zinc by preincubation with EDTA changed the decondensation kinetics (Fig. 4), making sperm nuclei more susceptible to the action of the mucopolysaccharide.

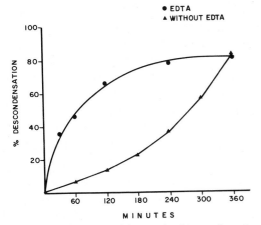

Figure 4. Time dependence of the reaction between heparin and swollen of spermatozoa nuclei ▲——▲ 5000 USP of heparin ●--● USP of heparin, pre-treated with EDTA 6 mM. (Delgado et al., unpublished observations).

3. SULFYDRYL GROUPS

3.1. *In nuclear decondensation*

Sulfydryl groups may indirectly be sustained by the recent discovery in epididymal and seminal plasma of a specific sulfydryl oxidase (Chang and Morton, 1975). This enzyme is different from the previously described thiol oxidases in that the product of its reaction is hydrogen peroxide and not water as is the case for the other two previously described enzymes (Aurbach and Jakoby, 1962). Realizing that the epididymal fluid enzyme is capable of utilizing mercaptoethanol, glutathione, cysteine and thioglycolate as substrates, thiol oxidase is inhibited by all these compounds except thiogly-colate. The enzyme from *Myrothecium verrucaria* is not capable of oxidizing thioglycolate (Mandels, 1956). Sulfydryl oxidase has been found in hamster testicular and epididymal sperm cells, hamster, guinea pig, dog and bull epididymal fluids and human seminal plasma and blood serum (Chang and Zirkin, 1978; Ellman, 1959). Although poten-tially dangerous, sulfydryl compounds may be nec-essary for the survival of spermatozoa. Sulfydryl is vital for sperm motility, sperm metabolism (Mann, 1964), and possibly for the binding of spermatozoa to the zona pellucida (Reyes et al., 1975a). How-ever, exogenous sulfydryls are capable of damaging sperm nuclear and tail structures. Although a crit-ical level of sulfydryls capable of supporting sperm survival needs to be maintained, it should be sufficiently low so that the sperm structure is not affected. The presence of disulfide-reducing and sulfydryl-oxidizing enzymes both in and around spermatozoa (Li, 1975; Chang and Morton, 1975) may maintain such sulfydryl concentration in the male reproductive tract.

3.2. *Sulfydryl oxidase*

The presence of sulfydryl-oxidase in the genital tract can easily be correlated with the increasing degree of disulfide binding occurring in the sperma-tozoa during epididymal maturation (Reyes et al., 1976). However, the highest activity of the enzyme is found in seminal vesicles (Chang and Zirkin, 1978). Therefore, this enzyme is necessary in the seminal plasma during and after ejaculation. This is possible if the enzyme participates in the mech-anisms of preservation of the chromatine structure during the presence of spermatozoa in seminal plasma (see above). The effective occurrence of spermatozoa attaching and binding to the zona pellucida, which is the initial step in the process of fertilization, requires the maintenance of a specific population of surface sulfydryl groups in the ejacu-lated, capacitated spermatozoa (Reyes et al., 1974). Protection of disulfide bonds against the possible interference of reductive agents (see above) that may induce the premature initiation of sperma-tozoa chromatin decondensation, may be accom-plished by the presence of sulfydryl oxidase in seminal plasma. These two complementary pro-cesses may depend on a carefully maintained equi-librium between oxidation and reduction of spec-ific populations of sulfydryl groups (Chang and Morton, 1975).

3.3. *Glutathione cycle*

Thiol compounds such as cysteine and glutathione protect the motility and glycolytic activity of spermatozoa in vitro against the inhibitory action of heavy metal ions and oxidizing agents. Other effective compounds are ergothionine and ascorbic acid present in the seminal plasma of some animal species (Mann, 1964). Oxidation of thiol groups occurs with senescence and during aging of sea urchin spermatozoa, when glutatione content decreases dramatically (Bäckström, 1958). Washed, ejaculated or epididymal spermatozoa from man, dog, ram and goat contain about 5 (1–13) nmoles of glutathione per 10^9 cells. In contrast, the total thiol content of the sperm samples is 350 (95–700) nmoles/10^9 cells, almost entirely protein-bound. The glutathione content of seminal plasma is less than 2 μM (Li, 1975). The spermatozoa containing glutathione also exhibit substantial glutathione reductase and glutathione peroxidase activities.

The physiological function of the glutathione cycle can best be characterized by an effective intracellular defense mechanism against a variety of oxidative damaging agents (Cohen and Hochstein, 1963). The compound H_2O_2 is highly toxic to mammalian spermatozoa and oxygenation of semen is deleterious to sperm function (MacLeod, 1943; Van Demark et al., 1949). H_2O_2 can be produced in seminal plasma by the activity of spermine oxidase, oxidative deamination of amine acids (Tosic and Walton, 1950), etc. Thus, the existence of an H_2O_2 removing mechanism — such as that formed by glutathione peroxidase which reduces H_2O_2, while the glutathione disulfide thus formed is converted back to glugathione by glutathione reductase — would not only be beneficial to sperm survival but would also contribute to the preservation of the important equilibrium between thiol and disulfide groups. This last preservative mechanism may also be accomplished through both the activity of glutathione S-transferase, and the enzyme activity present in significant amounts in mouse and human semen (Mukhtar et al., 1978).

4. LIPIDS

4.1. Decapacitation and lipid vesicles

Although spermatozoa of rabbits and rats must reside in the female tract for some time to acquire the capacity to fertilize the ovum (Chang, 1951; Austin, 1951) the presence of seminal plasma reverses capacitation and renders capacitated spermatozoa incapable of fertilization. Decapacitated spermatozoa can regain their capacity to fertilize if resubmitted to capacitating conditions (Reyes et al., 1975b).

This decapacitation factor is in fluids obtained from all levels of the male genital tract: seminiferous tubule, epididymis and in the seminal fluids from vasectomized animals. Decapacitation factor is also present in most studied mammalian species (Bedford, 1970; Chang et al., 1977). This ambiguity may result from more than one substance acting as the decapacitation factor. The molecular weight oscillates in the range between a few hundred (perhaps zinc[++] itself, Delgado et al., 1976) to hundreds of thousands. Since 1962, macromolecular dimensions in seminal plasma have been capable of reversibly blocking sperm fertilizing capacity (Bedford and Chang, 1962). The biochemical composition of this high molecular weight component is unknown. Some investigators consider it a glucoprotein (Davis and Niwa, 1974) whereas others have presented evidence that the antifertility activity is due to the presence of small membrane vesicles, approximately 50.7 nm in diameter (Davis, 1974).

Seminal plasma from fertile rabbits contain two classes of membrane vesicles that are capable of reversibly inhibiting the fertilizing capacity in uterine capacitated sperm cells. The less dense fraction (Fr. II) inhibits fertilization at concentrations between 20 and 72 μg protein/ml, while the more dense fraction (Fr. I) is less effective and requires much higher concentrations to inhibit the fertilizing capacity of spermatozoa capacitated in utero (Davis, 1978). Both kinds of vesicles also block fertilization in vitro of rat eggs by epididymal rat spermatozoa. This suggests a direct nonspecies-specific action of the vesicles on spermatozoa, preventing or inhibiting capacitation and/or fertilization.

The decapacitation activity of epididymal fluid and more importantly the need to capacitate epididymal spermatozoa before fetilization has been explained by Davis (1974) to be due to the high content of Fr. I-type vesicles in the epididymal secretion. These types of vesicles are not found in the seminal plasma of vasectomized animals which eliminates the accessory glands as possible sources. However, light vesicles are not present in epididymal fluid and are not eliminated from seminal plasma by vasectomy. Their formation could therefore be associated with the secretory activity of seminal vesicles and prostate (Davis, 1978). Membrane vesicles from rabbit seminal plasma contain a complex variety of proteins and lipids. Partial extraction of cholesterol and phospholipid significantly decreased decapacitation activity. Decapacitation was not affected by proteolytic digestion to remove surface proteins, or heating at 100° C for 3 min to cause enzyme inactivation. Vesicle lipids are clearly implicated in sperm decapacitation. Synthetic vesicles made of phosphatidylcholine and containing 10 to 40 (w/w) % cholesterol inhibited fertilization by uterine capacitated rabbit spermatozoa. Vesicles lacking the sterol were not inhibitory. The potency of cholesterol containing synthetic vesicles was comparable to that of membrane vesicles from seminal plasma (Davis, 1976).

4.2. Exchange of lipids between seminal plasma spermatozoa

Cholesterol and phospholipids are important constituents of cell membranes. The interaction of these lipid molecules to the physical characteristic changes of the membrane phospholipid bilayer which occurs when cholesterol is introduced has been studied. There is some relationship between the fluidity of this bilayer and the transport and enzymatic functions of the membrane.

Both cholesterol and phospholipids can be freely exchanged between the plasma membrane and its microenvironment. Nonuniform distribution of cholesterol exists on membranes and cholesterol may exist in specific pools within them. Studies on the erythrocyte-blood plasma relationship have shown that cholesterol either partially or totally exchanges (Hagerman and Gould, 1951; London and Schwarz, 1953) between erythrocyte membranes and plasma lipoproteins. Cholesterol and phospholipid content of normal and pathological seminal plasma have been studied to determine if this exchange is also present between sperm cells and seminal plasma.

Out of the 83 samples of human semen studied, 50 were obtained from patients seeking treatment for infertility and the rest from normal patients, including eight vasectomized who were chosen to match the age span of the group with reproductive pathology.

Spermatozoa from pathologic semen had similar concentrations of phospholipid-phosphorus and a significantly higher cholesterol concentration than spermatozoa from normal semen. However, only oligoasthenospermic spermatozoa showed a significantly higher cholesterol/phospholipid ratio (Table 3).

Lipids exchange freely between spermatozoa and seminal plasma in such a way that lipid composition of the spermatozoa membrane correlates with a high degree of statistical significance with the lipid composition of the seminal plasma (Fig. 5). These interrelations between sperm cells and their environment created by the secretions of the male genital tract are important.

Table 3. Lipid composition of normal and pathological human spermatozoa. The data express mean $\pm$ S.D. of the number of cases expressed in parentheses

	Normo-spermics (25)	Oligoastheno-spermics (15)	Astheno-spermics (23)
Cholesterol μmoles/10^9 cells	0.84 ± 0.33^a	1.86 ± 0.53^b	1.60 ± 0.63^b
Phospholipids μmoles/10^9 cells	1.10 ± 0.46^a	0.97 ± 0.38^a	1.48 ± 0.76^a
$\dfrac{\text{Cholesterol (moles)}}{\text{Phospholipids (moles)}}$	0.69 ± 0.34^a	1.85 ± 0.99^b	1.03 ± 0.71^a

In each line data with the same superscript are not statistically different (ANOVA analysis and Sheffe's test). (Huacuja and Delgado, unpublished observations).

4.3. Peroxidation and senescence

Molecular oxygen can be toxic not only to obligate anaerobes but also to other forms of life. This effect is mainly due to the possible formation of certain highly reactive free radicals, such as the peroxide anion radical O_2 and the hydroxyl radical OH. Oxidations produced by these radicals might produce organic peroxides, including the highly toxic lipid peroxides which are generated during the aerobic oxidation of unsaturated lipids.

Fifty years ago, Gray (1931) proposed that "senescence" of spermatozoa might be due to "auto-intoxication". The formation of lipid peroxides could at least be one of the causes of this auto-intoxication produced through "oxygen damage". The widespread distribution of unsaturated lipids in cell membranes and their lability in the presence

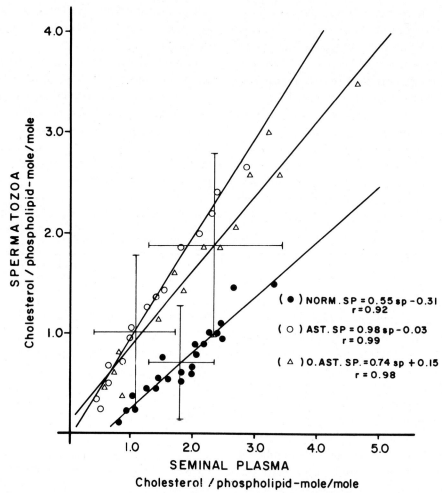

Figure 5. Regression lines obtained by comparing the lipid composition of spermatozoa (ordinates) and of seminal plasma (abscissae) of normal and pathological semen samples. The inserted values are the means of the cholesterol/phospholipid ratios in spermatozoa and seminal plasma. (Huacuja and Delgado, unpublished observations).

of oxygen correlates membrane lipid peroxidation with cellular damage. Hemolysis of erythrocytes (Tsen and Collier, 1960), blood platelet aggregation, swelling of mitochondria (Hunter et al., 1963; McKnight and Hunter, 1966), structural damage to DNA, loss of membrane integrity and inactivation of enzymes—particularly oxidative and respiratory enzymes — have all been ascribed to the formation of lipid peroxides. Lipid peroxides affect SH-containing proteins (Dubouloz and Fondarai, 1953; Willis 1972), and SH-containing enzymes are in generally more readily inhibited by lipid peroxides than other enzymes. Furthermore, sulfydryl compounds, such as reduced glutathione, confer some protection to the toxic effect of lipid peroxides.

In view of the high content of unsaturated fatty acids in the phospholipids of mammalian sperma-

tozoa, these fatty acids may undergo peroxidation (Darin-Bennet and White, 1977; Jones and Mann, 1976) which in turn, may adversely affect the viability of ejaculated spermatozoa. Under aerobic conditions, the lipids in spermatozoa — particularly, the plasmalogens — are susceptible to peroxidation. The peroxidation reaction takes place within the lipoprotein, and is associated with an increase in sperm agglutination and a decrease in motility and viability of spermatozoa (Fujihara and Howarth, 1978). Morphological observations revealed that peroxidation damages the plasma membrane, particularly in the region of the acrosome. Lipid peroxidation irreversibly abolishes the fructolytic and respiratory activity of spermatozoa (Jones and Mann, 1977a).

Although the amount of lipids in seminal plasma

is less than in spermatozoa, unsaturated plasmalogens, which form the natural substrate for peroxidation in spermatozoa, constitute as much as 30–40% of the seminal plasma phospholipids. Under certain conditions, these plasmalogens may be a potential source of organic peroxides. Within the general mechanism of lipid exchange between seminal plasma and spermatozoa, peroxidized or peroxidable lipids may preferentially be transferred from the seminal plasma to the spermatozoa membrane under conditions not yet completely understood. This may explain why ejaculated spermatozoa lose some of their capacity to resist cold shock, and also why spermatozoa from the epididymis survive longer than ejaculated ermatozoa in vitro (Jones and Mann, 1977). Of particular importance to the clinical aspects of sperm physiology are the following two facts. First, the phospholipids of abnormal spermatozoa peroxidize faster than those of normal spermatozoa (Jones et al., 1978; Diezel et al., 1980). Thus, immotile spermatozoa from necrospermic semen, or spermatozoa with an escessively high proportion of abnormal forms, peroxidize at a rate considerably higher than that of intact and fully motile sperm specimens (Jones et al., 1979). Second, the rate of endogenous lipid peroxidation exhibited by human spermatozoa is greatly depressed by the addition of seminal plasma to washed sperm suspensions. Both the endogenous peroxidation of sperm lipids and the concomitant decline of sperm motility can be effectively suppressed not only by antioxidants such as butylated hydroxyanisole (Jones and Mann, 1976), but also by human seminal plasma.

The protective action of seminal plasma is not confined to inhibiting peroxidation of endogenous phospholipids. The striking loss of motility experienced by spermatozoa upon exposure to exogenous peroxidized lipids is also preventable by seminal plasma (Jones et al., 1979). This protective action probably depends on the presence in seminal plasma not only of antioxidants, but also of specific binding mechanisms which will subtract peroxidized lipids from the environment, rendering them harmless.

Some pathological conditions in males might depend on excess lipid peroxidation due to abnormal lipid composition, either to an excess of intrinsic or extrinsic peroxidative activity, or to defects on the protective activity of seminal plasma. The beneficial effect of suspending washed spermatozoa, obtained from pathological semen, into cell-free seminal plasma obtained from normal ejaculates might explain the cause of infertility in some patients (Diezel et al., 1980). Cell and plasma components involved in the process of lipid peroxidation can be useful when included in the biochemical appraisal of sperm quality.

5. PROLACTIN AND CALCIUM IONS

5.1. Sperm number and metabolism

Adequate sperm and counts correlated well with higher prolactin levels in seminal plasma, whereas low semen prolactin levels were routinely found in pathological semen specimens (Sheth et al., 1975). Tzingounis and Aksu (1978), as well as Segal et al. (1978) found that oligozoospermic specimens show higher prolactin levels interfere with the testicular spermatogenic activity (Tzingounis and Aksu, 1978; Segal et al., 1978). The possible role of prolactin as a factor on serpmatozoa fertilizing capacity has been supported by its effects on various metabolic parameters of the human spermatozoa. Prolactin activates the ATPase activity of intact spermatozoa (Sheth et al., 1979a), increases cyclic AMP-accumulation, stimulates the utilization of fructose by the spermatozoa, and increases the $^{14}CO_2$ production from ^{14}C-glucose thus suggesting an increase in oxidative metabolism of the spermatozoa (Shah et al., 1976; Sheth and Rao, 1959). The activation of membrane-bound ATPase suggests the removal of some components bound to the spermatozoa plasma membrane, and also correlates with capacitation. A similar process, removal of tetracycline from human spermatozoa, is a good indicator of the initial steps of capacitation (Vaidya et al., 1969; Hicks et al., 1972). Prolactin causes a significant decrease in the tetracycline binding capacity of the spermatozoa. This decrease could be reversed by adding decapacitation factor prepared from human seminal plasma (Sheth and Shah, 1978).

5.2. Motility and capacitation

Prolactin participates in the mechanism by which the spermatozoa bind and/or transport calcium. Calcium ions are important regulators of spermatozoa metabolism (Peterson and Freund, 1976) and are also indispensable participants in the neurohormonal mechanism that controls spermatozoa motility (Nelson, 1978). Furthermore, Ca^{++} seems to be indispensable in all the processes related to cAMP activation, including capacitation and the acrosome reaction (Yanagimachi and Usui, 1974).

The role of prolactin on calcium binding and/or transport in ejaculated human spermatozoa has recently been studied (Reyes et al., 1979). Ca^{++} transport in these cells was little and dependent on a process which was already saturated after the first 15 min of incubation. Incubation in the presence of 50 ng of prolactin/ml was unable to modify this behavior, whereas concentrations of prolactin as high as 200 ng/ml induced an increase that was

PROLACTIN AND CALCIUM TRANSPORT IN
HUMAN SPERMATOZOA

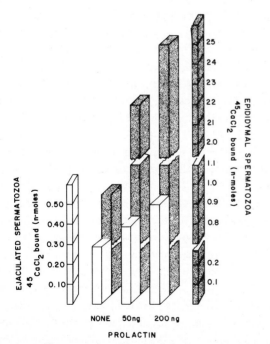

Figure 6. ^{45}Ca-labeled calcium chloride bound (nmoles/10^8 sperm) to epididymal (full bars) and ejaculated (empty bars) spermatozoa in the presence of different concentrations of prolactin. Values express the mean of six experiments. All results obtained with epididymal spermatozoa were significantly different from those obtained with ejaculated spermatozoa ($p < 0.001$). (Modified from Reyes et al., 1979).

expressed completely during the first 15 min of incubation. This lack of susceptibility of the ejaculated spermatozoa to prolactin is also reflected in the high concentration of this hormone (240 ng/ml) required to induce an increase in the accumulation of cyclic AMP in these cells (Sheth and Shah, 1978).

Human epididymal spermatozoa differed from ejaculated sperm cells in showing greater, time-dependent, calcium binding and/or transport under basal conditions and in being more susceptible to the stimulating action of prolactin upon this parameter. This differential susceptibility (Fig. 6) to the hormone may reflect an intrinsic property of the epididymal sperm cells.

Prolactin also increases the calcium uptake by the spermatozoa, especially at lower doses when the spermatozoa are exposed to the hormone for 20 min (Shah and Sheth, 1979). This influx of calcium was accompanied by efflux of Mg^{++}. Prolactin also produces a decrease in the concentration of Zn^{++} (Shah et al., 1980). In view of these effects of prolactin on the ionic equilibrium of spermatozoa it may not be surprising that many of the effects of prolactin signaled above may partially be due to this property. Although prolactin is present in human cervical mucus at levels 3 to 5 fold higher than serum levels (Sheth et al., 1976a), it may also affect the fertilizing potential of spermatozoa. Prolactin enters into seminal plasma by a selective secretory mechanism. Prolactin appears in seminal plasma at levels consistently higher than those existing in serum (Reyes et al., 1979) and in the absence of any correlation between serum prolactin concentration and that of seminal plasma, 30 min after the administration of LH-RH/TRH. Hyperprolactinemia induced in bonnet monkeys by acute and chronic treatment with chlorpromazine showed significantly higher prolactin levels in seminal plasma on the 8th and 16th days respectively, by which time the serum prolactin has already reached pretreatment levels (Sheth et al., 1979b).

Prolactin is apparently added to the seminal plasma at the moment of ejaculation. In the study of Reyes et al. (1979), human spermatozoa and fluid from the cauda epididymis were obtained from freshly post-mortem and semen from normal volunteers before vasectomy and 3 to 4 months after. The mean prolactin concentration in seminal plasma from euspermic and postvasectomy samples were not significantly different: 48 ± 12 and 50 ± 10.2 ng/ml, respectively. These values were 7 to 8 times higher than the prolactin concentration found in the blood serum (5.5–9.1 ng/ml) of the same volunteers. The prolactin concentration in human cauda epididymis fluid (7.1 ± 2.0 ng/ml) was similar to that found in male blood serum (5.5–9.1 ng/ml) yet significantly lower than the concentration of the hormone found in seminal plasma obtained from either euspermic or vasectomized volunteers.

6. OTHER FACTORS

6.1. Kinins

The participation of the kallikrein–kinin system in the regulation and stimulation of human sperm motility was first suggested by Schill et al. (1974), and subsequently confirmed by (Makler et al., 1980; Schirren, 1975). Physiologically, some components of the kinin system were present in male genital secretions. Seminal plasma possesses low amounts of kininogen and kininases (Schill and Haberland, 1974). In addition, the occurrence of seminal plasma kininogenases has been indirectly demonstrated: addition of low amounts of highly purified kininogen (0.1 mg per ml) to hypokynetic semen specimens induced a significant stimulation of spermatozoa motility (Makler et al., 1080).

Kinins are able to induce the following effects on the male genital system:

a) Increase the number of motile cells in hypokinetic specimens while increasing the mean velocity and the number of cells showing good forward progression (Schill, 1975a, b).

b) A slight improvement of spermatozoa viability accompanied by any stimulation of the fructose and oxygen consumption of the spermatozoa (Schill, 1975b).

The improvement of spermatozoa motility by kinins provided the theoretical basis for the therapeutical application of components of the kinin system. Systemic application of kallikrein (EC. 3.4.21.8), a kinin-liberating enzyme administered either parenterally or orally to asthenozoospermic or oligozoospermic men, induced a significant increase not only on spermatozoa motility (Schill et al., 1974; Schill, 1975c) but also in the mean number of ejaculated spermatozoa (Farris and Colton, 1958). This indirectly indicates the possible participation of the kinin system in the regulation of the spermatogenic function of the human testes.

The influence of kallikrein on cellular membrane permeability has been recently questioned. Makler et al. (1980) tested the effect of six metabolically active compounds, including kallikrein, on spermatozoa motility. There was no immediate or delayed effect on spermatozoa motility and velocity compared to the procedures and dosage of kallikrein used previously (Schill et al., 1974).

Aside from the presence of a specific seminal plasma kininogenase, acrosin behaves as a potent component kinin-liberating enzyme (Fritz et al., 1973). This finding raises the question whether acrosin plays a role as a kinin liberator participating in the mechanism of spermatozoa motility regulation. However, since large amounts of acrosin inhibitors are found in seminal plasma, it is doubtful whether acrosin present within the male secretions would be able to liberate kinins.

6.2. Polyamines

Until recently, no specific physiological function had been noted in the presence of unusually high concentrations of spermine in human semen. Polyamines in mammalian semen have now been related to two widely opposed ways of action. Products derived from spermine and spermidine through the action of diamine oxidase are toxic for a variety of cells, including spermatozoa (Tabor et al., 1964; Bachrach, 1970). These polyamines also participate as activators of spermatozoa metabolism and motility and as producers of capacitation (Pulkkinen et al., 1975).

Products arising from spermine and spermidine through the action of diamine oxidase could involve iminoaldehydes that are known as toxic substances for living cells (Tabor and Rosenthal, 1956). Iminoaldehydes are, however, very labile while undergoing B-elimination and polymerization (Kimes and Morris, 1971a; Kimes and Morris, 1971b). Diamino oxidase and a specific amine oxidase (spermin oxidase) are two enzymes in human semen that oxidize spermine (Zeller, 1941; Janne et al., 1973). About 5% of the total diamine oxidase activity of human semen is associated with the washed spermatozoa (Pulkkinen et al., 1975). In spite of the preferential location of spermine in seminal plasma, human spermatozoa, separated from the seminal plasma and washed extensively, contain appreciable amounts of spermine. Although the enzyme activity is fundamentally present in seminal plasma it is not known whether spermine functions by attaching itself to the outer membrane of the spermatozoa or binds more specifically to some intracellular component. Oxidation products formed from spermine also have a high affinity for human spermatozoa (Pulkkinen et al., 1975). Even in low concentrations, these oxidation products will completely inactivate human spermatozoa (Tabor et al., 1964). It seems unlikely however, that under normal physiological conditions, appreciable amounts of such products would be formed during the short period in which ejaculated spermatozoa remain in contact with seminal plasma. However, since both spermine and diamine oxidase are derived from the prostate gland (Jänne et al., 1973; Thakur et al., 1973), the ejaculated spermatozoa may make contact with preformed oxidation products. These products may influence the motility and fertilizing capacity of some spermatozoa.

As with polyamines, an important and usual characteristic of agents related to reproductive processes is their bifunctional activity, as under different conditions they may be either activators or inhibitors of the fundamental physiological processes.

Fair et al. (1972) found a correlation between the concentration of spermine in seminal plasma and the concentration and motility of spermatozoa in semen; however Jänne et al. (1973) could not confirm this. The presence of spermine induced motile spermatozoa, obtained from the vas deferens of mice, rats, guinea pigs and rabbits, to vibrate rapidly without forward motion (Tabor and Rosenthal, 1956). The addition of 1 to 10 mM spermine to epididymal sperm suspensions resulted in a 2 to 7 fold increase in the formation of labeled lactate from uniformly labeled fructose. The combination of spermine and calcium (1 mM), resulted in a striking synergistic stimulation in epididymal spermatozoa (Pulkkinen et al., 1975). The production of lactate from fructose in the presence of

spermine and Ca^{++} increased 5 to 30 fold over that in normal Ringer solution. While stimulating the aerobic pructolysis, the polyamines inhibited the formation of $^{14}CO_2$ from $2\text{-}^{14}C$-pyruvate, apparently interfering with the tricarboxylic acid cycle. Thus, these substances could conceivably belong to the factors responsible for the highly glycolytic metabolism of ejaculated spermatozoa (Sosa et al., 1972).

Cyclic AMP plays an important role in the metabolism and motility of human spermatozoa (Hicks et al., 1972; Rosado et al., 1975). Levels of cyclic AMP are regulated by the interplay of the enzyme adenylate cyclase which synthesizes it, and the enzyme phosphodiesterase which converts cyclic AMP into AMP. Spermine activates the enzyme acrosomal protease, which is vital for the penetration through the zona pellucida (Parrish and Polakoski, 1977). Polyamines inhibited the conversion of proacrosin to acrosin in both human and boar spermatozoa (Parrish et al., 1979).

The possible participation of polyamines in the process of spermatozoa capacitation may be due to the spermine reduction of the tetracycline-binding of spermatozoa (Shah and Sheth, 1979). This can also explain the initiation of capacitation (Hicks et al., 1972).

6.3. Catecholamines

Sperm motility partially depends on the environmental presence of motility factors. Some of these recently discovered factors, which are of protein origin, have been called "forward motility factors" (Hoskins et al., 1978) and are important components of epididymal secretions, forming part of the mechanism by which epididymal spermatozoa acquire the ability of progressive motility (Hoskins et al., 1978).

Another type of motility factor present in a variety of body fluids, including blood serum (Bavister, 1975), has been related not only to the stimulation of forward motility but also to the development of the "whiplash" type of movement called activation which is associated with sperm capacitation (Cornett and Meizel, 1978).

These protein free, low molecular weight agents also participate in the process of vesiculation of sperm head membranes which conduce capacitating spermatozoa towards the acrosome reaction (Bavister and Yanagimachi, 1977).

That these agents could be specifically catecholamines (CA) has been shown by:

1) The presence in adrenal extracts of high concentrations of these stimulator agents (Bavister et al., 1976). Spermatozoa preincubated for 3 h in a culture medium containing bovine serum albumin, and a protein-free ultrafiltrate of a bovine adrenal cortex preparation, were unable to fertilize cumulus-free eggs. In contrast, if the culture medium also contained a protein-free ultrafiltrate of a bovine adrenal medulla preparation, 92% of the inseminated eggs were fertilized within 2 h.

2) Catecholamines and α- and β-adrenergic agonists stimulate sperm capacitation activation and acrosome reaction (Cornett and Meizel, 1978; 1979). These effects are inhibited by α- and β-adrenergic antagonists (Cornett et al., 1979).

3) The presence of significant amounts of some monoamines, including norepinephrine, dopamine and 5-hydroxytriptamine in human seminal plasma and human follicular fluid (Sosa et al., in press) (Table 4).

6.4. Acethylcholine and calcium ions

Meizel and Working (1980) have presented evidence that stongly supports previous suggestions (Sosa et al., in press; Cornett and Meizel, 1978) that catecholamine stimulation of the sperm acrosome reaction occurs through a hormonal mechanism depending primarily on the interaction of specific adrenergic receptors present in the spermatozoa membrane. This is similar to spermatozoa motility which is regulated by the interaction of adrenergic and acetylcholinergic receptors, depending on the presence of activators and inhibitors of these systems present in seminal plasma.

Spermatozoa contain choline acetyltransferase, acetylcholinesterase and an acetylcholine receptor (Steward and Forrester, 1978a, 1978b). Acetylcholine may produce an increase in the ion permeability of a spermatozoa membrane system similar to what occurs at muscle end plates (Kaser-Glanzmann et al., 1978; Thorens, 1979).

Table 4. Presence of biogenic amines in human reproductive tract fluids. The data express the mean $\pm$ the standard deviation of the number of cases indicated in parentheses.

Neurotransmitter	Seminal plasma		Follicular fluid
	Normospermic	Azoospermic	
Dopamine (nM)	258 ± 36 (12)	345 ± 45[++] (6)	241 ± 22 (7)
Norepinephrine (nM)	272 ± 77 (12)	362 & 52[+] (6)	186 ± 17 (7)
5-Hydroxytryptamine (nM)	255 ± 40 (12)	417 ± 12[++] (6)	111 ± 10 (7)
5-Hydroxy-indole acetic acid (nM)	161 ± 15 (12)	173 ± 15 (6)	130 ± 10 (7)

[+]; [++] Unpaired "t" test indicates a significant difference ($p < 0.01$); $p < 0.001$ when compared with the same determination done in normospermic seminal plasma. (Sosa et al., in press).

REFERENCES

Atherton RW, Radany EW, Plaskoski KI (1978) Quantitation of human sperm motility. Biol Reprod 18: 624.

Aurbach GD, Jakoby WB (1962) The multiple functions of thiooxidase. J Biol Chem 237 565.

Austin CR (1951) Observations on the penetration of the sperm into the mammalian egg. Austr J Sci Res B4: 581.

Bachrach U (1970) Metabolism and function of spermidine and related polyamines. A Rev Microbiol 24: 109.

Bäckström S (1958) Glutathione in aging sperm and developing eggs of the sea urchin. Arkiv Zool II 11: 441.

Bavister BD (1975) Properties of the sperm motility-stimulating component derived from human serum. J Reprod Fert 43: 363.

Bavister BD, Yanagimachi R (1977) The effects of sperm extracts and energy sources on the motility and acrosome reaction of hamster spermatozoa in vitro. Biol Reprod 16: 228.

Bavister BD, Yanagimachi R, Teichman RJ (1976) Capacitation of hamster spermatozoa with adrenal gland extracts. Biol Reprod 14: 219.

Bedford JM (1970) Sperm capacitation and fertilization in mammals. Biol Reprod 2 Suppl: 128.

Bedford JM, Calvin HI (1974) The occurrence and possible functional significance of -S–S-crosslinks in sperm heads, with particular reference to eutherian mammals. J Exp Zool 188: 137.

Bedford JM, Chang MC (1962) Removal of decapacitation factor from seminal plasma by high speed centrifugation. Am J Physiol 202: 179.

Berridge MJ (1975) The interaction of cyclic nucleotides and calcium in the control of cellular activity. Adv Cyclic Nucl Res 6: 1.

Biswas S, Ferguson KM, Stedronska J, Baffoe G, Mansfield MD, Kosbad M (1978) Fructose and hormone levels in semen; their correlations with counts and motility. Fertil Steril 30: 200.

Calvin HI, Bedford JM (1971) Formation of disulphide bonds in the nucleus and accessory structures of mammalian spermatozoa during epididymal maturation. J Reprod Fertil Suppl 13: 65.

Chang MC, Austin CR, Bedford JM, Bracket BG, Hunter RHF, Yanagimachi R (1977) Capacitation of spermatozoa and fertilization in mammals. In Greep RO, Koblinsky MA, eds. Frontiers in reproduction and fertility control, pp 434–444. MIT Press.

Chang TSK, Morton B (1975) Epididymal sulfhydryl oxidase: a sperm-protective enzyme from the male reproductive tract. Biochem Biophys Res Comm 66: 309.

Chang TSK, Zirkin BR (1978) Distribution of sulfhydryl oxidase activity in the rat and hamster male reproductive tract. Biol Reprod 17: 745.

Cohen G, Hochstein P (1963) Glutathione peroxidase: the primary agent for the elimination of hydrogen peroxide in erythrocytes. Biochemistry 2: 1420.

Cornett LE, Bavister BD, Meizel S (1979) Adrenergic stimulation of fertilizing ability in hamster spermatozoa. Biol Reprod 20: 925.

Cornett LE, Meizel S (1978) Stimulation of in vitro activation and the acrosome reaction of hamster spermatozoa by catecholamines. Prod Natl Acad Sci USA 75: 4954.

Danscher G, Hammen R, Fjerdingstand E, Rebbe H (1978) Zinc content of human ejaculate and the motility of sperm cells. Int J Androl 1: 576.

Darin-Bennet A, White IG (1977) Influence of the cholesterol content of mammalian spermatozoa and susceptibility to cold shock. Cryobiology 14: 466.

Davis BK (1974) Decapaciation and recapacitation of rabbit spermatozoa treated with membrane vesicles from seminal plasma. J Reprod Fertil 41: 241.

Davis BK (1976) Inhibitory effect of synthetic phospholipid vesicles containing cholesterol on the fertilizing ability of rabbit spermatozoa. Proc Soc Exp Biol Med 152: 257.

Davis BK (1978) Inhibition of fertilizing capacity in mammalian spermatozoa by natural and synthetic vesicles. In: Symposium on the pharmacological effects of lipids, AOCS Monograph No 5 Chap 14: 145.

Davis BK, Niwa K (1974) Inhibition of mammalian fertilization in vitro by membrane vesicles from seminal plasma. Proc Soc Exp Biol Med 146: 11.

Delgado NM, Huacuja L, Merchant H, Reyes R, Rosado A (1980) Species specific decondensation of human spermatozoa nuclei by heparin. Arch Androl 4: 305.

Delgado NM, Huacuja L, Pancardo RM, Rosado A (1975) Modification of human sperm metabolism by the induced release of intracellular zinc. Life Sci 16: 1483.

Delgado NM, Huacuja L, Pancardo RM, Rosado A (1976) Selective utilization of endogenous phospholipids by zinc-depleted human spermatozoa. In Campos de Paz A, Drill VA, Hayashi M, Rodriguez W and Schally AV, eds. Recent advances in human reproduction, Amsterdam and Oxford: Excerpta Medica. New York: 325–328. American Elsevier.

Diezel W, Engel S, Sönnischsen N, Höhne WE (1980) Lipid peroxidation products in human spermatozoa: detection and pathogenic significance. Andrologia 12: 167.

Dubouloz P, Fondarai J (1953) Sur le métabolisme des peroxydes lipidiques II. Action des peroxydes lipidiques sur les groupements thiols protéïques. Bull Soc Chim Biol 35: 819.

Ellman GL (1959) Tissue sulfhydryl groups. Arch Biochem Biophys 82: 70.

Epel D (1978) Mechanism of activation of sperm and egg during fertilization of sea urchin gametes. Curr Top Dev Biol 12: 185.

Fair WR, Clark RB, Wehner N (1972) A correlation of seminal polyamine levels and semen analysis in human. Fertil Steril 23: 38.

Farris EJ, Colton SW (1958) Effects of L-thyroxine and listhyronine on spermatogenesis. J Urol 79: 863.

Franks S, Jacobs HS, Martin N, Nabarro JDN (1978) Hyperproleactinaemia and impotency. Clinical Endocrinol 8: 277.

Frenkel-Paz G, Sofer A, Homonnai ZT, Kraicer PF, (1977) Human semen analysis: seminal plasma and prostatic fluid compositions and their interrelations with sperm quality. Int J Fertil 22: 140.

Fritz H, Schiessler H, Schleuning WD (1973) Proteinases and proteinases inhibitors in the fertilization process. Adv Biosci 10: 271.

Fujihara N, Howarth B (1978) Lipid peroxidation in fowl spermatozoa. Poultry Sci 57: 1766.

Gray J (1931) The senescence of spermatozoa II. J Exp Biol 8: 202.

Guerin JF, Czyba JC (1977) Effets de la presion osmotique sur la mobilité et le métabolisme des spermatozoides. Cr Soc Biol Paris 171: 822.

Guerin JF, Czyba JC (1979) Effects of ions and K^+: Na^+ ratio on motility and oxygen consumption of human spermatozoa. Arch Androl 2: 295.

Hagerman JS, Gould RG (1951) The "in vitro" interchange of cholesterol between plasma and red cells. Proc Soc Exp Biol Med 78: 329.

Hernández-Montes H, Iglesias G, Mujica A (1973) Selective solubilization of mammalian spermatozoa structures. Exp Cell Res 76: 437.

Hernández O, Bello MA, Rosado A (1978) The human spermatozoa genome analysis by DNA reassociation kinetics. Biochim Biophys Acta 521: 557.

Hicks JJ, Martínez-Manautou J, Pedrón N, Rosado A (1972) Metabolic changes in human spermatozoa related to capacitation. Fertil Steril 23: 172.

Hoskins DD, Brand TH, Acott TS, (1978) Initiation of sperm motility in the mammalian epididymis. Fed Proc 37: 2534.

Huacuja L, Sosa A, Delgado NM, Rosado A (1973) A kinetic study of the participation of zinc in human spermatozoa metabolism. Life Sci 13: 1382.

Hunter FE, Gebicki JM, Hoffstein PE, Weinstein J, Scott A (1963) Swelling and lysis of rat liver mitochondria induced by ferrous ions. J Biol Chem 238: 828.

Jänne J, Holtta E, Haaranen P, Elfving K (1973) Polyamines and polyamine-metabolizing enzyme activities in human semen.

Clin Chim Acta 48: 393.

Janick J, Zeitz L, Whitmore WF (1971) Seminal fluid and spermatozoon zinc levels and their relationship to human spermatozoon motility. Fertil Steril 22: 573.

Johnson AL, Howards SS (1977) Hyperosmolality in intraluminal fluids from hamster testis and epididymis: a micropuncture study. Science 195: 492.

Jones R, Mann T (1976) Lipid peroxides in spermatozoa, formation, role of plasmalogen, and physiological significance. Proc R Soc Lond B 193: 317.

Jones R, Mann T (1977a) Toxicity of exogenous fatty acid peroxides towards spermatozoa. J Reprod Fertil 50: 255.

Jones R, Mann T (1977b) Damage to ram spermatozoa by peroxidation of endogenous phospholipids. J Reprod Fertil 50: 261.

Jones R, Mann T, Sherins R (1978) Adverse effects of peroxidized lipid on human spermatozoa. Proc Soc Lond B 201: 413.

Jones R, Mann T, Sherins R (1979) Peroxidative breakdown of phospholipids in human spermatozoa, spermicidal properties of fatty acid peroxides, and protective action seminal plasma. Fertil Steril 31: 531.

Jouannet P, Volochine B, Deguent P, Serrer C, David G (1977) Light scattering determination of various characteristic parameters of spermatozoa motility in a seris of human sperm. Andrologia 9: 36.

Kaser-Glanzmann R, Jakabora M, George JN, Luscher EF (1978) Further characterization of calcium-accumulating vesicles from human platelets. Biochim Biophys Acta 512: 1.

Kimes BW, Morris DR (1971a) Preparation and stability of oxidized polyamines. Biochim Biophys Acta 228: 223.

Kimes BW, Morris DR (1971b) Inhibition of nucleic acid and protein synthesis in *Escherichia coli* by oxidized polyamines and acrolein. Biochim Biophys Acta 228: 235.

Kvist U (1980a) Rapid post-ejaculatory inhibitory effect of seminal plasma on sperm nuclear chromatin decondensation ability in man. Acta Physiol Scand 109: 69.

Kvist U (1980b) Reversible inhibition of nuclear chromatin decondensation NCD ability of human spermatozoa induced by prostatic fluid. Acta Physiol Scand 109: 73.

Kvist U (1980c) Importance of spermatozoal zinc as temporary inhibitor of sperm nuclear chromatin decondensation ability in man. Acta Physiol Scand 109: 79.

Kvist U (1980d) Sperm nuclear chromatin decondensation ability. Acta Physiol Scand Suppl 486: 1.

Kvist U, Eliasson R (1980) Influence of seminal plasma an the chromatin stability of ejaculated human spermatozoa. Int J Androl 3: 130.

Li TK (1975) The glutathione and thiol content of mammalian spermatozoa and seminal plasma. Biol Reprod 12: 641.

Lindholmer C (1974) The importance of seminal plasma for human sperm motility. Biol Reprod 10: 533.

Lindholmer C, Eliasson R (1972) Zinc and magnesium in human spermatozoa. Int J Fertil 17: 153.

Lindholmer C, Eliasson R (1974a) Zinc and magnesium in human spermatozoa from different fractions of split ejaculates. Int J Fertil 19: 45.

Lindholmer C, Eliasson R (1974b) In vitro release and uptake of zinc magnesium by human spermatozoa. Int J Fertil 19: 56.

London IM, Schwarz H (1953) Erythrocyte metabolism. The metabolic behavior of the cholesterol of human erythrocytes. J Clin Invest 32: 1248.

MacLeod J (1943) The role of oxygen in the metabolism and motility of human spermatozoa. Am J Physiol 138: 512.

Makler A (1978) A new multiple exposure photography method for objective human spermatozoal motility determination. Fertil Steril 30: 192.

Makler A, Makler E, Itzkovitz, J, Brandes JM (1980) Factors affecting sperm motility. IV Incubation of human semen with caffeine kallikrein, and other metabolically active compounds. Fertil Steril 33: 624.

Mandels GR (1956) Properties and surface location of a sulfhydryl oxidizing enzyme in fungus spores. J Bacteriol 72: 230.

Mann T (1964) In: Biochemistry of semen and of the male reproductive tract. New York. John Wiley.

Marishige Y and Marushige K (1975) Transformation of sperm histone during formation and maturation of rat spermatozoa J Biol Chem 250: 39.

McKnight RC, Hunter FE (1966) Mitochondrial membrane ghost produced by ferrous ions. J Biol Chem 241: 2757.

Meizel S, Working PK (1980) Further evidence suggesting the hormonal stimulation of hamster sperm acrosome reactions by catecholamines in vitro. Biol Reprod 22: 211.

Mukhtar H, Lee IP, Bend JR (1978) Glutathione S-transferase activities in rat and mouse sperm and human semen. Biochem Biophys Res Commun 83: 1093.

Nelson L (1978) Chemistry and neurochemistry of sperm motility control. Federation Proc 37: 2543.

Parrish RF, Goodpasture JC, Zaneveld LJD, Polakoski KL (1979) Polyamine inhibition of the conversion of human proacrosin to acrosin. J Reprod Fertil 57: 239.

Parrish RF, Polakoski KL (1977) Effect of polyamines on the activity of acrosin and the activation of proacrosin. Biol Reprod 17: 417.

Peterson RN, Freund M (1976) Relationship between motility and the transport and binding of divalent cations to the plasma membrane of human spermatozoa. Fertil Steril 27: 1301.

Pulkkinen P, Sirkka Kanerva, Elfving K, Jänne J (1975) Association of spermine and diamine oxidase activity with human spermatozoa. J Reprod Fertil 43: 49.

Reyes A, Mercado E, Goicoechea B, Rosado A (1976) Participation of memebrane sulfhydryl groups in the epididymal maturation of human and rabbit spermatozoa. Fertil Steril 27:1452.

Reyes A, Mercado E, Rosado A (1975a) Inhibition of capacitation and of the fertilizing capacity of rabbit spermatozoa by blocking membrane sulfhydryl groups. In: Campos da Paz A, Drill VA, Hayashi M, Rodriguez W, Schally AV, eds. Recent advances in human reproduction, Amsterdam: Excerpta Medica. p 321.

Reyes A, Parra A, Chavarría ME, Goicoechea B, Rosado A (1979) Effect of prolactin on the calcium binding and/or transport of ejaculated and epididymal human spermatozoa. Fertil Steril 31:669.

Reyes A, Oliphant G, Brackett BG (1975b) Partial purification and identification of a reversible decapacitation factor from rabbit seminal plasma. Fertil Steril 26: 148.

Rosado A, Huacuja L, Delgado NM, Hicks JJ, Pancardo RM (1976) Cyclic-AMP receptors in the human spermatozoa membrane. Life Sci 17: 1707.

Rosado A, Huacuja L, Delgado NM, Merchant H, Pancardo RM (1977) Elemental composition of subcellular structures of human spermatozoa. A study by energy dispersive analysis of X-ray. Life Sci 20: 647.

Shah GV, Gunjikar AN, Sheth AR, Raut SJ (1980) Effect of prolactin and spermine on the zinc content of human spermatozoa. Andrologia 12: 207.

Shah GV, Sheth AR (1979) Is prolactin involved in sperm capacitation? Medical Hypotheses 5: 909.

52

Sheth AR, Shah GV (1978) Effect of prolactin on tetracycline binding to human spermatozoa. Fertil Steril 29: 431.

Sheth AR, Vaidya RA, Raikar ES (1976) Presence of prolactin in human cervical mucus. Fertil Steril 27: 397.

Schill WB (1975a) Caffeine and Kallikrein-induced stimulation of human sperm motility: a comparative study. Andrologia 7: 229.

Schill WB (1975b) Increased fructolysis of kallikrein-stimulated human spermatozoa. Andrologia 7: 105.

Schill WB (1975c) Improvement of sperm motility in patients with asthenozoospermia by kallikrein treatment. Int J Fertil 20: 61.

Schill WB, Braun-Fako O, Haberland GL (1974) The possible role of kinins in sperm motility. Int J Fertil 19: 163.

Schill WB, Haberland GL (1974) Kinin-induced enhancement of sperm motility. Hoppe-Seyler's Z Physiol Chem 335: 229.

Schirren C (1975) Experimental studies on the influence of Kallikrein on human sperm motility in vitro. In: Haberland GL, Rohen JW, Schirren C, Huber P, eds. Kininogens, Vol 2, p 59. Schauer, Stuttgart.

Segal S, Ron M, Laufer N, Ben DM (1978) Prolactin in seminal plasma of infertile men. Arch Androl 1: 49.

Shah GV, Desai RB, Shet AR (1976) Effect of prolactin on metabolism of human spermatozoa. Fertil Steril 27: 1292.

Shah GV, Shet AR (1979) Reduction of tetracycline binding capacity of human spermatozoa by spermine. Infertility 2: 99.

Shah GV, Sheth AR, Mugatwala PP, Rao SS (1975) Effect of spermine on adenyl cyclase activity of spermatozoa. Experientia 31: 631.

Sheth AR, Mugatwala PP, Shah GV, Rao SS (1975) Occurrence of prolactin in human semen. Fertil Steril 26: 905.

Sheth AR, Gunjikar AN, Shah GV (1979a) Effect of LH, prolactin and spermine on ATPase activity of human spermatozoa. Andrologia 11: 11.

Sheth AR, Hurkadly KS, Jayaran S (1979b) Relationship between serum and seminal plasma prolactin in bonnet monkeys. Andrologia 11: 305.

Sheth AR, Rao SS (1959) Fructose and fructolysis in human semen determined chromatographically. Experientia 15: 314.

Sheth AR, Shah GV, Rao SS (1976) Prostaglandins potentiating stimulatory effect of prolactin on human spermatozoal adenyl cyclase. Int J Biochem Biophys 13: 129.

Sheth AR, Wadadekar KB, Gadgil BA (1979) A note on in vitro effects of gonadotropins and spermine on phosphodiesterase activity of bull spermatozoa. Int J Anim Sci 49: 234.

Singh JP, Babcock DF, Lardy HA (1978) Increased calcium ion influx as a component of capacitation of spermatozoa. Biochem J 172: 549.

Sosa A, Altamirano E, Giner J, Rosdo A (1972) Adenine nucleotide concentration and redox value of human spermatozoa. Biol Reprod 7: 326.

Sosa A, Ortega-Corona B, Chargoy-Vera J, Vargas J, Rosado A (1981) Presence of biogenic amines in human reproductive tract secretions. Fert Steril (in press).

Stanković H, Mikac-Dević D, (1976) Zinc and copper in human semen. Clin Chim Acta 70: 123.

Stewart TA, Forrester IT (1978a) Acetylcholinesterase and choline acetyltransferase in ram spermatozoa. Biol Reprod 19: 271.

Stewart TA, Forrester IT (1978b) Identification of a cholinergic receptor in ram spermatozoa. Biol Reprod 19: 965.

Swarup D, Sekhon H (1976) Correlation of vitamin A and zinc concentration of seminal plasma to fertility of bovine semen. Nutr Rep Int 13: 37.

Tabor CW, Rosenthal SM (1956) Pharmacology of spermine and spermidine. Some effects on animals and bacteria. J Pharmac Exp Ther 116: 139.

Tabor CW, Tabor H, Bachrach U (1964) Identification of the aminoaldehydes produced by the oxidation of spermine and spermidine in purified plasma amine oxidase. J Biol Chem 239: 2194.

Thakur AN, Sheth AR, Rao SS (1973) Polyamines in the human semen and prostatic secretions. Int J Biochem and Biophys 10, 2: 136.

Thorens S (1979) Ca^{+2}-ATPase and Ca uptake without requirement for Mg^{+2} in membrane fractions of vascular smooth muscle. FEBS Lett 98: 177.

Tosic J, Walton A (1950) Metabolism of spermatozoa. The formation and elimination of hydrogen peroxide by spermatozoa and effects on motility and survival. Biochem J 47: 199.

Tsen CC, Collier HB (1960) The protective action of tocopherol against hemolysis of rat erythrocytes by dialuric acid. Canad J Biochem Physiol 38: 957.

Tzingounis VA, Aksu MF (1978) Prolactin levels in oligospermia. Presented at the 3rd Annual Meeting of the American Society of Andrology, Nashville, Tenn, p 81.

Vaidya RA, Bedford JM, Glass RH, Morris JM (1969) Evaluation of the removal of tetracycline fluorescence from spermatozoa as a test for capacitation in the rabbit. J Reprod Fertil 19: 483.

Van Demark NL, Salisbury GW, Bratton RW (1949) Oxygen damage to bull spermatozoa and its prevention by catalase. J Dairy Sci 32: 353.

Velázquez A, Pedrón N, Delgado NM, Rosado A (1977) Osmolality and conductance of normal and abnormal human seminal plasma. Int J Fertil 22: 92.

Walton A (1952) Flow orientation as a possible explanation of "wave-motion" and "rheotaxis" of spermatozoa. J Exp Biol 24: 520.

Westmoreland N, First NL, Hoekstra WG (1967) In vitro uptake of zinc by boar spermatozoa. J Reprod Fertil 13: 223.

Willis ED (1971) Effects of lipid peroxidation on membrane-bound enzymees of the endoplasmic reticulum. Biochem J 123: 983.

Yanagimachi R, Usui N (1974) Calcium dependence of the acrosome reaction and activation of guinea pig spermatozoa. Exp Cell Res 89: 161.

Zeller EA (1941) Ueber das Vorkommen der diamin-Oxydase in menschlichen Sperma. Helv Chim Acta 24: 117.

Author's address:
Dr A. Rosado
Sección de Enzimología
División de Bioquímica
Unidad de Investigación Biomédica, CMN
Apartado postal 73-231
México 73, D.F., México

6. FERTILIZING ABILITY AND MOTILITY OF SPERMATOZOA FROM FERTILE AND INFERTILE MEN AFTER EXPOSURE TO HETEROLOGOUS SEMINAL PLASMA

J. Cohen, M. Mooyaart, J.T.M. Vreeburg, R. Yanagimachi and G.H. Zeilmaker

Little is known of the effects of various fluids secreted by accessory sex organs on functional properties and fertilizing capacity of spermatozoa. In a variety of animals, epididymal spermatozoa liberated into simple salt solutions can fertilize eggs (Whittingham, 1979). Seminal plasma may adversely influence human sperm motility (Lindholmer, 1974; Lindholmer and Eliasson, 1974; Mann, 1964; Singh et al., 1969; Valezquez, 1977).

The low motility of spermatozoa derived from oligospermic semen was increased in 14 out of 17 cases by resuspension in seminal plasma obtained from semen with normal motility (Rozin, 1958, 1961). Conversely, the normal motility of spermatozoa of 17 out of 21 fertile men was reduced after resuspension in seminal plasma of oligozoospermic men (Rozin, 1958). Such findings have been confirmed (Eliasson et al., 1978; Polakoski et al., 1976; Polakoski and Zaneveld, 1977), while the use of heterologous seminal plasma has resulted in successful AIH (Rozin, 1958, 1961). In one study, no effect was seen of heterologous seminal plasma (Freund, 1962).

In view of abnormalities noted in seminal plasma of infertile men, it seems possible that such abnormalities could impair motility and fertilizing capacity of normal spermatozoa. This chapter mainly investigates whether spermatozoa from fertile men would be impaired in their motility and fertilizing capacity by incubation in seminal plasma from infertile males which was characterized by a high viscosity, the presence of a coagulum or a large volume of seminal plasma. The effects of seminal plasma from fertile men on spermatozoa derived from infertile men were also studied. Simultaneously, the influence of a simple defined culture medium on the motility of the spermatozoa was investigated.

A semi-automatic analysis of motility and the in vitro fertilizing capacity of human spermatozoa using zona-free hamster ova were used as techniques for measuring sperm characteristics. The use of zona-free hamster ova in studying human sperm fertilizing ability was first proposed by Yanagimachi et al. (1976) and later evaluated by others (Barros et al., 1978; 1979; Binor et al., 1980; Kanwar et al., 1979; Overstreet et al., 1980; Rogers et al., 1979). Various methods for objective assessment of sperm motility have been reported (Janik and McLeod, 1979; Makler, 1978; Milligan et al., 1978; Overstreeet al., 1979). In this study, the Multiple Exposure Photography (MEP) technique was used (Makler, 1978, 1980b). A semi-automatic analysis of motility using a digitizer–computer unit for computing sperm concentration, velocity and percentage (progressive) motility is presented. Moreover, by using all individual images of a sperm track, deviation from progression straight ahead and speed constancy can be calculated for each individual spermatozoon track. These two parameters determined for each photograph show a distinctive range of values and represent, together with the average velocity, a new system for objectivation of sperm characteristics.

1. METHODOLOGY

1.1. Resuspension of spermatozoa in heterologous and homologous seminal plasma

Eight normospermic patients who had been infertile from 3 to 8 years were studied. Sperm counts ranged from 22 to 61×10^6 per ml and only 10–20% of the sperms were motile. Abnormalities such as a large seminal plasma volume, high viscosity of seminal plasma and the presence of coagulum were commonly found in all semen samples of these

Hafez ESE & Semm K (Eds) Instrumental insemination.

infertile men. Semen of five men with proven fertility used in this experiment had a sperm concentration ranging from 53 to 116 × 10⁶ per ml and had a percentage motility ranging from 45 to 75%. Their seminal plasma never presented the abnormalities encountered in infertile men.

Semen samples were collected after a period of sexual abstinence of at least 72 h and allowed to liquefy at room temperature for 30–45 min. The samples were then poured into sterile 4 ml plastic tubes (2038, Falcon), and sperm concentration and percentage of motility were determined (Makler counting chamber, El-Op, Israel). Subsequently, the tubes were centrifuged for 30 min at 1500 g. Supernatant seminal plasma was carefully removed and checked for the presence of spermatozoa. The centrifugation step was repeated for samples having more than 10^5 spermatozoa per ml. The supernatant was frozen and maintained at $-20°$ C.

Several weeks later the specimens were thawed and left 1 h at room temperature. Debris, often containing some remaining spermatozoa, was pipetted from the seminal plasma.

At the same time, spermatozoa of fertile and infertile men were obtained by masturbation into sterile plastic containers (4013, Falcon) filled with 50 ml TMPA medium (360 mOsm) containing 0.3% BSA (Bevington, 1969). Masturbation into the medium was done to minimize the exposure of spermatozoa to homologous seminal plasma immediately after ejaculation. Five minutes later the samples were filtered through a single layer of tissue (Kleenex, Kimberly-Clark, England). Each sample was collected in four sterile 15 ml conical centrifuge tubes (2095, Falcon) and centrifuged at 600 g for 5 min at room temperature. The supernatant was removed and the pellets were dissolved in 3 ml medium. The four suspensions were pooled and centrifuged again. The supernatants were removed and the pellets were immediately resuspended in a small aliquot of homologous or heterologous seminal plasma or a solution of 5% polivinyl-pyrrolidone (M = 24000) in TMPA medium.

Five donors were used for eight matched experiments. At least three samples for each semen studied were used and a total of 42 different suspensions were obtained. Since sperm concentrations higher than $100 × 10^6$ per ml inhibit the speed of the sperma-

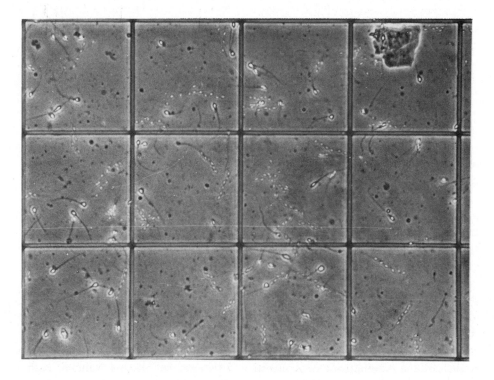

Figure 1. Photomicrograph of an undiluted semen sample. Each square of the grid engraved in the cover glass of the chamber is 0.1 × 0.1 mm². Motile spermatozoa are visible as strings of six beads. Nonmotile spermatozoa are clearly visible.

tozoa (unpublished observations), the sperm concentrations were adjusted to values ranging from 50 to 90 × 10⁶ per ml. These samples were incubated at 37° C for 7 h. After 1, 3, 5 and 7 h, all suspensions were studied by multiple exposure photography.

1.2. Multiple exposure photography

A drop of sperm was placed with a pasteur pipette between the upper and lower disc of a Makler counting chamber. From each specimen, 2–4 viewing areas covering 0.50 mm × 0.35 mm² of the counting chamber were photographed after the nonmotile spermatozoa had come to a complete standstill. The focus was set on the motile spermatozoa. A phase-contrast microscope (Zeiss) and a registration camera (Leica, MD-2) with 22 din film (Kodak plus-X pan) were used. A revolving stroboscope (38 rpm motor) was placed between the condensor and the light source. The film was exposed six times during 1 s while the sample was illuminated by six stroboscopically induced light pulses as originally described by Makler (1978). The corners of an area corresponding to 12 squares on the grid of the counting chamber were marked on each photograph. Mostly this area measured 190–220 mm and 140–165 mm. Motile spermatozoa are depicted as a string composed of maximally 6 or 7 beads (Fig. 1). All motile but non-progressive spermatozoa are seen as blurred images on the photograph and therefore separately marked.

1.3. Motility analysis using a digitizer-computer system

Photographs were fixed on the co-ordinates plate of a digitizer unit (developed by the Technische Hogeschool Delft) connected with an 11/70 digital computer. The XY coordinates were recorded on RMO3 discs pack. For each photograph, the following information was teletyped on the terminal: a file name corresponding to the negative and film number, the name or code of the individual studied, the date of the experiment, and additional remarks. The desired number of digitizable squares of the counting chamber grid was computed as well. Three different sperm images were digitized for each photograph: progressive motile spermatozoa indicated by clear displacements of the sperma-

tozoa, non-motile spermatozoa and motile but non-progressive spermatozoa (moving less than 10 μm/s). Moreover, other cells visible on the photograph could be recorded separately. All dots of a given track were touched according to the swimming sequence by the recording pen attached to the digitizer. In this way, a maximum of seven XY coordinates were stored for each motile spermatozoon. Every non-motile spermatozoon or non-progressive motile spermatozoon was computed as a single coordinate pair. The following variables were determined.

A) The *sperm concentration* (× 10⁶ per ml), the *percentage motility* (fraction of progressive and non-progressive motile spermatozoa) and the *percentage progressive motility* were computed.

B) The *average velocity* in μm/s was calculated according to the formula presented by Makler (1978). The distance covered by each spermatozoon during 1 s was determined by connecting each successive head image of a track (Figs 2a, 2b and 2c).

C) The deviation from straight-ahead progression was determined by calculating an ideal progression track for each digitized track. This was done by computing the least squares fit to a straight line for each trace using a Linfit program (Bevington, 1969). The Straight Line Approach was computed using the formula D_L/D_R in which D_L is the ideal distance between two end points of the straight line, while D_R is the total distance between the images of a trace (Fig. 3). Theoretically, the

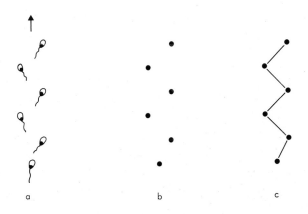

Figure 2. Determination of the distance covered by one spermatozoon during a 1 s exposure. The sperm images are marked with dot(s). These dots are digitized (b) and the coordinates are connected by straight lines according to the swimming sequence (c).

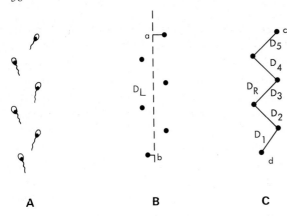

Figure 3. Determination of the straight line approach. Marked images (A) are digitized. The least square fit to a straight line is determined (– – – –) representing an ideal progression (B). The distance between a and b (B) is the ideal distance D_L, while D_R is the distance found by connecting the images of the spermatozoa (C). The speed constancy is calculated by determining the intermediate distances. D1 to D5: See text.

Straight Line Approach will range between 0 (extremely shaking spermatozoon) and 1 (representing a spermatozoon moving straight ahead). The *Average Straight Line Approach* of the progressive motile spermatozoa of an analyzed sperm sample was used as a standard semen parameter.

D) The Speed Constancy was computed using the following formula:

$$\text{Speed Constancy} = 1 \quad - \quad \frac{\sum\limits_{1}^{n} \left| \frac{D_R}{n} - D_i \right|}{D_R}$$

in which n is the number of distances between the images of a track (Fig. 3) and D_R/n is the distance between two successive images of a track from a motile spermatozoon progressing with a constant speed. The recorded distances between successive images of one track are given by D_1, D_2 ... D_L. The Speed Constancy, like the Straight Line Approach, will range between 0 and 1. The *Average Speed Constancy* of the motile spermatozoa was determined and used as a parameter of motility. In addition, a plotter image of the digitized spermatozoa was also printed (Fig. 4).

1.4. In vitro fertilization using zona-free hamster ova

All matched donor/patient reversal sperm suspensions were used (29 samples). After 2 h incubation

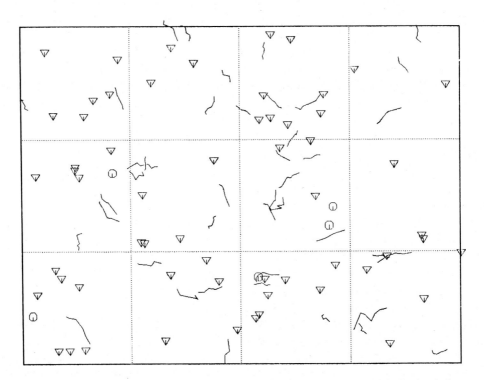

Figure 4. Plotter image of the sperm images visible in Fig. 1. This printer/plotter image is routinely obtained and allows a comparison with the position of the sperm on the original photomicrograph. Triangles: nonmotile spermatozoa; hexagons: nonmotile spermatozoa with moving head; squiggly lines: motile spermatozoa visible as traces.

at 37° C the sperm suspensions were poured into sterile 15 ml Falcon Tubes. TMPA medium was added to each sample to obtain a total volume of 15 ml. Samples were washed in TMPA three times by centrifugation at 600 g for 5 min. The final pellets were resuspended in 0.1 ml of TMPA containing 3% BSA. The concentration of spermatozoa was adjusted to 2×10^6 progressively motile sperm per ml with TMPA containing 3% BSA. From each sample 0.2 ml aliquots were transferred to plastic sterile petri dishes (3001, Falcon), covered with mineral oil (Squibb & Sons) and preincubated at 37° C for 2 h in air.

Adult female hamsters were induced to superovulate by an intraperitoneal injection of 25–30 IU of pregnant mare's serum (Gestyl, Organon Holland) on day 1 of the cycle (= day of postestrous vaginal discharge)) followed by an intraperitoneal injection of 25 IU of hCG (Pregnyl, Organon Holland) on the evening of day 3. The animals were killed on day 4, 15–16 h after the last injection. The oviducts were removed and placed in TMPA containing 0.1% hyaluronidase (ICN, Cleveland). To prevent damage to the eggs, the manipulations were performed as much as possible in the dark (Hirao et al., 1979c). The cumulus clots were extruded into the medium and the cumulus masses dispersed over 10 min incubation at room temperature. The eggs were washed four times in medium and transferred for 1 min to a TMPA droplet containing 0.1% trypsin (ICN, Pharmaceut) at room temperature. Immediately after zona dissolution the eggs were washed another three times and transferred to the incubated sperm suspensions. After 5 h of incubation in air at 37° C the eggs were rinsed twice in medium and pressed between a cover slip and a slide. The eggs were studied with a phase-contrast microscope. The presence of at least one swelling sperm head or male pronucleus with a sperm tail visible in the cytoplasm were criteria for penetration (Fig. 5). All eggs were fixed overnight with a mixture of ethanol/acetic acid (3:1) and stained with 0.25% acetocarmin. A definite fertilization percentage was obtained after the fixed and stained eggs were studied again.

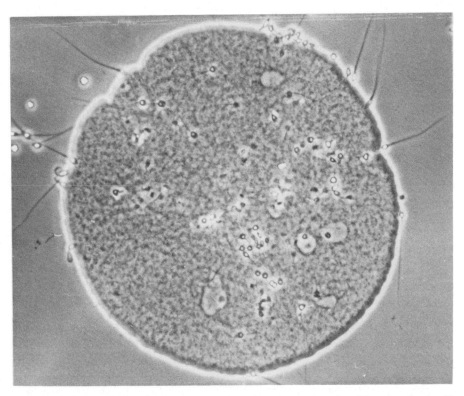

Figure 5. Zona-free hamster egg showing several attached spermatozoa on the ovum surface. More than four swelling sperm heads are visible in the ooplasma (phase contrast × 750).

2. EFFECTS OF REVERSAL SEMINAL PLASMA AND MEDIUM ON MOTILITY

The motility of spermatozoa was objectively determined by using the method developed by Makler (1978). With the aid of a digitizer–computer system information about sperm concentration, percentage motility and spermatozoal velocity was obtained. The MEP method differs from other time lapse exposure techniques in that very distinct intermittent images of moving sperm appear on the film. The different images can be recorded accurately by a high resolution digitizer. Thus, sperm movements can be described by two parameters concerning progression straight ahead and speed constancy.

A total of 168 aliquots were photographed and analyzed by the digitizer–computer unit. All samples were photographed after 1, 3, 5 and 7 h of incubation. Since the results after 1, 3, 5 and 7 h were essentially the same and since the most important physiologically significant data are expected to be derived from the analyses of photographs made after 1 h of incubation, only the data obtained after 1 h are reported. The effects of incubating spermatozoa in heterologous or homologous seminal plasma or medium on different motility parameters are shown in Table 1. The average percentage motility of spermatozoa from fertile men in homologous seminal plasma was 45%, while the average percentage motility of comparable sperm incubated in seminal plasma from infertile men was 42%. No stimulating effects on the average percentage motility could be demonstrated if spermatozoa from infertile men (22%) were brought into seminal plasma of fertile men (16%). However, significant differences were demonstrated between the Average Speed Constancies of spermatozoa from infertile and fertile men incubated in reversal seminal plasma, showing a stimulating effect of seminal plasma from fertile men on the Average Speed Constancy of spermatozoa from infertile men and vice versa (Table 1). These findings corroborate those obtained by Rozin (1958; 1961). In the latter work (1958) the use of oligozoospermic semen may have added a complicating factor because of the presence of abnormal sperm. In the present study, seminal plasma from normozoospermic ejaculates had a small but significant effect on the motility of the spermatozoa.

Differences between the present results and those obtained by other workers may be due to differences in the handling of the ejaculates. Thus, in the present work, the exposure of spermatozoa to homologous seminal plasma after ejaculation was minimized by the method of ejaculation into medium and the use of thawed sperm-free seminal plasma. In the experiments of Freund (1962) and Rozin (1958), seminal plasma was added to the sperm pellets as long as 30 min after centrifugation.

Although the value of parameters expressing speed constancy and deviation from progression straight ahead (straight line approach) remains to be demonstrated, the data presented here show differences of these variables between spermatozoa

Table 1. Influence of seminal plasma and medium on different motility variables of spermatozoa from fertile and infertile men after 1 h of incubation at $37°C$ (mean $\pm$ SD).

Motility variable	Spermatozoa from	Suspended in seminal plasma from		Suspended in medium
		Fertile men	Infertile men	
% motility	Fertile men	45 ± 7	42 ± 9	61 ± 6^a
	Infertile men	16 ± 2	22 ± 3	23 ± 4
% progressive motility	Fertile	43 ± 8	40 ± 7	53 ± 8^a
	Infertile	16 ± 3	19 ± 4	20 ± 3
Average straight line approach	Fertile	0.64 ± 0.05	0.64 ± 0.08	0.76 ± 0.04^a
	Infertile	0.76 ± 0.10	0.53 ± 0.03	0.75 ± 0.07^a
Average velocity	Fertile	25 ± 1	32 ± 3	36 ± 5^a
	Infertile	27 ± 3	23 ± 8	35 ± 2
Average speed constancy	Fertile	0.74 ± 0.03	0.67 ± 0.02^a	0.72 ± 0.01
	Infertile	0.65 ± 0.03^a	0.58 ± 0.06	0.73 ± 0.02^a

[a] Significant differences between these suspensions and the homologous spermatozoa suspensions for $p < 0.05$, dependent Student t-test.

from fertile and infertile men. The average straight line approach and the average speed constancy of sperm from infertile men were lower than in fertile men. The expression of different motility parameters into percentiles based on similar data obtained from other analyzed samples with comparable sperm concentration, will make the automation of sperm analysis more practical by enabling the observer to compare specimens with different sperm concentrations. The velocity is usually determined by employing methods in which the beginning and the end of a track are connected by a straight line (Makler, 1980b; Overstreet et al., 1979). The present method uses intermediary images as components of a velocity determination.

Although spermatozoa from only five fertile men were used and despite the extensive washing procedure, the average percentage of motile sperm (45%) (Table 1) and the average velocity (25 μm/s) were remarkably similar to those found by Makler et al. in 100 normozoospermic specimens: percentage of motile spermatozoa was 45% and speed of motile spermatozoa 30.3 μm/s (Makler et al., 1979b). The Makler method is an easy and objective method for motility estimation. Incubation of spermatozoa from fertile men in medium resulted in a significant increase in most of the variables determined (Table 1).

These data confirm the observations that a simple medium with a relatively low viscosity stimulates sperm motility (Makler et al., 1979a; Pauldon and Polanski, 1977). This phenomenon was not so distinct if spermatozoa from infertile men were incubated in medium and compared to

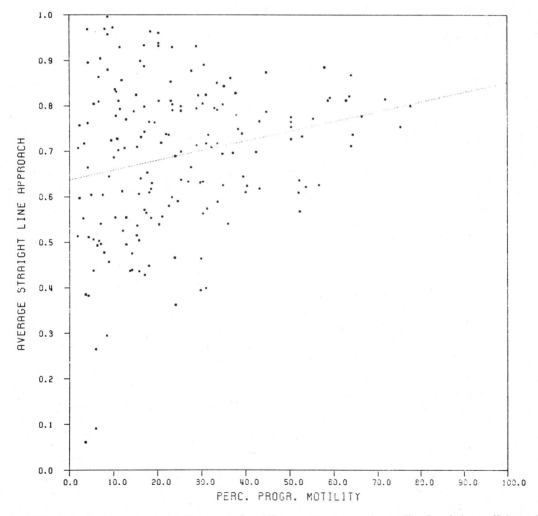

Figure 6. Relation between the average straight line approach and the percentage progressive motility. Correlation coefficient $+0.22$ for 168 data points.

spermatozoa in homologous suspensions. Although the Average Straight Line Approach and the Average Speed Constancy of these spermatozoa increased significantly (Table 1), no effects on the percentage motility and the average velocity could be demonstrated.

Despite the lack of an overall improvement in motility parameters when spermatozoa of infertile men were brought into seminal plasma of fertile men, individual changes in motility of the spermatozoa from the infertile men may occur. Individual evaluation of the different motility variables in the eight infertile men demonstrated a stimulating effect of heterologous seminal plasma on the motility in three out of eight cases after 1 h of incubation, the changes ranging from 5 to 20% for all motility parameters.

A high viscosity of the seminal plasma was found in two out of the latter three men and the removal of this abnormal plasma may explain the improvement in sperm motility. From analyses made the samples that had a high percentage progressive motility tended to contain more spermatozoa that moved straight ahead; this may be seen when the values of the Average Straight Line Approach are plotted against the percentage progressive motility (Fig. 6, correlation coefficient $+0.22$). A similar relationship was found between the average velocity and the percentage progressive motility (correlation coefficient 0.19). The Average Straight Line Approach determined for this experiment ranged from 0.1 to 0.95 and the Average Speed Constancy ranged from 0.35 to 0.90.

3. EFFECTS OF REVERSAL SEMINAL PLASMA ON THE IN VITRO FERTILIZATION

The average in vitro fertilization percentage of spermatozoa from the eight infertile men studied here, after a pre-incubation period of 2 h in homologous seminal plasma, using zona-free hamster ova, was 4% (range 0–19%). The average in vitro fertilization percentage of spermatozoa derived from the five fertile men studied here was 54% (range 20–93%) (see Table 2). The average in vitro fertilization percentage of spermatozoa from infertile men was not changed after pre-incubation in seminal plasma from fertile men (4%). Thus, there was no beneficial effect of heterologous seminal plasma on the in vitro fertilizing capacity of human spermatozoa. The average in vitro fertilization percentage of spermatozoa from fertile men was not altered by pre-incubation in seminal plasma of infertile men (58%). However, in two individual instances, the in vitro fertilization percentage of sperm samples from fertile men were reduced after pre-incubation in seminal plasma of infertile men

Table 2. Fertilization of zona-free hamster eggs by spermatozoa obtained from fertile and infertile men and preincubated in homologous or heterologous seminal plasma.

Code	Spermatozoa from infertile men preincubated in		Code	Spermatozoa from fertile men preincubated in	
	Homologous seminal plasma	Heterologous seminal plasma (code)		Homologous seminal plasma	Heterologous seminal plasma (code)
L	9/48 (19%)	11/48 (22%) (A)	A	22/46 (47%)	16/38 (42%) (L)
M	0/75 (0%)	0/31 (0%) (A)			19/33 (58%) (M)
N	4/46 (9%)	0/39 (0%) (B)	B	50/54 (93%)	24/28 (86%) (N)
O	2/50 (4%)	0/32 (0%) (B)			34/48 (71%) (O)
P	0/45 (0%)	1/33 (3%) (B)			45/48 (94%) (P)
Q	1/51 (2%)	2/47 (4%) (C)	C	7/35 (20%)	14/46 (30%) (Q)
R	0/32 (0%)	0/40 (0%) (D)	D	24/32 (76%)	32/44 (73%) (R)
S	0/29 (0%)	0/39 (0%) (E)	E	12/36 (33%)	4/44 (10%) (S)
Mean (±S.D.) in vitro fertilization percentages	4.3 ± 2.4	3.6 ± 2.7		53.6 ± 13.4	58.0 ± 10.2

(Table 2). The in vitro fertilization percentage of spermatozoa from one donor decreased from 93 to 71% under influence of seminal plasma obtained from one patient, while a similar decrease was found if spermatozoa from another donor were pre-incubated in seminal plasma from another patient (from 33% to 10%). Both patients possessed seminal plasma with a high viscosity. In one patient, a deleterious effect of the seminal plasma on sperm motility and the in vitro fertilizing potential was demonstrated simultaneously.

The reproducibility of the in vitro fertilization assay using zona-free hamster ova appears to be very high in this study. Semen samples obtained over long periods of time in other studies also showed only minor fluctuations of the fertilization percentages (Rogers et al., 1979).

The fertilization rates of the infertile and fertile men do not overlap in the present investigation. The infertile men were preselected for seminal plasma abnormalities.

It is important to evaluate the in vitro fertilizing system with sperm from infertile men with other dysfunctions, such as oligospermia and terato-spermia. Spermatozoa from infertile men can in some cases penetrate hamster eggs as efficiently as those from fertile men (Cohen et al., in press). How-ever, in a previous study (Rogers et al., 1979) using normozoospermic infertile patients the fertilization rate was always lower than in a group of fertile men. In cases where infertility is due to different causes, the interaction with the hamster egg is probably not necessarily affected.

4. CONCLUDING REMARKS

The effect of seminal plasma on sperm motility and hamster egg penetration was studied by resuspen-sion of spermatozoa obtained from a selected group of eight infertile men in seminal plasma of five fertile men and vice versa. The infertile men were preselected for visual seminal plasma abnormalities and concentrations of spermatozoa exceeding 20×10^6 per ml.

A semi-automatic motility analysis based upon the Multiple Exposure Technique (MEP) was used, in which intermittent images of motile spermatozoa

were stored in a computer. Two new parameters quantifying straight line progression and speed constancy are presented. No overall stimulating or inhibiting effect of heterologous seminal plasma on the average sperm motility could be found except for a change in the average speed constancy. In three out of eight cases motility increased 5-20% after incubation in seminal plasma from fertile men. These changes in motility are explained in two out of three cases since these men had highly viscous seminal plasma. The average in vitro fertilizing capacity of spermatozoa after exposure to heterol-ogous seminal plasma did not change. In two out of eight cases, the fertilizing capacity of spermatozoa from fertile men decreased by this treatment. These two patients possessed seminal plasma with a high viscosity.

ACKNOWLEDGEMENTS

We gratefully acknowledge the following persons for their advice: Dr J.C.M. van der Vijver, Dr R.F.A. Weber P.E. Schenck, Koos Slob and Professor J.J. van der Werff ten Bosch. Paula van der Vaart, Henny Wolffensperger, Rob Euser Anneke Bot, Petra Landsmeer and the second class students (class 1979) are acknowledged for their enthusiastic contributions.

REFERENCES

Barros C, Gonzales J, Herrera E, Bustos-Obregon E (1978) Fertilizing capacity of human spermatozoa evaluated by actual penetration of foreign eggs. Contraception 17:87.

Barros C, Gonzales J, Herrera E, Bustos-Obregon E (1979) Human sperm penetration into zona-free hamster ova as a test to evaluate the sperm fertilizing capacity. Andrologia 11:197.

Bevington PR (1969) Data reduction and error analysis for the physical sciences, pp 92–118. New York: McGraw-Hill.

Binor Z, Sokolosko JE, Wolf DP (1980) Penetration of the zona-free hamster egg by human sperm. Fertil Steril 33:321.

Cohen J, Weber RFA, Van der Vijver JCM, Zeilmaker GH: Fertil Steril: in press.

Eliasson E, Arver S, Johnson Q, Kvist U, Lindholmer C (1978) Some effect of human seminal plasma on the spermatozoa. P Serono Sy 14:215.

Freund M (1962) Interrelationships among the characteristics of human semen and factors affecting semen-specimen quality. J Reprod Fertil 4: 143.

Hirao Y, Yanagimachi R (1978) Detrimental effects of visible light on meiosis of mammalian eggs in vitro. J Exp Zool 206: 365.

Janik J, McLeod J (1979) Measurement of human spermatozoa motility. Fertil Steril 21: 140.

Kanwar KC, Yanagimachi R, Lopata A (1979) Effects of human seminal plasma on fertilizing capacity of human spermatozoa. Fertil Steril 31: 321.

Lindholmer C (1974) The importance of seminal plasma for human sperm motility. Biol Reprod 10: 533.

Lindholmer C, Eliasson R (1974) The effects of albumin and zinc on human sperm survival in different fraction of split ejaculates. Fertil Steril 25: 424.

Makler A (1978) A new multiple exposure photography method for objective human spermatozoal motility determination. Fertil Steril 30: 192.

Makler A (1980a) The improved ten-micrometer chamber for rapid sperm count and motility evaluation. Fertil Steril 33: 337.

Makler A (1980b) The use of the elaborated Multiple Exposure Photography MEP method in routine sperm motility analysis and for research purposes. Fertil Steril 33: 160.

Makler A, Blumenfeld Z, Brandes JM, Paldi E (1979a) Factors affecting sperm motility. II. Human sperm velocity and percentage of motility as influenced by semen dilution. Fertil Steril 32: 443.

Makler A, Itskovitz J, Brandes JM, Paldi E (1979b) Sperm velocity and percentage of motility in 100 normospermic specimens analysed by the Multiple Exposure Photography MEP method. Fertil Steril 31: 155.

Makler A, Zaidise I, Brandes JM (1979c) Elimination of errors induced during a routine human sperm motility analysis. Arch Androl 3: 201.

Mann T (1964) Biochemistry of semen and of the male reproductive tract. London: Wiley.

Milligan MD, Harris SJ, Dennis KJ (1978) The effect of temperature on the velocity of human spermatozoa as measured by time lapse photography. Fertil Steril 30: 592.

Overstreet JW Katz DF, Hanson FW, Fonseca JB (1979) A simple inexpensive method for objective assessment of human sperm movement characteristics. Fertil Steril 31: 162.

Overstreet JW, Yanagimachi R, Katz DF, Hayashi K, Hansou FW (1980) Penetration of human spermatozoa into the human zona pellucida and the zona-free hamster egg: a study of fertile donors and infertile patients. Fertil Steril 33: 534.

Pauldon JD, Polanski KL (1977) Preparation of human semen by glass wool columns. In: Hafez ESE, ed. Techniques of human andrology, p 11. Amsterdam: North-Holland.

Polakoski KL, Syner FN, Zaneveld LJD (1976) Biochemistry of human seminal plasma. In: Hafez ESE, ed. Human semen end fertility regulation in the male. p 133. St. Louis: Mosby.

Polakosko KL, Zaneveld LJD (1977) Biochemical examination of the human ejaculate. In: Hafez ESE, ed. Techniques of human andrology, p 265. Amsterdam: Norht-Holland.

Rogers BJ, Van Campen H, Ueno M, Lambert H, Bronson R, Hale R (1979) Analysis of human spermatozoal fertilizing ability using zona-free ova. Fertil Steril 32: 664.

Rozin S (1958) The role of seminal plasma in motility of spermatozoa. Acta Med Orient 17: 24.

Rozin S (1961) Studies on seminal plasma. Int J Fertil 6: 169.

Singh B, Mahapatro BB, Sadhu DP (1969) Chemical composition of cattle and buffalo spermatozoa and seminal plasma under different climatic conditions. J Reprod Fertil 20: 175.

Velazquez A, Pedron N, Delgado NM, Rosado A (1977) Osmolality and conductance of normal and abnormal seminal plasma. Int J Fertil 22: 92.

Whittingham DG (1979) In vitro fertilization, embryo transfer and storage. Br Med Bull 35: 105.

Yanagimachi R, Yanagimachi H, Rogers BJ (1976) The use of zona-free animal ova as a test-system for the assessment of the fertilizing capacity of human spermatozoa. Biol Reprod 15: 471.

Author's address:
Dr J. Cohen
Dept. Endocrinology, Growth and Reproduction
Erasmus University, P.O. Box 1738
3000 DR Rotterdam, The Netherlands

7. ACQUISITION OF FERTILIZING CAPACITY OF SPERMATOZOA IN THE HUMAN EPIDIDYMIS

M.J. HINRICHSEN and J.A. BLAQUIER

Mammalian spermatozoa undergo maturation during their passage through the epididymis, which results in the development of fertilizing capacity (Bedford, 1975). The epididymis actively contributes to sperm maturation with factors produced by the epithelium under the influence of androgens (Orgebin-Crist, 1975).

Technical and ethical difficulties have precluded the performance of experiments to ascertain whether sperm maturation occurs in man. The motility of spermatozoa from different epididymal segments has been examined (Belonoschkin, 1942; Bedford et al., 1973) and an increased capacity for progressive motility was found as spermatozoa pass through the epididymis. An increase was also noted (Bedford et al., 1973) in the formation of S–S bonds and changes in the ability to bind positively charged colloidal ferric oxide to the surface of spermatozoa of different segments of the epididymis in man. These changes are similar to those that occur in laboratory and domestic animals and are considered a facet of sperm maturation (Bedford, 1975).

In contrast, Young (1970) reported fertility in patients with obstructive azoospermia after anastomosis of the vas deferens to the caput epididymis, suggesting that spermatozoa are already fertile in the caput epididymis, or that maturation can occur in the vas deferens. However, both of these possibilities seem unlikely in view of the results obtained from laboratory animals, where spermatozoa artificially retained in the caput epididymis failed to develop fertilizing capacity (Gaddum and Glover, 1965; Bedford, 1967; Cummins, 1976). Furthermore, the environment of the vas deferens is not conducive to sperm survival in the hamster (Lubicz-Nawrocki and Chang, 1978).

The existence of sperm maturation in man was therefore re-examined by using the techniques recently developed to assess the ability of human spermatozoa to penetrate zona-free hamster oocytes (Yanagimachi et al., 1976; Barros et al., 1978). This presumably provides a more meaningful measure of maturation than previous observations.

1. METHODOLOGY

The epididymides were obtained from patients with testicular cysts (patient 1, age 26), prostatic carcinoma (patient 2, age 63), carcinoma of the penis (patient 3, age 49) or para-epididymal cysts (patients 4 and 5, ages 54 and 57, respectively). Immediately after removal, the epididymides were placed in sterile culture medium at room temperature. The tissues were carefully dissected and divided into three segments: caput, corpus and cauda (segments 2a, 2b; segment 3b and segments 4b, 4c, respectively) (Holstein, 1969). The caput and corpus epididymides were minced in tubes containing 1 ml of a modified Tyrode's medium (TMPA) (Barros et al., 1979). The tissues were allowed to sediment and the supernatant containing spermatozoa was aspirated. Spermatozoa from the cauda epididymis were obtained by retrograde washing by introducing a needle into the vas deferens. Sperm suspensions, diluted to a concentration between 1 and 2×10^6 per ml, were incubated 1 h prior to addition of zona-free golden hamster oocytes.

1.1. Penetration of zona-free hamster oocytes by human epididymal spermatozoa

The results regarding the ability of human spermatozoa to attach to zona-less hamster oocytes are indicated in Table 1.

No penetration of oocytes occurred after the

Hafez ESE & Semm K (Eds) Instrumental insemination.
© *1982 Martinus Nijhoff Publishers, The Hague/Boston/London. ISBN 90-247-2530-5. Printed in the Netherlands.*

Table 1. Attachment of spermatozoa recovered from different segments of the human epididymis to zona-free hamster oocytes. (Oocytes were obtained from adult female hamsters super-ovulated by PMSG and HCG, freed from the cumulus cells and the zona pellucida, and incubated with the sperm suspensions for 5–7 h at 37° C, in small Petri dishes, covered with mineral oil.)

Spermatozoa from	Number of oocytes	% of oocytes with		
		1–5	5–10	>10
		spermatozoa		
Caput	53	83	11	6
Corpus	62	64	23	8
Cauda	99	38	27	34

incubation with either caput or corpus spermatozoa, whereas caudal spermatozoa penetrated 26% of the eggs (Table 2) as judged by the observation of the sperm chromatin dispersion within the oocyte (Hinrichsen and Blaquier, 1980). Of the 26 oocytes penetrated, eight had less than five spermatozoa attached, nine had 5–10, and nine others had more than 10 attached spermatozoa. Contrary to what was observed for spermatozoa obtained from the caput and corpus epididymis, caudal spermatozoa showed a marked increase in their forward motility during the period of incubation.

In several mammalian species, some mature spermatozoa are detectable in proximal segments of the epididymis (Bedford, 1975), but most of

Table 2. Penetration of zona-free hamster oocytes by human spermatozoa recovered from the cauda epididymis. (Oocytes were obtained and incubated with spermatozoa as described in Table 1. Penetration was considered when one or more dispersed sperm nuclei were observed within the oocyte.)

Experiment	1	2	3	4	5	$\bar{x} \pm s.e.$
No occytes penetrated/ total oocytes	8/35	2/12	7/18	5/13	4/21	26/99
% penetrated oocytes	23	17	39	38	19	27 ± 5.27*

* Significantly different from caput and corpus ($p < 0.001$).

the sperm population develops fertilizing ability abruptly in the distal regions, as in the rabbit (Orgebin-Crist, 1969), hamster (Horan and Bedford, 1972) and rat (Blandau and Rumery, 1964). A similar phenomenon might occur in man and imply the existence of a maturation process, as was suspected from previous observations (Bedford et al., 1973).

The percentage of penetration of zona-less oocytes by cauda epididymis spermatozoa (26%, Table 2) resembles that obtained by Barros et al. (1979) (25%) using ejaculated spermatozoa from normal men, and thus suggests that spermatozoa have fully matured by the time they reach the cauda epididymis, as judged by the present tests.

There is an apparent absence of correlation between penetration of the ova and the number of spermatozoa attached to them. However, there is a marked increase in the number of ova with a larger number of sperm attached, as spermatozoa were tested from the successive epididymal segments (Table 1). This would indicate the gradual acquisition by spermatozoa, of the morphological and functional characteristics needed for sperm–egg interaction to occur. Sperm–egg fusion only takes place after spermatozoa have undergone the acrosome reaction (Cummins, 1976; Yanagimachi et al. 1976). This reaction involves complete capacitation (Chang and Hunter 1975; Cummins, 1976). Therefore, human spermatozoa acquire the ability to capacitate as they reach the caudal portion of the epididymis. In laboratory animals, this ability to capacitate is one of the changes undergone by spermatozoa during their maturation (Cummins, 1976; Overstreet, 1970).

ACKNOWLEDGMENTS

The authors wish to aknowledge the help of Dr Claudio Barros in setting up the technique used in this study. This work was supported by Grant 780-0349 from the Ford Foundation. J.A. Blaquier is a Research Career Awardee from the National Research Council (Argentina).

REFERENCES

Barros C, Gonzales J, Herrera E, Bustos-Obregon E (1978) Fertilizing capacity of human spermatozoa evaluated by actual penetration of foreign eggs. Contraception 17: 87.

Barros C, Gonzales J, Herrera E, Bustos-Obregon E (1979) Human sperm penetration into zona-free hamster oocytes, as a test to evaluate the sperm fertilizing ability. Andrologia 11: 197.

Bedford JM (1967) Effects of duct ligation on the fertilizing ability of spermatozoa from different regions of the rabbit epididymis. J Exp Zool 176: 271.

Bedford JM (1975) Maturation, transport and fate of spermatozoa in the epididymis. In: Hamilton DW, Greep RO, Handbook of physiology, Section 7, Vol V, p 303. Washington, DC: Am Physiol Soc.

Bedford JM, Calvin H, Cooper GW (1973) The maturation of spermatozoa in the human epididymis. J Reprod Fertil 28: 477.

Belonoschkin B (1942) Biologic der Spermatozoen in menschlichen Hoden und Nebenhoden. Arch Gynaecol 174: 357.

Blandau RJ, Rumery RE (1964) The relationship of swimming movements of epididymal spermatozoa to their fertilizing capacity. Fertil Steril 15: 571.

Cummins JM (1976) Effects of epididymal occlusion on sperm maturation in the hamster. J Exp Zool 197: 187.

Chang MC, Hunter RHF (1975) Capacitation of mammalian sperm: biological and experimental aspects. In: Hamilton DW, Greep RO, eds. Handbook of physiology, Section 7, Vol V, p 339. Washington, DC: Am Physiol Soc.

Gaddum P, Glover TD (1965) Some reactions of rabbit spermatozoa to ligation of the epididymis. J Reprod Fertil 9: 119.

Hinrichsen MJ, Blaquier JA (1980) Evidence supporting the existence of sperm maturation in the human epididymis. J Reprod Fertil 60: 291.

Holstein AF (1969) Morphologische Studien am Nebenhoden des Menschen. Zwanglose Abhandlung aus dem Gebiet der normalen und pathologischen Anatomie. Barrmann W, Doerr W, eds. Stuttgart: Georg Thieme Verlag.

Horan AH, Bedford JM (1972) Development of fertilizing ability of spermatozoa in the epididymis of the Syrian hamster. J Reprod Fertil 30: 417.

Lubicz-Nawrocki CM, Chang MC (1978) The influence of the testis on the fertilizing life of spermatozoa in the ligated vas deferens of the golden hamster. J Reprod Fertil 53: 147.

Orgebin-Crist MC (1969) Studies on the function of the epididymis. Biol Reprod Suppl 1: 155.

Orgebin-Christ MC, Danzo BJ, Davies J (1975) Endocrine control of the development and maintainance of sperm fertilizing ability in the epididymis. In: Hamilton DW, Greep RO eds. Handbook of physiology Section 7, Vol V, p 319, Washington DC: Am Physiol Soc.

Overstreet JW (1970) Fertilizing capacity of epididymal spermatozoa. J Reprod Fertil 21: 423.

Yanagimachi R, Yanagimachi H, Rogers BJ (1976) The use of zona-free animal ova as a test system for the assessment of fertilizing capacity of human spermatozoa. Biol Reprod 15: 471.

Young D (1970) Surgical treatment of male infertility. J Reprod Fertil 23: 541.

Authors' addresses:
Dr M.J. Hinrichsen
I. Frauenkliniek und Hebammenschule der Universität München
Maistrasse 11, 8000 München, FRG

Dr J.A. Blaquier
Instituto de Biología y Medicina Experimental
Obligado 2490, 1428 Buenos Aires, Argentina

8. EFFECT OF KALLIKREIN ON SPERM MOTILITY: IN VITRO TESTING OF EJACULATE VS IN VIVO TREATMENT

B. Schütte and C. Schirren

The use of kallikrein has been investigated in several clinical and experimental studies (Hofmann and Hornstein, 1975; Schill, 1975, 1977, 1978; Schirren, 1977, 1978; Hofmann, 1978; Lunglmayr and Maier, 1978; Meyhöfer and Krause, 1978; Steiner et al., 1978; Maier et al., 1980). Clinical trials of the application of kallikrein to male infertility at three andrological centers (Düsseldorf, Hamburg, Munich) give evidence of a statistically significant effect on various parameters of the ejaculate. In particular, the polypeptides, kallidin, bradykinin and kinin inactivating enzymes have a positive effect on the motility, density and morphology of spermatozoa (Schill and Haberland, 1974; Schill, 1977). Kallikrein is andrologically used with patients having either oligozoospermia or asthenozoospermia.

1. KALLIKREIN TREATMENT

Before kallikrein treatment, all risk factors must be eliminated: (1) any influence of nicotine must be excluded, since nicotine inhibits spermatozoal motility; (2) in the presence of a varicose condition, a varicocelectomy with high-level ligation of the spermatic vein must be performed; and (3) any other toxins such as alcohol and any drugs must be strictly avoided. Treatment with kallikrein may not be effective if these precautions are disregarded (Schirren, 1975, 1977, 1978).

The following two studies were conducted: (1) The influence of kallikrein on sperm motility in vitro was studied in 48 patients with reduced sperm motility; 42 of whom also had a reduced spermatozoa density. (2) The influence of kallikrein in vitro on sperm motility was studied after long-term treatment (15–32 months).

For in vitro testing, 1 unit of kallikrein was applied to 1 ml of ejaculate and motility was examined microscopically from 15 min to 4 h of incubation time at 37° C. The native ejaculate was used as control. While testing kallikrein in vitro of 48 patients, the sperm motility mostly increased after 2 h (44 patients out of a total of 48 patients) followed by a small decrease up to 4 h. These results are similar to those of Schill (1975) and Maier et al. (1980). Four patients showed no effect on kallikrein.

Expressing the increase of the sperm motility in percentages, kallikrein enhanced the motility mostly at 5 and 10%. In 44 patients, the motility (in addition of 5 and 10%) amounted to 80% after 2 h (Fig. 1). The results of this in vitro investigation question the possibility of transferring these results to in vivo conditions.

Because the influence on sperm motility can be rated as an immediate effect (Schill, 1975, 1977, 1978; Schirren, 1977, 1978; Hofmann, 1978; Lunglmayr and Maier, 1978; Meyhöfer and Krause, 1978; Steiner et al., 1980), the patients were initially treated with kallikrein (oral dosage 6 × 100 units daily) for 4 months. In low patients, the sperm motility increased about 10%. The results after 4 months of treatment in vivo were different. Five

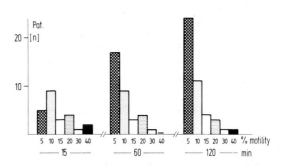

Figure 1. Survey of the number (n) of patients with an increase of sperm motility (in %) by kallikrein (applied in vitro: 1 unit of kallikrein/1 ml ejaculate). Incubation time: 15, 60 and 120 min.

Hafez ESE & Semm K (Eds) Instrumental insemination.

patients showed a positive effect and three even showed a negative effect.

A testis biopsy was performed in one patient who had a necrozoospermia which was neither in vitro nor in vivo influenced by kallikrein, and was also performed on one patient whose sperm motility decreased about 15% after kallikrein treatment. The semi-thin slide revealed that all spermatids had protoplasm-like appendages at the heads, which is a sign of defects in the axonema. Electron microscopical examinations by Professor Holstein confirmed these defects. It is a morphological abnormality that leads to the question of whether the origin of the so-called therapy failures of long-term treatment with kallikrein rests in the defects of axonema in the spermatozoa tails, and this cannot be influenced by drugs.

The ejaculates of 24 patients who received kallikrein for 15 to 32 months were examined. In low patients, the motility of the spermatozoa was unchanged; however, by testing one unit of kallikrein in vitro, an increase of the motility could be observed. Five patients showed no effect and only one showed a decrease. There was a decrease of motility in vitro in six patients who showed a decrease of sperm motility by kallikrein treatment. Out of eight patients, however, with a positive effect after kallikrein treatment in vitro, an increase of sperm motility was observed in five cases.

2. CONCLUDING REMARKS

The influence of kallikrein in vitro was tested in the ejaculate of 48 patients with reduced sperm motility. The highest increase of the motility was observed in 44 patients two hours after application. Therefore, these patients were treated with kallikrein (oral dosage 6 × 100 units daily) initially for four months. The results proved different: most of the patients resulted in an increase of sperm motility but there were also cases where sperm motility decreased. Testis biopsy was performed in two patients. Electron microscopy revealed morphological defects of the spermatozoa tails, especially of the axonema. These abnormalities cannot be influenced by drugs and may be the reason for so-called therapy failures in treatment with kallikrein.

REFERENCES

Hofmann N, Hornstein OP (1975) The influence of kallikrein on the semen of subfertile men with particular regard to sperm morphology. In: Haberland GL, Roben JW, Schirren C, Huber P, eds. Kininogenases. Kallikrein 2, p 147. Stuttgart and New York: Schattauer.

Hofmann H (1978) Klinisch-pathologische Untersuchungen zur Kallikrein-Therapie subfertiler Männer. Fortschritte der Andrologie 6: 39.

Lunglmayr G, Maier O (1978) Therapie der Subfertilität mit Kallikrein. Fortschritte der Andrologie 6: 73.

Maier U, Grünberger W, Stackl W, Lunglmayr G (1980) Aktivierung der Spermienmotilität vor homologer Insemination mit Nativ- und Kryosperma. Fortschritte der Fertilitätsforschung 8: 216.

Meyhöfer W, Krause W (1978) Therapeutische Erfahrungen mit Kallikrein bei Astheno- und Oligozoospermie. Fortschritte der Andrologie 6: 49.

Schill WB, Haberland GL (1974) Kinin-induced enhancement of sperm motility. Hoppe Seylers Z Physiol Chem 355: 229.

Schill WB (1975) Influence of the kallikrein-kinin system on human sperm motility in vitro. In: Haberland GL, Rohen JW, Schirren C, Huber P, eds. Kininogenases. Kallikrein 2, p 47. Stuttgart and New York: Schattauer.

Schill WB (1977) Kallikrein as a therapeutical means in the treatment of male infertility. In: Haberland GL, Rohen JW, Suzuki T, eds. Kininogenases. Kallikrein 4, p 251. Stuttgart and New York: Schattauer.

Schill WB (1978) Klinische Erfahrungen mit Kallikrein bei der Therapie der Oligo- und Asthenozoospermie. Fortschritte der Andrologie 6: 52.

Schirren C (1975) Experimental studies on the influence of kallikrein on the human sperm motility in vitro. In: Haberland GL, Rohen JW, Schirren C, Huber P, eds. Kininogenases. Kallikrein 2, p 59. Stuttgart and New York: Schattauer.

Schirren C (1977) Clinical experiences with kallikrein on subfertile males. In: Haberland GL, Rohen JW, Suzuki T, eds. Kininogenases. Kallikrein 4, p 247. Stuttgart and New York: Schattauer.

Schirren C (1978) Klinische Ergebnisse der Kallikrein-Anwendung bei Fertilitätsstörungen des Mannes. Fortschritte der Andrologie 6: 76.

Author's address:
Dr B. Schütte
Abteilung für Andrologie der Universität Hamburg
Martinistrasse 52
D-2000 Hamburg 20, FRG

9. ENHANCEMENT OF MOTILITY IN FRESH AND CRYO-PRESERVED SEMEN BY KALLIKREIN AND CAFFEINE

R. KADEN and K. GROSSGEBAUER

Motility in sperm is an important factor in estimating fertility. In cryopreserved sperm, motility of spermatozoa is usually further reduced due to freezing procedures, and great effort is required to enhance motility (Kaden, 1979). Kallikrein and caffeine are effective agents in fresh and cryo-preserved sperm (Schill et al., 1976, 1979). However, the concentration rate of these agents in sperm and the freezing schedule as well as the timing of their addition remained questionable. Some selected concentrations of kallikrein and caffeine and their effects on cryopreserved sperm were investigated; the effect of kallikrein added *before freezing* was compared with kallikrein added *after thawing*.

There were 45 human semen specimens of oligozoospermatic ejaculates used for kallikrein and 24 for caffeine experiments.

1. KALLIKREIN EXPERIMENTS

Five different groups of semen specimens were distinguished. The first group was just fresh sperm after liquefaction used as control. The second group was a solution of porcine pancreatic kallikrein (highly purified, specific activity 1180 kallikrein units (KU)/mg; Bayropharm GmbH, FRG) added to fresh sperm to a final concentration of 10 KU/ml kallikrein. The third group was just cryosperm after thawing, used as control. In the fourth group, kallikrein was added to cryosperm *after thawing* to a final concentration of 10 KU/ml kallikrein. In the fifth group, kallikrein was added to cryosperm *before freezing* to a final concentration of 10 KU/ml kallikrein. After freezing, storage in liquid nitrogen at −196°C for about 1 month, and thawing, the samples are ready for examination. To prepare sperm for cryopreservation, a protective medium of glycerol and egg yolk extender with antibiotics is added in a ratio of 1 to 1 (Sherman, 1978; Kaden et al., 1974). The preparation is named cryosperm.

2. CAFFEINE EXPERIMENTS

Three different groups of semen specimens were distinguished. The first group was just fresh sperm after liquefaction and was used as control. In the second group, a solution of caffeine (DAB 7) was added to fresh sperm to a final concentration of 50 mM caffeine. In the third group, a solution of caffeine was added to cryosperm after thawing, to a final concentration of 50 mM caffeine.

3. TECHNIQUES FOR CRYOPRESERVATION

The method used was based on the relatively simple liquid-nitrogen-vapor freezing technique (Sherman, 1978) involving cryosperm, the use of plastic straws (minitubes) with a volume of 0.25 ml, a freezing schedule of 8 min, a semiautomatic biological freezer, and liquid nitrogen for frozen storage (Kaden et al., 1976). All experiments were performed in plastic material and siliconized glassware.

Table 1. Improvement of motility. Percentage of sperm and cryossperm samples showing improved motility after 1 h incubation following kallikrein addition.

Response	Sperm		Cryopreserved sperm	
	Number	*%*	*Number*	*%*
Improvement	26	58	14	39
No improvement	19	42	22	61

Hafez ESE & Semm K (Eds) Instrumental insemination.

4. READING MODALITIES

The readings of motility in fresh sperm were taken immediately after liquefaction, and in cryosperm right after thawing and after 60 min incubation. To calculate the motility in sperm, the number of motile spermatozoa was determined using a hemocytometer.

5. EFFECT OF KALLIKREIN

Among the individual samples, the effect of kallikrein 10 KU/ml on motility in sperm and cryosperm varied. Of 45 sperm specimens examined, 26 (58%) samples demonstrated improvement of motility with kallikrein after 1 h incubation. Of 36 cryosperm specimens examined, only 14 (39%) samples demonstrated improvement (Table 1). In these 45 sperm specimens, the average motility was 41%. After 1 incubation, the sperm samples with kallikrein added showed a motility of 39% the control sperm samples a motility of 35%. According to the Wilcoxon matched pairs signed rank test, this difference is statistically highly significant

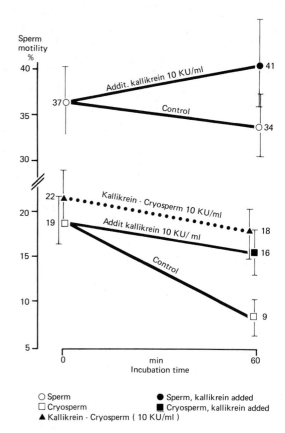

Figure 2. Effect of kallikrein on motility in sperm and its cryosperm. Selection of sensitive sperm samples. Mean values (± SEM) of 26 results.

(p < 0.001). In the 45 cryosperm specimens, the average motility after thawing was 19%. This value means a 53% retained motility or 47% survival rate. After 1 h incubation, the cryosperm samples with kallikrein added after thawing showed a motility of 17% the control 13%. In the 45 kallikrein-cryosperm specimens, the average motility right after thawing was 22%. This value means a 46% retained motility or 54% survival rate. After 1 h incubation, the kallikrein-cryosperm samples showed a motility of 18%. Kallikrein-cryosperm showed a 16% better motility than cryosperm with kallikrein added after thawing (Fig. 1).

In the selection of sensitive samples, restricted to those samples demonstrating improvement of motility by kallikrein stimulation, major differences were found. Kallikrein raised motility in sperm from 37% to 41%, while the control fell from 37% to 34% after 60 min. This difference is statistically significant. In cryosperm, motility fell from 19% to 16%; control from 19% to 9%; kallikrein-cryosperm from 22% to 18% (Fig. 2). The addition of kalli-

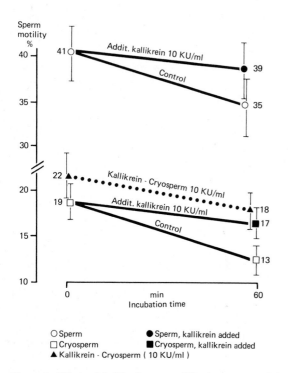

Figure 1. Effect of kallikrein on motility in sperm and its cryosperm. Mean values (± SEM) of 45 results.

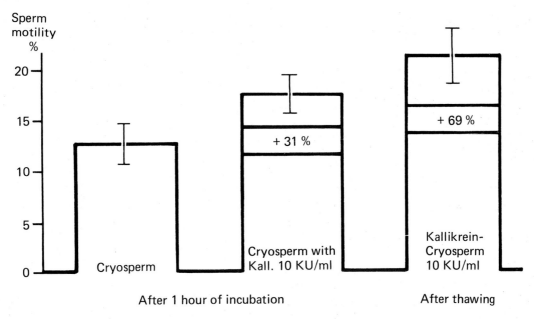

Figure 3. Enhancement of motility by kallikrein in cryosperm. Mean values ($\pm$ SEM) of 45 results.

krein to cryosperm resulted in an average enhancement of motility of 31% after 1 h incubation, compared to 69% for kallikrein-cryosperm right thawing. Only the result for kallikrein-cryosperm is statistically highly significant ($p < 0.001$) (Fig. 3).In sensitive sperm samples, there were major and statistically significant differences in the enhancement of motility for both cryosperm with kallikrein

(78%) and kallikrein-cryosperm (as much as 144%) (Fig. 4).

6. EFFECT OF CAFFEINE

Out of 24 ejaculates, the average motility in sperm was 44%, and in cryosperm, 31%. This value means

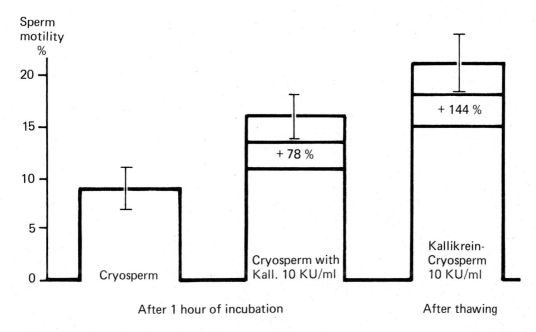

Figure 4. Enhancement of motility by kallikrein in cryosperm. Selection of sensitive sperm samples. Mean values ($\pm$SEM) of 26 results.

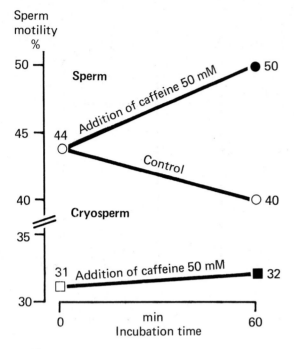

Figure 5. Effect of caffeine 50 mM on motility in sperm and its cryosperm. Mean values of 24 results.

proved effective even in a final concentration of 50 mM instead of 5 mM caffeine, which has been recommended for obtaining a maximum stimulation effect. The caffeine experiments were discontinued as it is now suspected that caffeine interferes in the repair mechanisms of DNA in cases of defects.

a 30% decrease of mortility due to freezing, storage, and thawing. After an incubation time of 60 min, sperm with the addition of 50 mM caffeine showed 50% motility; just sperm as control, 40%. The motility of cryosperm with caffeine added ranged from 31% to 32% (Fig. 5).

In accordance with reports on the enhancement of motility in sperm and cryosperm by kallikrein or caffeine (Schill, 1975), the results of our investigations confirmed this improving effect in sperm and cryosperm of oligozoospermatic ejaculates. In sperm and cryosperm, a final concentration of 10 KU/ml kallikrein has yielded more modest results than 5 KU/ml kallikrein. In kallikrein-cryosperm, 10 KU/ml has proven to be the optimal concentration (Fig. 6).

The observation of a statistically significant improvement of motility in kallikrein-cryosperm suggests a routine addition of kallikrein to cryosperm *before* freezing in a final concentration of 10 KU/ml kallikrein or to fresh sperm in a final concentration of 5 KU/ml kallikrein. Caffeine has

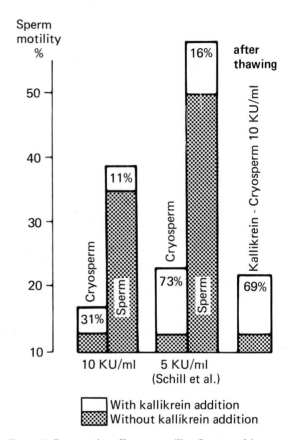

Figure 6. Comparative effect on motility. Sperm and its cryosperm with addition of kallikrein 10 KU/ml, and 5 KU/ml (Schill, 1975; Schill et al., 1979), respectively, after 1 h incubation; kallikrein-cryosperm 10 KU/ml after thawing.

ACKNOWLEDGMENTS

The highly purified porcine pancreatic kallikrein was granted by Bayropharm GmbH. The careful technical assistance of Miss Dorothee von Arnoldi is gratefully acknowledged. We are indebted to Dipl.-Ing. Katharina Schmidt, Institut Medizin. Statistik und Dokumentation, for the calculations of significance.

REFERENCES

Kaden R (1979) Die Renaissance eines Enzyms. Sex Med 8: 211.

Kaden R, Grossgebauer K, Rohloff D, Sokol K (1974) Konservierbarkeit von Sperma im Alter. In: Proceedings Congr Urology and Nephrology, Budapest, p 407.

Kaden R, Grossgebauer K, Grund S, Rohloff D, Sokol K, Sperling K (1976) Spermakonservierung der interdisziplinären Arbeitsgruppe "Kryospermforschung". In: Fortschr Fertil Forschung III. Berlin: Grosse-Verlag.

Schill WB (1975) Caffeine- and kallikrein-induced stimulation of human sperm motility: a comparative study. Andrologia 7: 229.

Schill WB, Pritsch W (1976) Kinin-induced enhancement of sperm motility in cryopreserved human spermatozoa. In: Proceedings VIII Internat Congr Anim Reprod Artif Insem, Krakow. Vol IV, p 1071.

Schill WB, Pritsch W, Preissler G (1979) Effect of caffeine and kallikrein on cryo-preserved human spermatozoa. Int J Fertil 24: 27.

Sherman JK (1978) Banks for frozen human semen; current status and prospects. In: Proceedings Round-table Conference: The integrity of frozen spermatozoa, p 78. Nat Acad Sciences Washington.

Author's address:
Prof Dr R. Kaden
Hautkliniek/Andrologie
Freie Universität
Hindenburgdamm 30
D-1000 Berlin 45, FRG

10. EFFECT OF KININS (KALLIKREIN) ON RECOVERY OF MOTILITY IN FROZEN SPERMATOZOA

A.P. Chong, W. Cappiello and S. Weinrieb

The use of frozen sperm for artificial insemination in man has increased substantially in the last few decades as a result of better techniques for recovery and preservation of motile sperm. As of today, thousands of successful inseminations have been accomplished, and the clinical use of frozen-stored human semen has proven to be safe and quite effective. In clinical practice, stored frozen sperm represents a clear advantage over fresh specimens because of the readily available samples with wide phenotypic characteristics. However, one of the problems that remains to be solved is that of freezing and thawing. Even with the best results reported so far (Behrman and Ackerman, 1969; Sawada and Ackerman, 1968; Schill, 1975a; Smith and Steinberger, 1973; Steinberger and Smith, 1973), a decline in the percentage of recovered viable spermatozoa is inevitable.

Recently, the idea of improving pharmacologically the recovery of frozen-stored human semen has been investigated. Kallikrein, a kinin-releasing proteinase, enhances in vitro motility of fresh human sperm in samples from oligo or asthenospermic men (Schill, 1975b, 1975c).

Since the kallikrein-kinin enzymatic system plays a physiologic role in the regulation of human sperm motility (Fritz, 1975), the present study was designed to examine the effect of this agent on semen from healthy fertile donors on recovery of frozen-stored specimens and to see if the damage to sperm by the freezing and thawing process could be reversible by the use of kallikrein.

1. METHODOLOGY

Specimens were frozen using the cryofreezer developed by Ricor (Cryo Sperm Freezer, CSF-16, RICOR Cryogenic and Vacuum Systems, Israel), which consists of a freezing chamber mounted on a vessel containing liquid nitrogen. Pressure in this vessel forces a controlled flow of liquid nitrogen through a cryogenic solenoid valve until the desired temperature is reached. The solenoid valve then closes and the liquid nitrogen evaporates in the freezing chamber, cooling a freezer plate which has recesses shaped to form sperm pellets and is suitably coated to prevent sticking.

Semen from ten healthy, fertile donors were frozen. Acceptable criteria for inclusion of a specimen included a concentration of at least 40.0×10^6 cells/cm, 50% or greater motile forms, 60% or greater normal morphology and a forward progression of greater than 8^+. Assessment of forward progression and motility was done microscopically; forward progression was rated subjectively by the observer on a scale of 0 to 10^+, and percentage motility was ascertained by obtaining a differential count on at least 200 cells.

The effects of kallikrein addition (highly purified hog pancreatic kallikrein, supplied by Bayer AG, Leverkesein, Federal Republic of Germany) were examined before freezing and after thawing. Before freezing, aliquots of semen of 0.15 cm³ were mixed at room temperature (22° C) with differing amounts of kallikrein containing the following initial specific activities: 0 (control), 0.25 KU, 0.5 KU, 1.0 KU, 5.0 KU and 10.0 KU. Treatment was carried out within 15 min of semen liquefaction.

Following treatment, the mixture was warmed to 36° C and was mixed with an equal volume of protective medium which had been warmed to the same temperature. Composition of the protective medium was a slight modification of that described by Barkay (1974), and consisted of sodium citrate (3% solution), 4.0 ml; glycerol, 1.25 ml; fresh egg yolk, 4.0 ml; crystalline penicillin, 100,000 U in 0.1 ml; streptomycin, 10 mg in 0.05 ml.

Hafez ESE & Semm K (Eds) Instrumental insemination.

Following the addition of equal volumes of protective medium, the final specific activities (in KU/ml) of each experimental unit were as follows: 0, 0.78, 1.47, 2.67, 4.44, 7.40 and 9.50. The entire mixture was then placed in a refrigerator at 4° C for 15 min so that an initial gradual lowering of temperature would be obtained.

After refrigeration, the mixture was frozen in pellets on the cryofreezer plate, which had already been cooled to −75° C. Pellets formed within seconds and were then transferred to plastic tubes and stored in a liquid nitrogen sperm bank at a temperature of −196° C. Storage was maintained for a period of one week. At the end of that time, thawing was carried out by removing the tubes from the liquid nitrogen and transferring them to a 35° C water bath until completely thawed, which took approximately 5 min.

Assessment of motility, including percentage of motile forms and forward progression, was then carried out at 0, 2, 4, 6 and 24 h post-thaw. For inclusion in the study, an initial recovery index (% final recovery/% initial recovery × 100) of at least 30% was required for control values.

In the second series of experiments, the effect of kallikrein addition immediately after thawing was examined. Aliquots of semen of 0.5 cm³ were mixed with equal amounts of protective medium frozen and stored as previously described. Again, storage was for one week. Then, 0.15 cm³ portions of the mixture were removed and treated at room temperature with identical amounts of kallikrein as described in the first experiment. After addition of the kallikrein, the final specific activities (in KU/ml)

Table 1. Individual characteristics of semen specimens.

Donor	Concentration (× 10⁶/cm³)	Initial motility (%)	Initial forward progression	Recovery index*
1	99	64	10$	90
2.	80	68	8$	57
3	48	82	9$	56
4	91	86	9$	58
5	125	65	9$	64
6	128	64	9$	51
7	158	66	9$	65
8	109	50	8$	58
9	41	53	9$	62
10	75	70	9$	51

* Control value after one week freeze-storage.

of each experimental unit were 0, 2.28, 4.2, 7.28, 11.4, 17.5 and 21.0.

Final specific activities of prefreezing-treated and post-thawing-treated specimens were slightly different. This was necessary because of restrictions imposed by the limited and varying volume of semen available and by the need to keep dilution factors at a minimum in order to avoid impairment of microscopic observation and collection of data. Percentage motility and forward progression were evaluated after 0, 2, 4, 6 and 24 h.

Two-way analysis of variance was used in evaluating concentration of enzyme and donor effects on recovery index and on forward progression. Testing was done separately for both prefreezing treatment data and post-thawing treatment data. This two-way analysis is necessary because of the inherent variability in donors (Table 1), and this form of statistical testing removes the donor effect in order to examine the effect of concentration of enzyme.

Table 2. Recovery index vs concentration of kallikrein used in prefreezing treatment. Mean recovery index:*
$\frac{\text{\% final motility}}{\text{\% initial motility}} \times 100 \pm$ standard deviation.

Specific activity of kalikrein (KU/ml)	Post-thaw time (h)				
	0	2	4	6	24
0 (control)	61 ± 11	48 ± 17	46 ± 15	38 ± 16	15 ± 2
0.8	60 ± 10	48 ± 15	44 ± 14	38 ± 17	15 ± 11
1.5	57 ± 11	50 ± 14	46 ± 15	41 ± 16	15 ± 11
2.7	59 ± 12	45 ± 18	41 ± 18	37 ± 19	14 ± 10
4.5	56 ± 15	44 ± 16	37 ± 18	30 ± 23	13 ± 11
7.4	45 ± 20	34 ± 32	27 ± 16	21 ± 17	9 ± 8
9.5	30 ± 17	20 ± 13	13 ± 8	13 ± 8	6 ± 4

*N = 10.

Table 3. Forward progression vs concentration of kallikrein used in prefreezing treatment. Mean forward progression* ± standard deviation.

Specific activity of kallikrein (KU/ml)	Post-thaw time (h)				
	0	2	4	6	24
0 (control)	6.7 ± 1.2	6.6 ± 1.2	6.5 ± 1.0	6.0 ± 1.3	2.9 ± .7
0.8	6.9 ± 1.4	6.6 ± 1.2	6.6 ± 1.0	6.0 ± 1.5	3.1 ± 1.1
1.5	6.9 ± 1.3	6.7 ± 1.3	6.4 ± 1.1	6.0 ± 1.2	3.2 ± 1.0
2.7	7.1 ± 1.3	6.7 ± 1.3	6.1 ± 1.2	5.8 ± 1.3	2.9 ± 1.0
4.5	7.0 ± 1.3	6.6 ± 1.5	6.2 ± 1.2	5.6 ± 1.3	2.9 ± 1.0
7.4	6.5 ± 1.1	6.1 ± 1.5	5.0 ± 1.2	4.9 ± 1.2	2.6 ± 1.2
9.5	5.9 ± 1.4	5.3 ± 1.4	4.4 ± 1.2	4.0 ± 1.2	2.0 ± 1.3

* N = 10.

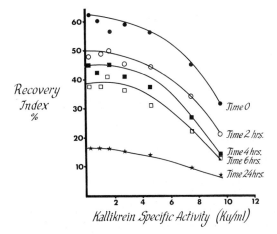

Figure 1. Recovery index vs concentration of kallikrein used in prefreezing treatment.

2. THE KALLIKREIN EFFECT

In the pre-freezing treatment group, recovery indices and forward progressions are listed in Tables 2 and 3. Statistical testing demonstrates that there is a significant difference ($P = <0.01$) within each group for effect of concentration on both recovery index and forward progression for all time periods. At one specific post-thawing time there was non-homogeneity of groups for different concentrations of enzyme; i.e. treatment effect was significant in all cases. The kallikrein effect was a decrease in motility at the higher ranges of concentration used (Figs. 1 and 2).

For most post-thaw times, the significant decrease in motility of treated samples from controls occurred at the higher ranges of kallikrein specific activity used; treatment effect became significant at an activity of 4–5 KU/ml or above. In general, the higher the concentration of the enzyme, the greater the decrease in motility.

The post-thawing treatment groups reflects the results for the prefreezing group; at every post-thaw time there was a significant difference (less than 0.5 in every case and less than 0.1 in most cases) for effect of concentration on recovery index and forward progression (Tables 4 and 5). Although the range of kallikrein specific activities was slightly higher than in the prefreezing treatment group, the higher concentrations used (usually above 15 KU/ml) proved to cause the significant decreases in recovery over control values (Figs. 3 and 4). The slight rises in forward progression at most times at the enzyme activity of 7.28 KU/ml are not significant. In general, there was a gradual decrease in motility over time in all cases.

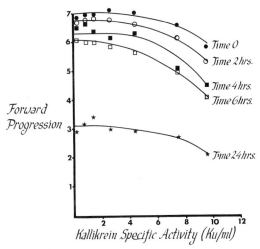

Figure 2. Forward progression vs concentration of kallikrein used in prefreezing treatment.

Table 4. Recovery index vs concentration of kallikrein used in post-thawing treatment. Mean recovery index* ± standard deviation.

Specific activity of kallikrein (ml)	Post-thaw time (h)				
	0	2	4	6	24
0 (control)	62 ± 12	50 ± 16	44 ± 16	37 ± 15	16 ± 8
2.3	60 ± 11	53 ± 15	44 ± 17	38 ± 13	17 ± 9
4.2	63 ± 8	53 ± 9	42 ± 18	40 ± 16	18 ± 8
7.3	61 ± 11	49 ± 15	40 ± 18	41 ± 13	15 ± 11
11.4	55 ± 11	39 ± 15	37 ± 22	35 ± 13	16 ± 12
17.5	40 ± 12	50 ± 15	26 ± 15	25 ± 11	10 ± 7
21.0	29 ± 11	19 ± 10	14 ± 8	12 ± 4	8 ± 7

* N = 10.

In no case did treatment with kallikrein cause a significant improvement in recovery index or forward progression. Although statistical comparison between prefreezing and post-thawing results cannot be made because of differences in the treatment group, the same effect of kallikrein was observed, in general. However, in the post-thawing groups, the decrease in motility was seen at somewhat higher specific activities of kallikrein.

3. FUTURE USES

In most series, the pregnancy success rate with frozen semen for therapeutic (artificial) donor insemination (TDI) has been 10% to 30% lower than results obtained by using fresh samples (Behrman, 1959; Chong and Taymor, 1975; Haman, 1959; Kleegman, 1954; Korne and Lieberman, 1976). Freezing and thawing produce significant decreases in motility (Behrman and Sawada, 1966; Smith and Steinberger, 1973; Steinberger and Smith, 1973) in

"normal" sperm samples. How the process of freezing adversely alters this motility is not well understood; however, compromise in fructose utilization and changes in basic metabolic pathway (Ackerman, 1971, 1968), sperm respiration (Behrman, 1959) and damage to adenyl-cyclase-cAMP system (Casillas and Hoskins, 1971, 1979; Garbers et al., 1971; Schill, 1975d; Wallner et al., 1975) seem to play important roles.

Recently, stimulation of human sperm motility by kinins has been demonstrated (Schill and Haberland, 1974). Kallikrein, a kinin-releasing proteinase, improved sperm motility in the presence of kininogen up to an observation period of 24 h at 22° C (Schill and Haberland, 1974). Stimulation of sperm metabolism by kinins is also demonstrated by an increase in fructolysis (Schill, 1975d). In addition to other systems (cAMP, prostaglandins, etc.), the kallikrein–kinin system is involved in regulation of sperm motility.

Definite improvement of sperm motility in patients with asthenospermia and oligospermia has

Table 5. Forward progression vs concentration of kallikrein used in post-thawing treatment. Mean forward progression* ± standard deviation.

Specific activity of kallikrein (KU/ml)	Post-thaw time (h)				
	0)	2	4	6	24
0 (control)	7.1 ± 1.3	6.8 ± 1.2	6.2 ± 1.4	5.7 ± 1.2	2.8 ± 0.6
2.3	7.2 ± 1.5	6.9 ± 1.3	6.3 ± 1.5	5.7 ± 1.2	2.9 ± 0.9
4.2	6.8 ± 2.1	6.9 ± 1.2	6.3 ± 1.5	5.7 ± 1.2	3.0 ± 0.8
7.3	7.5 ± 1.6	6.9 ± 1.1	6.5 ± 1.5	5.9 ± 1.2	3.2 ± 1.3
11.4	7.6 ± 1.5	6.9 ± 1.4	6.5 ± 1.8	6.0 ± 1.1	3.0 ± 0.8
17.5	6.8 ± 1.4	6.3 ± 1.2	5.7 ± 1.5	5.8 ± 0.9	2.5 ± 1.1
21.0	6.3 ± 1.4	5.0 ± 1.5	4.6 ± 1.1	4.5 ± 1.0	2.3 ± 0.9

* N = 10.

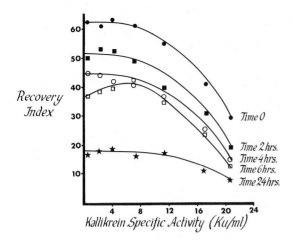

Figure 3. Recovery index vs concentration of kallikrein used in post-thawing treatment.

been observed after treatment with kallikrein (Schill, 1975c). The addition of kallikrein causes a significant increase of in vitro penetration of sperm through ovulatory cervical mucus (Wallner et al., 1975).

The possibility that extreme low temperatures or the "cryo shock", among other processes, could damage the kallikrein–kinin system was examined. The presumptive "used up" enzyme was added to see if the damage to sperm motility was reversible and was self-limiting to this specific enzymatic

system. Multifactorial systems regulate sperm motility, and the damage that is produced by the freezing and thawing process is not reversible by the addition of kallikrein alone.

Further studies to improve percentage motility recovery of frozen human sperm is needed since the use of frozen samples rather than fresh samples in artificial donor insemination is easier and more practical for the practicing gynecologist.

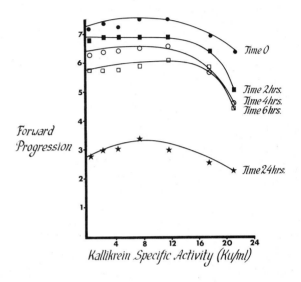

Figure 4. Forward progression vs concentration of kallikrein used in post-thawing treatment.

REFERENCES

Ackerman DR (1971) Variation due to freezing in the citric acid content of human semen. Fertil Steril 22: 58.

Ackerman DR (1968) The effect of cooling and freezing on the aerobic and anaerobic lactic acid production of human semen. Fertil Steril 19: 123.

Barkay J, Zuckerman H, Heiman M (1974) A new, practical method of freezing and storing human sperm and a preliminary report on its use. Fertil Steril 25: 399.

Behrman SJ (1959) Artificial insemination. Fertil Steril 10: 248.

Behrman SJ, Ackerman DR (1969) Freeze preservation of human sperm. Am J Obst Gynec 103: 654.

Behrman SJ, Sawada V (1966) Heterologous and homologous inseminations with human semen frozen and stored in a liquid nitrogen refrigerator. Fertil Steril 17: 457.

Casillas ER, Hoskins DD (1979) Activation of monkey spermatozoal adenyl cyclase by thyroxine and triiodothyronine. Biochem Biophys Res Commun 40: 255.

Casillas ER, Hoskins DD (1971) Adenyl cyclase activity and cyclic 3', 5' AMP content of ejaculated monkey spermatozoa. Archs Biochem Biophys pp 147, 148.

Chong AP, Taymor ML (1975) Sixteen years' experience with therapeutic donor insemination. Fertil Steril 26: 791.

Friedman S (1977) Artificial insemination with frozen human semen. Fertil Steril 28: 1230.

Fritz H (1975) The kallikrein–kinin system in reproduction — biochemical aspects. In: eds. Haberland GL, Rohen JW, Schirren C, Huber P, Kininogenases 2: 9. Stuttgart and New York: Schattauer.

Garbers DL, First NL, Sullivan JJ, Fardy HA (1971) Effects of phosphodiesterase inhibitors and cyclic nucleotides on sperm respiration and motility. Biochemistry 10: 1825.

Haman JO (1959) Herapeutic donor insemination: review of 440 cases. Calif Med 90: 130.

Kleegman SJ (1954) Therapeutic donor insemination. Fertil Steril 5: 7.

Koren Z, Lieberman R (1976) Fifteen years' experience with artificial insemination. Int J Fertil 21: 119.

Menkin MF, Lusis P, Azikis JP, Rock J (1964) Refrigerant preservation of human spermatozoa II. Factors influencing recovery in oligo- and euspermic semen. Fertil Steril 15: 511.

Sawada Y, Ackerman DR (1968) Use of frozen human semen. In: Bhrman SJ, Kistner RW, eds. Progress in infertility, p 731. Boston: Little, Brown.

Sawada Y, Ackerman DR, Behrman SJ (1976) Motility and respiration of human spermatozoa after cooling to various low temperatures. Fertil Steril 18: 775.

Schill WB (1975) Influence of the kallikrein–kinin system on

80

human sperm motility in vitro. In: Haberland GL, Rohen JW, Schirren C, Huber P, eds. Kininogenases 2: 47, Stuttgart and New York: Schattauer.

Schill WB (1975b) Influence of kallikrein on sperm count and sperm motility in patients with infertility problems: preliminary results during parenteral and oral application with special reference to asthenozoospermia and oligozoospermia. In: Haberland GL, Rohen JW, Schirren C, Huber P, eds. Kininogenases 2: 129. Stuttgart and New York: Schattauer.

Schill WB (1975c) Increased fructolysis of kallikrein-stimulated human spermatozoa. Andrologia 7: 105.

Schill WB (1975d) Stimulation of sperm motility by kinins in fresh and 24 hour aged human ejaculate. Andrologia 7: 135.

Schill WB, Haberland GL (1974) Induced enhancement of sperm motility. Hoppe-Seyler's F Physiol Chem 355: 229.

Sherman JK (1973) Synopsis of the use of frozen human semen since 1964: state of the art of human semen banking. Fertil Steril 24: 397.

Smith KD, Steinberger E (1973) Survival of spermatozoa in a human sperm bank. JAMA 223: 774.

Steinberger E, Smith KD (1973) Artificial insemination with fresh or frozen semen. A comparative study. JAMA 223: 778.

Tash JS, Mann T (1973) Adenosine 3′:5′-cyclic monophosphate in relation to motility and senescence of spermatozoa. Proc R Soc Fond B 184: 109.

Wallner O, Schiil WB, Grosser A, Fritz H (1975) Participation of the kallikrein–kinin system in sperm penetration through cervical mucus — in vitro studies. In: Haberland GL, Rohen JW, Schirren C, Huber P, eds. Kininogenases 2: 63. Stuttgart and New York: Schattauer.

Author's address:
Dr A.P. Chong
675 Tower Avenue
Hartford, CT 06112, USA

11. MICROORGANISMS IN SEMEN

J.D. PAULSON, S. LETO and F. FRENSELLI

Micro-organisms have long been recognized as being associated with infertility. Research in this field between 1930 and 1970 was not prolific, but set the stage for the abundance of research performed since 1970. Certain strains of bacteria produce sperm agglutination (Rosenthal, 1931). Experiments were performed which grew spermicidal bacteria in women with long-standing infertility (Matthews and Buxton, 1951), and treatment of these individuals demonstrated marked improvement in their fertility rate (Buxton and Wong, 1952). Routine examination on semen ejaculates of males from infertile couples and those of routine artifical insemination specimens demonstrated that 50% of 375 samples were contaminated by bacteria and 50% were sterile (Wu, 1957); of those contaminated, 44% cultured a spermicidal bacteria. Bacteria such as *Staphylococcus aureus*, *Streptococcus hemolyticus* and *viridans*, and *E. coli* are highly spermicidal; but other organisms such as *Micrococcus*, *Enterococcus*, *Staphylococcus albus*, *Diphtheroid*, and non-hemolytic *Streptococcus* are also slightly spermicidal when the concentrations of these organisms reach certain levels. Increased pregnancy rates ensue when the ejaculate is treated with antibiotics and then artificially inseminated. Others have treated men who had both genital infections and infertility and have increased pregnancy rates in the couples (Quesada et al., 1968). Appropriate antibiotic treatment in women, men, and the ejaculate itself has increased conceptions in certain circumstances of symptomatic and asymptomatic individuals.

There are two types of infections which must be considered when dealing with possible male reproductive tract infections and the effect of fertility. The first of these types of infections is one that is acute and systemic (Derrick and Dahlberg, 1976; Moberg et al., 1979; Appell and Evans, 1978). The second and most difficult to diagnose and treat are those of subclinical infections (silent type of bacteriospermia) (Swenson et al., 1980; Nikkanen et al., 1979).

The organisms found in semen have included bacteria (Wu, 1957; Swenson et al., 1980; Appell and Evans, 1978; Derrick and Dahlberg, 1976), mycoplasmas (Barile, 1978; Lapido and Osoba, 1979; Swenson et al., 1979; Matthews et al., 1978; Idriss et al., 1978; Toth et al., 1978; Friberg, 1980; Derrick and Dahlberg, 1976), and viruses (Lang, 1978; Barile, 1978; Derrick and Dahlberg, 1976). Male genital tract infections can also be contributory in male infertility. Mumps orchitis is rarely seen to be a prepubertal problem; however, postpubertal orchitis can cause testicular atrophy and fibrosis leading to diminished fertility or sterility. Post-inflammatory obstructions of the male reproductive tract are also associated with bacterial infection. Urethritis, prostatitis, and orchiepididymitis are often found in association with venereal disease while genital tuberculosis may lead to destruction of the entire epididymis. Mycoplasmas and viruses have been found in equal or greater numbers in fertile men in some studies and a great deal of controversy exists as to their role in male fertility.

1. MICROORGANISMS

1.1. Bacteria

A reconfirmation of the ealier examinations on semen ejaculates which demonstrated almost 50% contamination rate by bacteria in semen ejaculates (Wu, 1957) was performed (Swenson et al., 1980). Of 109 examined semen specimens, not one was sterile. In fact, 107 of the 109 samples contained

Hafez ESE & Semm K (Eds) Instrumental insemination.

Table 1. Microorganisms isolated from the semen of 109 infertile men (adapted from Swenson et al., 1980).

Microorganism	Positive specimens		Microorganism	Positive specimens	
Aerobic and facultative	No.	%	Anaerobic	No.	%
Staphylococcus epidermidis	86	78.8	Peptococcus asaccharolyticus	31	28.4
Viridans streptococci	75	68.8	Veillonella parvula	15	13.7
Diphtheroids	70	64.2	Propionibacterium sp.	14	12.8
Streptococcus fecalis	27	24.7	Peptococcus magnus	13	11.9
Beta-hemolytic streptococci	12	11.0	Bacteroides sp.	9	8.2
Neisseria subflava	9	8.2	Bacteroides corrodens	7	6.4
Escherichacoli	9	8.2	Eubacterium lentum	5	4.6
Klebsiella sp.	5	4.6	Bifidobacterium sp.	3	2.7
Enterobacter aerogenes	4	3.6	Peptococcus saccharolyticus	3	2.7
Proteus mirabilis	4	!3.6	Eikenella sp.	3	2.7
Acinetobacter calcoaceticus	4	3.6	Bacteroides melaninogenicus	2	1.8
Lactobacillus sp.	3	2.7	Fusobacterium nucleatum	1	0.9
Staphylococcus aureus	2	1.8	Eubacterium alactolyticum	1	0.9
Proteus morganii	1	0.9	Peptococcus prevotii	1	0.9
Proteus vulgaris	1	0.9			
Pseudomonas sp.	1	0.9			

two or more different bacterial species; 63% of the specimens also had anaerobic organisms. Many of the organisms isolated are spermicidal in vitro, confirming previous work (Wu, 1957). When freshly ejaculated spermatozoa are mixed with *E. coli*, agglutination and decreased motility are noted when bacterial concentrations are greater than 10^6/ml (Teague et al., 1971). Changes in motility and agglutination at concentrations of 10^6/ml or greater are seen with *E. coli* in semen solutions, but a period of several hours or longer is required for these changes to occur (Wu, 1957; Del Porto et al., 1975). In addition to agglutination by various bacterial organisms, it has also been demonstrated that low molecular weight spermatozoal immobilization factors exist and have been isolated from bacterial cultures (Paulson and Polakoski, 1977a, 1977b). This factor is stable to heat, freezing and lyophilization and rather than being spermicidal, it has the ability to immobilize spermatozoa. Spermatozoal survival of 70% or more of the sperm for at least 8 h is important to a good conception rate. Many different species have been found in specimens examined in infertility patients (Tables 1 and 2). These studies suggest that, unlike previous reports where it was concluded that in healthy men, few, if any, microorganisms are present, a bacterial flora in semen exists which is as varied as the vaginal flora (Corbishley, 1977). The large percentage of anaerobes (Swenson et al., 1980) suggests that while

relatively little is known about their significance in the male reproductive tract, evidence is emerging that links them to gynecological infections as improved isolation techniques become more available. There is some suggestion that *Peptococcus*, *Bacteroides*, and *Eubacterium* may find their way into the upper female reproductive tract by attaching to spermatozoa. Thus, treatment should include both partners when reproductive tract infections exist in either. Other reports support the above conclusions (Moberg et al., 1979). Aerobic and anaerobic bacterial flora were studied in infertile couples and it was demonstrated that mutual bacterial species were isolated in cervical mucus cultures and in semen cultures in 22% of the couples studied.

Table 2. Bacteria isolated in infertile men utilizing standard growth techniques (adapted from Wu, 1957).

Microorganism	Positive specimens	%
Escherichia coli	15	6.5
Staphylococcus aureus	54	23.4
Streptococcus hemolyticus	30	13.0
Streptococcus viridans	15	6.5
Enterococcus	9	3.9
Micrococcus	51	22.0
Staphylococcus albus	33	14.3
Streptococcus nonhemolyticus	9	3.9
Paracolobacterium	6	2.6
Diphtheroid	6	2.6
Bacillus	3	1.3

Studies have demonstrated enhanced agglutination and decreased motility when bacterial concentrations were equal or greater than 10^6/ml (Fig. 1) (Wu, 1957; Derrick and Dahlberg, 1956; Teague et al., 1971). The decrease in spermatozoal motility has been partially attributed to the bacterial growth and partially contributed to by-products of bacterial metabolism (Paulson and Polakoski, 1977b). An additional factor related to the time and temperature to which the spermatozoa are exposed is independent of the presence of bacteria (Appell and Evans, 1978). The observation of delayed motility at room temperature over a 24 h period frequently leads to the finding of bacterial growth under essentially anaerobic conditions (Leto et al., 1980). When these specimens are examined and found to have bacterial growth, agglutination and immobilization are invariably present. This growth is found on occasion that samples of the ejaculate which have heavy contamination with bacteria and large numbers of white blood cells showing poor initial spermatozoal motility and a rapid further diminution of motility over several hours.

1.2. Trichomonas vaginalis

Trichomonas vaginalis is a common disease in women. In men, however, symptoms can range from hematospermia and epididymitis to asymptomatic states. Most commonly the affected male is symptom-free. This organism has been associated with male infertility and can interfere with motility and viability of spermatozoa (Argenziano et al., 1967; Schmor, 1970; Walther, 1973). Spermatozoal motility was decreased by the addition to spermatozoal ejaculates of preparations of Trichomonas vaginalis (Paulson and Leto, 1980). The effect was more marked upon specimens with lower spermatozoal density. Fructose levels were seen to decrease in direct correlation to the decrease of motility of

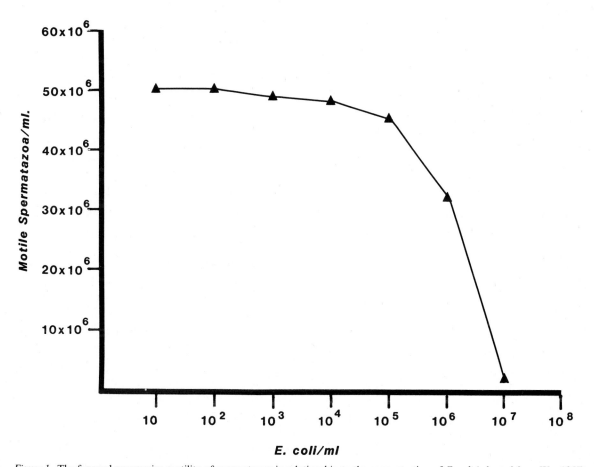

Figure 1. The forward progressive motility of spermatozoa in relationship to the concentration of E. coli (adapted from Wu, 1957).

the sample; the addition of fructose to samples with low motility after exposure to trichomonas showed a marked improvement in the motility of the spermatozoa. The addition of metronidazole to the specimen of *Trichomonas* prior to the addition of this mixture to the ejaculate eradicated the immobilizing effects of *Trichomonas* on the motility of the semen specimen. The effect of *Trichomonas* on the motility of the spermatozoa may be due to its effect on the metabolism of fructose and the need for that hexose in the metabolism of sperm motility.

1.3. Ureaplasmas (mycoplasmas)

Many reports have appeared recently implicating a group of organisms known as mycoplasmas in nonbacterial infections. Several species have been isolated from man (Barile, 1978). Positive cultures of mycoplasma are directly related to sexual activity; men with little or no sexual contact are virtually free of genital mycoplasma; therefore, sexual transmission of genital mycoplasmas has been postulated.

Large percentages of these organisms have been found in both fertile and infertile couplies (De Louvois et al., 1974; Harrison et al., 1975; Graber et al., 1979; Gnarpe and Friberg, 1972; Toth et al., 1978). Long-term antibiotic therapy showed a decreased trend in the observed abnormalities of both coiled and fuzzy tails while overall semen quality improved (Toth et al., 1970). Improved forward progression in motility with a concomitant decrease in coiled tails and fuzzy or granular tail segments in patients sucessfully treated with tetracycline or

doxycycline is seen after treatment (Swenson et al., 1979). Despite the overwhelming evidence of the presence of mycoplasma in male and female reproductive tracts, there is still no agreement as to the role mycoplasma plays in human infertility. Table 3 demonstrates the isolation rates of mycoplasma in healthy pregnant women. A newly developed media M-9 facilitates laboratory growth and allows for easier detection (Sheppard, 1980). In selected cases where these organisms are present, therapy should be instituted especially where it has been shown that semen quality is below accepted normals and the morphology is such that there are changes in the tail structure, despite current reports that such treatment has not resulted in significant improvement in all reports. The presence of these organisms, although in high numbers in the normal population, is not part of the normal reproductive tract environment; therefore, they should be eliminated because of the recent reports of finding urealyticum in significantly more samples from the endometrium in patients with habitual abortions. There is a considerably higher incidence of post-abortal fever observed among the patients having positive cultures for ureaplasma cultured at the time compared to ones with negative cultures (Stray-Pederson et al., 1978; Stray-Pederson et al., 1979).

1.4. Viruses

Several viruses have been unequivocally isolated in semen: *cytomegalovirus* (CMV) and *hepatitis virus* (surface antigens of hepatitis BHBsAG). Both of these viruses are capable of establishing persistent infections. *Herpes virus*, hominis type 2, is also well documented by epidemiological evidence to be sexually transmitted; however, despite recovery from urethral swabs, prostatic fluid, and vas deferens, documentation of actual virus presence in semen has not occured. Contamination probably occurs with direct skin and mucous membrane contact with the friction of coitus upon the lesions in an active infection. Transmission, therefore, is possible from one heterosexual or homosexual partner to the other (Lang, 1978).

In mice, infectious virus was recovered from epididymal sperm, seminal vesicles and uterine sperm from mated females. It could not be determined whether the spermatozoa were infected or

Table 3. Mycoplasma isolation in healthy pregnant women (adapted from DeLouvois et al., 1974).

Workers	M. hominis isolations	T-mycoplasma isolations
Braun et al. (1970)	22/568 (39%)	403/568 (71%)
Gnarpe and Friberg (1972)	3/40 (8%)	9/40 (23%)
Kundsin and Driscoll (1970)	10/50 (20%)	21/50 (42%)
Mardh and Westrom (1970)	2/50 (4%)	22/50 (44%)
DeLouvois et al. (1974)	22/92 (24%)	51/92 (55%)

whether the virions were extracellular or associated with other seminal components. However, the virus was excreted with sperm, suggesting sexual transmission. There was a reduction of the fertilization rate without any apparent effects on spermatozoal motility. This reduction of fertilization and litter size in mice warrants similar research in the human. Investigation into the modes of transmission and immediate affect on reproductive functions and the fetus if pregnancy occurs is necessary. The effects on subsequent pregnancies as a result of transmission of the virions is also an important step in elucidating the role of the viruses in infertility.

2. CONCLUDING REMARKS

Although long being recognized as being associated with infertility, new research has demonstrated a broader spectrum of microorganisms in the pathophysiology of the spermatozoa's inability to fertilize an ovum. With increasing isolation techniques, not only bacteria but also other microorganisms are being investigated. Spermicidal, agglutinating and immobilization factors are now well documented, but there is much controversy surrounding certain aspects and areas. One fact is important – it is necessary to investigate microorganisms in the semen if there is any suggestion or thought of its detrimental affect on the spermatozoa or its ability to fertilize.

REFERENCES

Appell RA, Evans PR (1978) The effect of temperature on sperm motility. II Is bacterial growth a factor? Fertil Steril 30: 436.

Argenziano D, Deluca M, Rossi A (1967) Relationship between trichomonas and male infertility. Prinerva Dermatol 42: 388.

Barile MF (1978) Mycoplasma contamination of human spermatozoa. The integrity of frozen spermatozoa, pp 226–237. National Academy of Sciences.

Braun P, Klein JO, Lee YH, Kass EH (1970) Methodologic investigations and prevalence of genital mycoplasmas in pregnancies. J Infect Dis 121: 391.

Buxton CL, Wong MB (1952) Spermicidal bacteria in the cervix as a cause of sterility. Am J Obstet Gynecol 64: 628.

Corbishley CM (1977) Microbial flora of the vagina and cervix. J Clin Path 30: 745.

DeLouvois J, Blades M, Harrison RF, Hurley R, Stanley VC (1974) Frequency of mycoplasma in fertile and infertile couples. Lancet: I 1073.

DelPorto GB, Derrick FC Jr, Bannister ER (1975) Bacterial effect on sperm motility. Urology 5: 638.

Derrick FC Jr, Dahlberg B (1976) Male genital tract infections and sperm motility. In: Hafez ESE, ed Human semen and fertility regulation in men, p 389. St. Louis: Mosby.

Friberg J (1980) Mycoplasmas and ureaplasmas in infertility and abortion. Fertil Steril 33: 351.

Gnarpe H, Friberg J (1972) Mycoplasma and human reproductive failure: 1, The occurrence of different mycoplasma in couples with reproductive failure. Am J Obstet Gynec 114: 727.

Graber CD, Creticos P, Valicenti J, Williamson HO (1979) T-mycoplasma in human reproductive failure. Obstet Gynec 54: 558.

Harrison RF, DeLouvois J, Blades M, Hurley R (1975) Doxycycline treatment and human infertility. Lancet 1: 605.

Idriss WM, Patton WC, Taymor ML (1978) On the etiologic role of ureaplasma urealyticum (T-mycoplasma) infection in infertility. Fertil Steril 30: 293.

Kundsin RB, Driscoll SG (1970) Mycoplasmas and human reproductive failure. Surg Gynec Obstet 131: 89.

Lang DJ (1978) Viruses in human semen. The integrity of frozen spermatozoa, pp 237–250. Washington, DC: National Academy of Sciences.

Lapido OA, Osoba AO (1979) T-mycoplasma and reproductive failure. Infertility 2 (2): 135.

Leto S, Frenselli F, Paulson JD (1980) Personal communication.

Mardh PA, Westrom L (1970) Tubal and cervical cultures in acute salpingitis with special reference to *Mycoplasma hominis* and t-strain mycoplasma. Br J Vener Dis 46: 179.

Matthews CD, Clapp KH, Tansing JA, Cox LW (1978) T-mycoplasma genital infection: the effect of doxycycline therapy on human unexplained infertility. Fertil Steril 30: 98.

Matthews CS, Buxton CL (1951) Bacteriology of the cervix in cases of infertility. Fertil Steril 2: 45.

Moberg PJ, Eneroth P, Ljung A, Nord CE (1979) Bacterial growth in samples from cer-vix and semen from infertile couples. Int J Fertil 24: 157.

Nikkanen V, Gronroos M, Suominen J, Multamaki S (1979) Silent infection in male accessory genital organs and male infertility. Andrologia 11: 236.

Paulson JD, Leto S (1980) The effects of trichomonas on spermatozoal motility. Presented at the World Congress of Embryo Transfer and Instrumental Insemination, Kiel, FRG, September 1980.

Paulson JD, Polakoski KL (1977a) Isolation of a spermatozoal immobilization factor from *Escherichia coli* filtrates: Fertil Steril 28: 182.

Paulson JD, Polakoski KL (1977b) Further characterization of the spermatozoal immobilization factor from *Escherichia coli*. Fertil Steril 28: 315.

Quesada EM, Dukes CD, Dean GH, Franklin RR (1968) Genital infection and sperm agglutinating antibodies in infertile man. J Urol 99: 106.

Rosenthal L (1931) Spermagglutination by bacteria. Proc Soc Exp. Biol Med 28: 827.

Schmoor J (1970) Sterility in urogenital trichomoniasis. Wien Med Wochenschr 120: 808.

Sheppard MC (1980) Standard fluid medium 10 for cultivation and maintenance of *Ureaplasma urelyticum*. The American Type Culture Collection, 14th eds, p 552 Media 943.

Stray-Pedersen B, Bruu AZ, Molne K (1979) Infertility and

uterine colonization with *Ureaplasma urealyticum*. Am J Obstet Gynecol. In press.

Stray-Pedersen B, Eng J, Reikvam T (1978) Uterine t-mycoplasma colonization in reproductive failure. Am J Obstet Gynecol 130: 307.

Swenson CE, Toth A, O'Leary WM (1979) Ureaplasma urealyticum and human infertility: the effect of antibiotic therapy on semen quality. Fertil Steril 31: 660.

Swenson CE, Toth C, Wolfgruber L, O'Leary WM (1980) Asymptomatic bacteriospermia in infertile men. Andrologia 12: 7.

Teague NS, Borarsky J, Glenn JF (1978) Interference of human spermatozoa motility by *E. coli*. Fertil Steril 22: 281.

Toth A, Swenson CE, O'Leary WM (1978) Light microscopy as an aid in predicting *Ureaplasma* infection in human semen. Fertil Steril 30: 586.

Walther H (1973) Trichomonas infection, clinical picture; therapy and significance to fertility and sterility. Z Hautkr 48: 553.

Wu DH (1957) Bacteriological studies on the semen and experimental studies on the influences of antibiotics, crystalline penicillin, potassium, dehydrostreptomycin sulfate and terramycin hydrochloride upon the semen. Keizo J Med 34: 509.

Author's address:
Dr J.D. Paulson
4801 Kenmore Avenue
Alexandria, VA 22304, USA

12. MICROBIOLOGICAL ANALYSIS OF SEMEN FROM INFERTILE MEN

K. GROSSGEBAUER and R. KADEN

Infections of the male reproductive tract may cause infertility (Deture et al., 1978; Eneroth et al., 1978; Friberg, 1980; Grossgebauer, 1978; Kaden and Grossgebauer, 1978; Moberg et al., 1979; Moberg et al., 1980; Rehewy et al., 1979; Swenson et al., 1980). The effects of certain acute and systemic infections on human reproduction are well known, but the influence of asymptomatic forms, their natural course and possible role for chronic inflammatory disease of the male accessory genital glands and the effect of bacteriospermia is not yet understood. Comprehensive microbiological and microscopical analysis of semen from infertile men as a causative correlation between microorganisms and an infectious process and/or between microorganisms and the infertility proves difficult.

1. QUANTITATIVE ANALYSIS OF SEMEN SAMPLES

1.1. Microbiological analysis

There is as yet no consensus concerning the composition of a "normal" bacterial flora in semen. The microorganisms may originate in the bulbourethral glands, the urethra or could be a contamination. It may be difficult to assess whether isolated bacteria are actually pathogens or whether they just colonize the genital tract when there is damage from some other cause (non-specific, opportunistic microorganisms; secondary infection). Local cleansing of the urethral and periurethral region is critical to reduce contamination. The culture of midstream urine samples indicates that the type of cleansing agent is not so critical. Quantitative microbiological analysis of semen is necessary to separate contamination from an infectious process. Some controversy has been generated concerning the question of the level of colony count and the number of leukocytes that constitutes "significant" bacteriospermia and/or genital infection. However, these difficulties are also well known in cases of other patient specimens that pass the urethra, e.g. urine and expressed prostatic fluid. Such specimens contain non-specific, potentially pathogenic microorganisms and are also indicators of an asymptomatic, subclinical or symptomatic infection or of a simple contamination. This mainly depends on the local cleansing of the urethral and periurethral region, the optimal transport of the specimens, the number of the polymorphonuclear granulocytes, the clinical data and the chosen dividing line between contamination and infection.

1.2. Classification of microbial isolates

Established bacterial pathogens, normal bacterial flora, occasional bacterial invaders and possible pathogens of the genital tract are classified according to the proposals of Danielsson (1976). This chapter does not include a systematic search for anaerobic bacteria.

1. *Normal bacterial flora.* Bacterial isolates in low colony counts ($< 10^3$ colony forming units/ml), often inhabits the distal urethra or contamination and is microscopically less than ten inflammatory cells (average number based on observations in 10 microscopic fields; $\times 400$).

2. *Potentially pathogenic flora.* Bacteria and yeasts which belong to this group reveal more than 10^3 colony forming units/ml and more than ten inflammatory cells. Pus-forming non-specific bacteria include *Staphylococcus aureus*, *E. coli*, *Klebsiella* sp., *Proteus* sp., *Pseudomonas aeruginosa* and *Streptococcus* sp.

3. *Pathogenic flora.* The detection of a few pathogenic ("specific") microorganisms indicates an infectious process.

Hafez ESE & Semm K (Eds) Instrumental insemination.

1.3. Microscopical analysis

The microscopic analysis of the semen indicates the known variations in the rate of excretion of leukocytes. Arbitrary standards have been empirically set to demarcate normal from abnormal numbers of leukocytes, but these arbitrary values (5 per high power field, etc.) have no valid or factual basis. Although the presence of high number of leukocytes by any definition generally means that infection is present, the absence of these cells is of no diagnostic value in eliminating the possibility of bacteriospermia and/or asymptomatic or symptomatic infection.

2. MICROSCOPICAL AND MICROBIOLOGICAL ANALYSIS OF SEMEN FROM INFERTILE MEN

2.1 Patients and collection of semen

Quantitative microbiological analysis of 720 semen specimens were performed. The men and their wives displayed no overt symptoms of genital infections and belonged to a group with primary sterility in marriage. The samples were collected in sterile glass containers under aseptic conditions by masturbation after thorough washing of the hands and penis.

2.2. Microscopical analysis.

The samples were processed within two hours

Table 1. Microbiological analysis of 720 semen samples of infertile, asymptomatic men.*

A	Growth of bacterial flora	82%
B	Normal bacterial flora	64%
C	Potentially pathogenic flora:	
	Ureaplasma urealyticum	8%
	Mycoplasma hominis	2%
	Candida albicans	2%
	Pus-forming bacteria (nonspecific)	4%
D	Pathogenic flora:	
	Trichomonas vaginalis	1%
	Chlamydia trachomatis	1%
	Neisseria gonorrhoeae	0%
	Herpes simplex-viruses	**

* Anaerobic bacteria are excluded.
** Two cases, overt infections.
Colony counts and number of leukocytes chosen to separate contamination and infection (see 2.2.).

and analyzed microscopically for: a) polymorphonuclear granulocytes, b) erythrocytes, c) pathological forms, especially "coiling forms", or spermatozoa, d) bacteria and fungi, e) epithelia, and f) *Trichomonas vaginalis*. The specimens were mixed with DAPI-fluorochrome (4′, 6-diamidino-2-phenylindole, Serva Feinbiochemica, Heidelberg) 1 + 1 (end concentration of the fluorochrome 10 μg/ml), held for 10 min at room temperature and examined by a fluorescence microscope under oil immersion. Type: standard 18, HBO 50 W with incident illumination; filter combination: KP 490, KP 500, Rfl 510, and LP 528. Microscopical analysis was performed with white light and ultraviolet light in order to identify vital and devitalized cells.

2.3. Microbiological analysis

Each specimen was cultured to isolate: a) extracellular, pus-forming bacteria, b) *Candida albicans*, c) *Ureaplasma urealyticum*, d) *Chlamydia trachomatis*, and e) *Herpes* simplex-viruses. Media used were blood agar, Endoagar, Sabouraud's agar, Mycoplasma (Table 1, Fig. 1) media MPI, McCoy-cells and chorioallantoic membranes of embryonated eggs. To achieve quantitative results, especially in cases of non-specific bacteria, a 0.01 ml pipette was used. *Chlamydia trachomatis* was identified with both Giemsa staining and DAPI-Technique (Grossgebauer, 1979).

Results of the study are summarized in Table 1. Of the 720 ejaculated cultured, 82% revealed the growth of bacterial flora (64% as normal bacterial flora). Among the potentially pathogenic microorganisms, *Ureaplasma urealyticum* could be cultured most frequently.

1. *Bacterial isolates*. The semen samples contained various kinds of bacteria. Mixed bacterial flora were isolated. The highest percentage of the semen samples of this randomly chosen group of asymptomatic infertile men contained bacteria normally present in the urethra. These could be found in low colony counts and can be considered as normal flora and nonpathogenic. Pus-forming bacteria, e.g. *Staphylococcus aureus*, *E. coli*, *Klebsiella* sp., *Proteus* sp. and *Pseudomonas aeruginosa* were present in low colony counts (contamination, colonization of the urethra and/or periurethral region) and in high colony counts (indicative for a

Figure 1. Correlations between microorganisms, bacteriospermia infection and infertility.

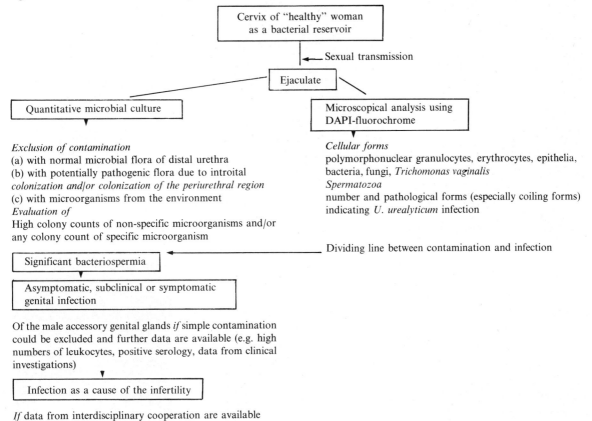

chronic prostatitis). No cases of gonorrhea were found.

2. *Special forms of bacteria. Ureaplasma urealyticum* was detected by using the DAPI-technique. A seminal ureaplasma infection was predicted with an accuracy of 60% (devitalized spermatozoa with coiled tails and swollen necks). More than 80% of the cultures grew out from the spermatozoa. Using transmission electron microscopy, ureaplasms were localized in the junction between the sperm head and the middle piece and at the sperm heads (Grossgebauer et al., 1977).

Chlamydia trachomatis was cultured in around 1% of all cases. Concerning the pathogenic flora of the genital tract, the isolation of *Chlamydia trachomatis* is of special interest. These obligatory intracellular bacteria could also be found in the urethra of "healthy" sexual active individuals. There is no convincing evidence that *Chlamydia* persists in the intact host in a non-replicating form, but it is more likely that latent or subclinical infections represent persistent low levels of multiplication held in check by host defense mechanisms (Taylor-Robinson and Thomas, 1980). Using the DAPI-technique to identify *Chlamydia*-induced inclusions, it was also possible to detect early forms of chlamydial development (Grossgebauer, 1979). The microscopical analysis of the ejaculates also revealed *Trichomonas vaginalis* in around 1% of the cases. *Candida albicans* was cultivated in around 2% of cases, and in two cases, *Herpes* simplex-viruses could be demonstrated (overt infections of the urethra).

3. CONCLUDING REMARKS

Quantitative microbiological analysis of 720 semen samples of a randomly chosen group of asymptomatic infertile men were performed. Of the 720 semen samples cultured, 82% revealed the growth of bacterial flora (64%) as normal bacterial flora, 8% *Ureaplasma urealyticum*, 4% non-specific pus-

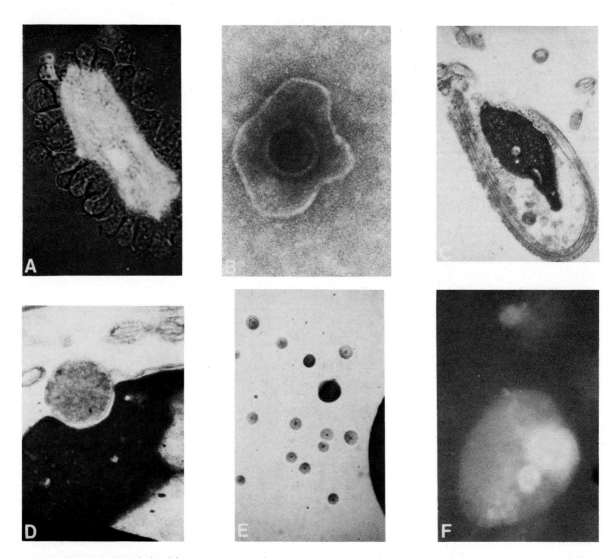

Figure 2. Microorganisms isolated from semen. A: *Trichomonas vaginalis:* DAPI-stained. Devitalized epithelia (yellow fluorescence) surrounded with living, unstained trichomonads; × 530. B: *Herpes* simplex-virus: transmission electron microscopy; virus size 110 nm. C: Spermatozoon: transmission electron microscopy; typical "coiling form" possibly due to a ureaplasma infection; × 9350. D: Spermatozoon: transmission electron microscopy; ureaplasma-induced changes of the head region × 22000. E: *Ureaplasma urealyticum:* colonies ("fried eggs") on agar medium; × 132. F: *Chlamydia trachomatis:* DAPI-stained McCoy cell. Green-yellow fluorescent cell nucleus with nucleoli and an intensive yellow fluorescent *Chlamydia*-induced intracytoplasmatic inclusion; × 660.

forming bacteria, 2% *Mycoplasma hominis*, 2% *Candida albicans*, 1% *Trichomonas vaginalis*, and 1% *Chlamydia trachomatis*). In two cases, *Herpes* simplex viruses could be cultivated (overt infection). The results mainly depend on the local cleansing of the urethral and periurethral region, the optimal transport of the specimens, the number of the polymorphonuclear granulocytes and the chosen dividing line between contamination and infection (in cases of nonspecific microorganisms,

more than 10^3 colony forming units/ml and more than ten inflammatory cells – observations in ten microsopic fields, average number, 400 ×).

A seminal ureaplasma infection was predicted with an accuracy of 60% (devitalized spermatozoa with coiled tails and swollen necks). Even with quantitative analysis of semen samples from infertile men, it is still difficult to prove a causative correlation between microorganisms and an infectious process and/or between microorganisms and infertility. To achieve a comparison of microbiological and microscopical results with that of other laboratories, it is essential to define the building-stones of "significant" bacteriospermia, "significant" leukocyto-spermia, asymptomatic infection and symptomatic infection.

REFERENCES

Danielsson D (1976) Infections of the male genital tract. Int J Androl Suppl 1: 36.

Deture FA, Drylie DM, Kaufman HE, Centifanto Y (1978) Herpes virus type 2: study of semen in male subjects with recurrent infections. J Urol 120: 449.

Eneroth P, Ljungh-Wadström A, Moberg PJ, Nord C (1978) Studies on the bacterial flora in semen from males in infertile relations. Int J Androl 1: 105.

Friberg J (1980) Mycoplasmas and ureaplasmas in infertility and abortion. Fertil Steril 33: 351.

Grossgebauer K (1978) Mikrobiologische Untersuchungen bei ProstatoUrethritis. Münch Med Wschr 120: 1599.

Grossgebauer K (1979) Der Einsatz eines neueren Fluorochromes DAPI in der diagnostisch-medizinischen Mikrobiologie. Tagung der Dtsch Ges Hyg Mikrobiol 1–3 Oct 1979 in Berlin West FRG.

Grossgebauer K, Henning A, Hartmann D (1977) Mykoplasmenbedingte Spermatozoenkopfschäden bei infertilen Männern. Hautarzt 28: 299.

Kaden R, Grossgebauer K (1978) Neues fluoreszenzoptisches Verfahren zur Darstellung menschlicher Spermatozoen. Andrologia 10: 327.

Moberg PJ, Eneroth P, Ljungh A, Nord CE (1979) Bacterial growth in samples from cervix and semen from infertile couples. Int J Fertil 24: 157.

Moberg PJ, Eneroth P, Ljungh A, Nord CE (1980) Bacterial flora in semen before and after Doxycycline treatment of infertile couples. Int J Androl 3: 46.

Rehewy MSE, Hafez ESE, Thomas A, Brown WJ (1979) Aerobic and anaerobic bacterial flora in semen from fertile and infertile groups of men. Arch Androl 2: 263.

Swenson CE, Toth A, Wolfgruber L, O'Leary W (1980) Asymptomatic bacteriospermia in infertile men. Andrologia 12: 7.

Taylor-Robinson D, Thomas BJ (1980)The role of *Chlamydia trachomatis* in genital tract and associated diseases. J Clin Pathol 33: 205.

Author's address:
Dr K. Grossgebauer
Institute for Medical Microbiology
Hindenburgdamm 27
D-1000 Berlin 45, FRG

13. MUTATION IN MAMMALIAN CELLS AFTER DEEP FREEZING

Evelyn Zeindl and K. Sperling

Many years of experience in cryoconservation of human sperm with freezing periods of up to ten years revealed good insemination results, notwithstanding a minor loss of motility (Behrman and Ackerman, 1969). The occurrence of congenital malformations among the newborn even seems to range below that of the population in general (Karow, 1979). However, this does not exclude the possibility of certain genetic damages which may manifest themselves in future generations.

A variety of ultrastructural alterations have been observed after deep freezing (Sherman and Liu, 1973; Gasser et al., 1976; Sherman, 1972, Persidsky, 1971; Peddersen and Lebech, 1971). As these include membrane alterations of the lysosomes (Allison and Paton, 1965; Persidsky, 1971; Persidsky and Ellett, 1971), which might lead to a release of lysosomal enzymes, especially DNase, an impairment of the genetic material cannot be ruled out.

Changes in the genetic material induced by environ- mental hazards can be broadly classified into chromosome and gene mutations (Fig. 1).

We have studied the effect of deep freezing, at a rate of $1° C$ min to $-30° C$ immediately followed by storage at $-80° C$ and $-196° C$ respectively, on: 1) the rate of chromosomal aberrations and the frequency of satellite associations in human lymphocytes, and 2) the number of gene mutations producing resistance to 6-thioguanine in Chinese hamster ovary (CHO) cells. Also using CHO cells, we investigated 3) the number of sister chromatid exchanges (SCEs), most probably a sensitive indicator of DNA repair (Perry and Evans, 1975; Galloway, 1977; Carrano et al., 1978).

1. CHROMOSOMAL ABERRATIONS AND SATELLITE ASSOCIATIONS IN HUMAN LYMPHOCYTES AFTER CRYOCONSERVATION

After storage at $-80° C$ or $-196° C$, from two days to several months, isolated human lymphocytes were grown in Ham's F10 medium, containing 10% fetal calf serum, phytohaemagglutinin (Difco) and the usual amount of antibiotics. First mitoses were collected after 50 h in $-80° C$ treated cells, and after 70 h in $-196° C$ treated cells. Colcemid (0.08 ug/ml) was added 4 h before harvesting. Air-dried slides were prepared as usual. In all series, including untreated controls and dimethylsulphoxide-treated controls, the frequency of satellite associations between the acrocentric D and G chromosomes and the rate of chromosomal aberrations were determined (Fig. 2A).

About 600 lymphocyte metaphases, in the first mitotic division after recovery from the frozen state, were scored for structural chromosome aberrations (Table 1). No increase in the average frequency of damaged cells or certain types of

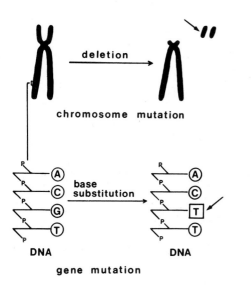

Figure 1. Schematic figure of chromosome — and gene — mutation.

Hafez ESE & Semm K (Eds) Instrumental insemination.

Table 1. Frequency of chromosomal aberrations in human lymphocytes after deep freezing at $-80°$ C or $-196°$ C for different lengths of time.

| Experimental groups | CI | CII | $-80°$ C Storage time (days) | | | | | $-196°$ C | |
			2	7	14	30	270	2	14
Mitoses analysed	106	100	90	91	100	74	59	100	100
Chromatid breaks	2	1	1	1	1	—	1	4	3
Exchange figures	—	1	—	—	—	—	—	—	1
Dicentric chromosomes	—	—	—	1	—	—	—	—	—
Total number of breakage events*	2	3	1	3	1	—	1	4	5

CI = untreated control, CII = control, incubated with 10% DMSO at 4° C.
* The total number of breakage events is calculated from the number of chromatid breaks, so translocations and dicentric chromosomes were counted twice.

chromosomal aberrations could be found ($P = 0.9$). This is in accordance with the findings of Ashwood-Smith and Friedmann (1979) that after cryoconservation the frequency of micronuclei (an indicator of chromosomal aberrations) was not elevated.

There was, however, a significant increase ($P < 0.0027$) in the number of chromosomes involved in satellite associations (Fig. 3). This points to an enhanced rate of ribosomal RNA synthesis, probably to compensate for the cytoplasmic proteins which have been damaged by the freezing procedure.

2. GENE MUTATIONS AT THE HGPRT-LOCUS AFTER CRYOCONSERVATION

For the gene mutational assay, we utilised resistance to the purine analogue thioguanine, which is usually accompanied by alterations in the enzyme hypoxanthine-guanine-phosphoribosyltransferase (HGPRT). Mutant colonies of cells, deficient in the enzyme HGPRT, were selected by their ability to grow in medium containing the cytotoxic 6-thioguanine (Shapiro and Vershaver, 1975; O'Neill et al., 1977; Abbondandolo, 1977).

CHO cells, grown in Eagle's MEM supplemented

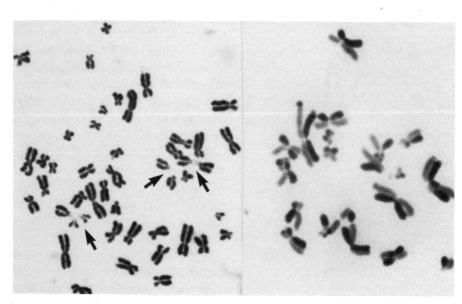

Figure 2. A: Human lymphocyte metaphase. → satellite associations between acrocentric D- and G-chromosomes. B: CHO metaphase after two rounds of replication in the presence of BUdR showing 8 SCEs.

Comparison of the frequency (%) of human lymphocyte mitoses with and without satellite associations after deep freezing at −80°C and −196°C

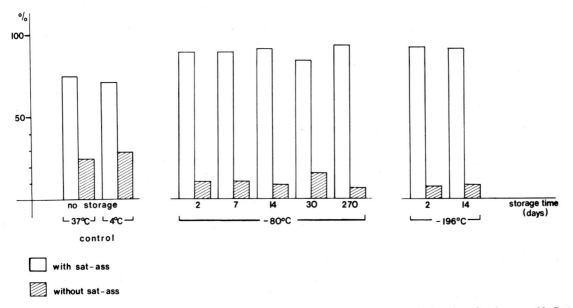

Figure 3. Number of acrocentric chromosomes participating in satellite associations (sat-ass) after deep freezing at −80° C or −196° C for different lengths of time. Control: one untreated, one incubated with 10% DMSO at 4° C.

with 10% fetal calf serum, were stored at −80° C or −196° C for 2 and 14 days. After thawing, the cells were plated into 10 cm petri dishes at a concentration of 10^5 cells per dish (5 plates/group) for a 72 h growth period. Thereafter, 10^5 cells were plated into 10 cm petri dishes (10 plates = 10^6 cells in total) with selective medium containing 20 μg/ml 6-thioguanine. For estimating the cloning efficiency 100 cells were plated in non-selective medium (20 plates = 2000 cells in total). After 12 days of incubation the surviving colonies were fixed, stained and counted. (Fig. 4).

There was only a slight difference between the average number of spontaneously occurring 6-thioguanine resistant colonies and those after deep freezing (Table 2). Thus we found no significant difference in the rate of gene mutations after cryo-conservation ($P > 0.05$). The considerable variability in the number of resistant colonies in parallel experiments is characteristic of spontaneous mutations. In accordance with this, no increase was observed after cryoconservation in the rate of gene mutations from the auxotrophic to the prototrophic state in *E. coli* (Ashwood-Smith, 1965).

The stability of phenotypic change to 6-thio-

guanine resistance was determined by cultivating isolated colonies (10 colonies per experiment) in selective and normal medium alternatively. The cloning efficiency in normal and selective medium was determined for passage I, III, VI and IX, by inoculating each of the five plates with 300 cells, which were then incubated for another 12 days. No phenocopies were detected within the 6-thioguanine resistant clones.

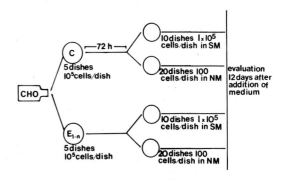

Figure 4. Schematic figure of the experimental procedure for detection of gene mutation at the HGPRT locus. NM = normal medium (MEM + 10% fetal calf serum); SM = selective medium (addition of 20 μg/ml 6-thioguanine). C = untreated control, E = experimental series, storage at −80° C or −196° C for two and 14 days.

Table 2. Number of 6-thioguanine resistant colonies of CHO cells after deep freezing at $-80°$ C or $-196°$ C for different length of time.

Experiment no.	Number of resistant colonies				
		$-80°$ C		$-196°$ C	
	Untreated control	Storage time (days)			
		2	14	2	14
1	11	14	12	—	9
2	17	3	10	3	7
3	6	2	15	25	4
4	6	6	11	2	8
5	14	20	3	11	4
6	26	6	9	7	11
Total no.	80	51	60	48	43
Average no. of colonies/10^6 cells	13,3	8,5	10,0	9,6	7,1

Each set of experiment involved 10 plates. The number of cells per plate was 10^5.

3. SISTER CHROMATID EXCHANGES AFTER CRYOCONSERVATION

For determining the rate of sister chromatid exchanges (SCEs), CHO cells were grown for two rounds of replication in the presence of bromodeoxyuridine (BUdR) at a final concentration of 10^{-5} M. During the first cell cycle, the cells were synchronized by N_2O (8 h at 4.2 kp/cm^2) at mitosis,

frozen in the following S-phase and stored at $-80°$ C or $-196°$ C for two and 14 days. This experiment included an untreated and a DMSO-treated control group.

After thawing and reincubation, the frequency of SCEs was determined in the following mitosis (Fig. 2B). SCEs in the centromeric region were not recorded because of the difficulty in distinguishing between true exchanges and twisting of chromatids.

The results of the analysis of SCEs in the CHO cells (Fig. 5) show a remarkably constant frequency of SCEs between single experimental groups (265 cells analysed in total) and the controls (189 cells analysed in total).

Our investigations on deep frozen and long-term preserved human and rodent material did not, however, reveal an increase of chromosome aberrations and gene mutations at the HGPRT-locus. There was also no indication (by means of the SCE rate) of an increased repair of genetic damage in CHO cells after cryoconservation. It was striking, however, that the average number of satellite associations per cell increases after cold storage.

REFERENCES

Abbondandolo A (1977) Prospects for evaluating genetic damage in mammalian cells in culture. Mut Res 42: 279.

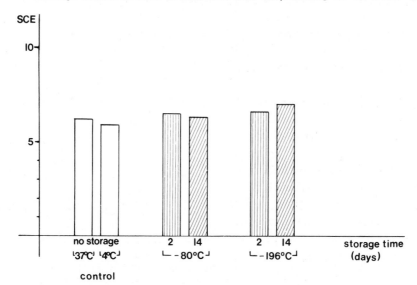

Average number of SCEs in CHO cells after deep freezing at -80°C and -196°C

Figure 5. Frequency of sister chromatid exchanges (SCEs) in CHO cells after deep freezing at $-80°$ C or $-196°$ C for different lengths of time. Control: one untreated, one incubated with 10% DMSO at $4°$ C.

Allison AC, Paton GR (1965) Chromosome damage in human diploid cells following activation of lysosomal enzymes. Nature 207: 1170.

Ashwood-Smith MJ, Friedmann EB (1979) Lethal and chromosomal effects of freezing, thawing, storage time, and X-irradiation on mammalian cells preserved at −196° C in DMSO. Cryobiology 16: 132.

Behrman SJ, Ackerman DR (1969) Freeze preservation of human sperm. Am J Obst Gynec 103: 654.

Carrano AV, Thompson LH, Lindl PA, Minkler JL (1978) Sister chromatid exchange as an indicator of mutagenesis. Nature 271: 551.

Galloway SM (1977) What are sister chromatid exchanges? In: Nichols WW, Murphy DG eds. DNA-repair processes.

Gasser G, Kaspar L, Klaushofer K, Mayr HG, Mossig H (1976) Kryobiologie aufgetauter Spermadepots. In: Kaden R, Lübke F, Schirren C, eds. Fortschritte der Fertilitätsforschung III, Berlin: Gosse. 243.

Karow A (1979) Cited in New Scientist 81: 238.

O'Neill PJ, Brimer PA, Machanof R, Hirsch GP, Hsie AW (1977) A quantitative assay of mutation induction at the HGPRT locus in Chinese hamster ovary cells (CHO/HGPRT-system): development and definition of the system. Mut Res 45: 91.

Peddersen H, Lebech PE (1971) Ultrastructural changes in the human spermatozoon after freezing for artificial insemination. Fert Steril 22: 125.

Perry P, Evans HJ (1975) Cytological detection of mutagen–carcinogen exposure by sister chromatid exchanges. Nature 258: 121.

Persidsky MD (1971) Lysosomes a primary target of cryoinjurie. Cryobiology 8: 482.

Persidsky MD, Ellett MH (1971) Lysosomes and cell cryoinjurie. Cryobiology 8: 345.

Shapiro NI, Vershaver NB (1975) Mutagenesis in cultured mammalian cells. In: Prescott DM, ed. Methods in cell biology, Vol 10, p 209.

Sherman JK (1979) Comparision of in vitro and in situ ultrastructural cryoinjury and cryoprotection of mitochondria. Cryobiology 9: 112.

Sherman JK, Liu KC (1973) Ultrastructural cryoinjury and cryoprotection of rough endoplasmic reticulum. Cryobiology 10: 104.

Author's address:
Dr Evelyn Zeindl
Institut für Hümangenetik
Heubnerweg 6
D-1000 Berlin 19, FRG

II. TECHNOLOGY OF INSEMINATION

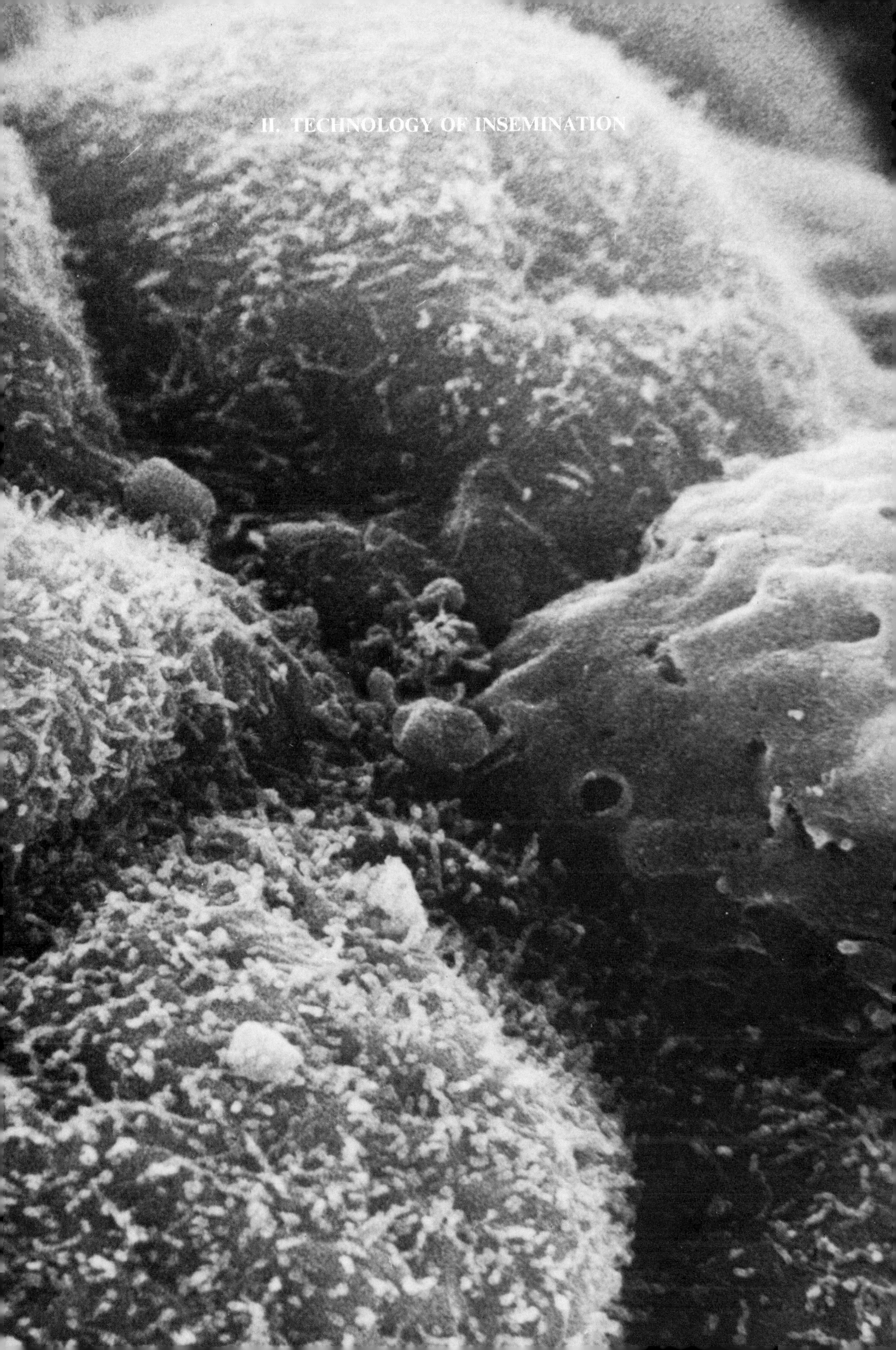

14. SELECTION AND ASSESSMENT OF DONOR AND RECIPIENT FOR AID

U. HERMANNS and E.S.E. HAFEZ

Insemination was first documented in the Hebraic Talmud, dating from the second century, followed by records in 1322, when an Arab artificially inseminated a mare. Table 1 summarizes the highlights in the development of artificial insemination. Until recently, artificial insemination by donor semen (AID) was generally a subject of either ignorance or disapproval. There is, however, a growing acceptance by clients, as AID offers the only means of achieving pregnancy for about 25% of all infertile couples (Joyce, 1979). During the last 5 to 10 years, AID practice has dramatically increased in nearly every country of the developed world. The exact number of inseminations is unknown, as AID is not registered in any country, mainly due to the uncertain legal status of the procedure (McLaren, 1973). According to estimations in the U.S.A., 5000 to 10000 babies are born annually after AID (Curie-Cohen et al., 1979). The increased demand for instrumental insemination can be attributed to the liberalization of attitudes towards sexual relationships and to the relative scarcity of babies for adoption which has followed by legalization of induced abortion in many countries.

The indications for AID include: azoospermia, unsuccessful insemination with husband's sperm (AIH) in case of severe oligozoospermia, genetic errors and Rh-incompatibility. The most common indication is the untreatable infertility of the husband (95%).

A nationwide study of the practice of AID in the U.S.A. revealed that 10% of the physicians performed AID on single women wishing to have a child, this being the third most cited reason for AID (Curie-Cohen, 1979). Since the first births following AID were recorded, several papers have been published describing the experiences of individual physicians or AID clinics. Whereas acceptable technology for storage of semen and insemination techniques seems to be available, various questions concerning the selection and assessment of donor and recipient for AID still remain unanswered.

1. THE DONOR

The selection of a suitable donor for a couple undergoing AID may be done by their private physician, an infertility clinic or a sperm bank. The

Table 1. Development of instrumental insemination.

Invention	Name	Year of discovery
First AIH in man	Hunter	End of the 18th century
First low-temperature observation of human semen	Spallanzani	1776
Ten successful cases of AIH in France	Girault	1833
First successful case of AIH in the U.S.A.	Sims	1866
First suggestion of a bank for frozen semen	Mantegazza	1866
First AID in man	Dickinson	1890
Use of glycerol as cryoprotective agent	Polge et al.	1949
First pregnancy from stored spermatozoa	Bunge et al.	1954
Four births with nitrogen-vapor store technique	Perloff et al.	1964
Pregnancy with plastic-straw store technique	Matheson, Trelford and Mueller	1969
First progeny from semen after 10 years of storage	Sherman	1972–1973
About 1500 AID births worldwide	Sherman	1976

Hafez ESE & Semm K (Eds) Instrumental insemination.
© *1982 Martinus Nijhoff Publishers, The Hague/Boston/London. ISBN 90-247-2530-5. Printed in the Netherlands.*

couple is only involved in the last step of the selection procedure — the matching. Although from a medico-legal standpoint standardization of donor screening would be advantageous, there are no uniform guidelines among various countries.

1.1. Recruitment

Medical students are the most common source of human donors for both fresh and frozen-stored semen, especially in university based banks. The select group is considered to assure the couple of some degree of health and intelligence, although this assumption remains somewhat questionable. Physicians might give medical students far more credit than they deserve for reliability, honesty, and knowledge of their family history. Some authors consider it "preferable" if the donor is a father of healthy children (Pollock, 1967; Goss, 1975). Several centers advocate approaching husbands of obstetric patients to ensure their fertility (Schoysman, 1975). There may be some criticism about using single donors without previous fertility records; however, it is difficult to find married fathers who are willing to become donors (Beck, 1977). There has been an increased tendency to accept healthy men up to the ages of 30 to 35 years. This age limit should be considered in order to minimize possible hazards for the following age-related effects:

1. Aging is associated with several degenerative changes in the testes causing decreases in the quality of the ejaculate (Hafez, 1976).

2. There is indirect evidence that the early fetal death rate increases not only with maternal age, but also with the age of the father (Guerrero, 1975).

3. Stillbirth is rather common when the father is older than 40 years, regardless of the age of the mother (Parson and Sommers, 1978).

4. The incidence of some human genetic abnormalities increases with advancing paternal age, including four autosomal dominant disorders: (a) achondroplasia (Penrose and Camb, 1955; Murdoch et al., 1970), (b) Apert syndrome (Blank, 1960; Erickson and Cohen, 1974), (c) Marfan syndrome (Lynas, 1958; Smith, 1972), and (d) myositis ossificans progressiva (Tunte et al., 1967). Three other disorders are still under discussion: bilateral retinoblastoma (Tunte, 1972), hemophilia (Herrman, 1966), and Duchenne's muscular dystrophy (Hutton and Thompson, 1970).

1.2. Investigation

The use of a select donor pool without further investigation is unsatisfactory for the following reasons: 1) More than 20% in the select group of male students have sperm densities of 20 million/ml or less, the level generally defined as functional sterility. 2) Less than 20% of the general male population willing to become semen donors fulfill the minimum demands of donor recruitment (Witherington et al., 1977; Hansen et al., 1979). 3) Previously fertile men may have inadequate spermatozoa for insemination. This may be a temporary phenomenon because semen quality varies at different times throughout analysis, but it should not justify the use of unscreened donors. 4) The incidence of asymptomatic gonorrhea is 10 to 20% (Godden, 1973; Portnoy et al., 1974). As venereal disease is not limited in any group or subgroup, select donor pools such as "young healthy medical students" have to be screened carefully.

Investigational procedures vary considerably among centers and countries, ranging from a minimum of personal and family history with physical examination and semen analysis, to protocols including genetic analyses with karyotyping, and various special tests for potential pathogens (Joyce, 1979). A proper donor selection should include personal, physical and genetic history, physical examination, and in-depth andrological analysis.

Personal history, particularly intelligence, personality traits, talents, and occupation are of interest to the recipient couple. The characteristics of somatotype are recorded in order to allow the inseminating doctor a close match between husband and donor. A full history of the donor and his family is obtained to limit the risks of genetic or family diseases and of venereal infections. The medical history will also reveal illnesses affecting the genital area to denote any probable decrease of fertility. Donors taking any kind of drugs should not be considered because of the inhibiting effect on the motility and metabolism of spermatozoa (Peterson and Freund, 1976).

Donor selection should be based on the following criteria from laboratory analysis:

1. *Blood grouping and Rh-typing*. Both blood type and Rh-factor are routinely determined because Rh-negative women must not receive semen

Table 2. Summary of major parameters to be considered in the assessment of donors for AID.

Parameters	Factors to be considered
1. History	
a) Personal history	Personality characteristics Intelligence Special talents, attitudes, interests Occupation
b) Physical history	1. Physical appearance (height, weight, eye color, hair color, racial group, body type). 2. Illnesses affecting genital organs (orchitis, epididymitis, prostatitis, urethritis, mumps with testicular involvement, urogenital tuberculosis, venereal diseases, varicocele, hydrocele, undescended testicule, inguinal hernia operation, injury to testicles). 3. Proven fertility: children, pregnancy of any women. 4. Drugs; alcohol; cigarettes
c) Family history	Cancer, diabetes, epilepsy, heart disease, congenital defects.
d) Genetic history (three- generation family history)	Birth defects Diseases of the various body systems } of Habitual abortions } family Fertility problems } members Ages and causes of deaths
2. Physical investigation	
a) Physical defects	
b) Present physical diseases	
c) Genital organs	Penis, testes: size, consistency, hydrocele, spermatocele Epididymis: consistency Prostate and seminal vesicle
3. Special investigations	
a) Blood analyses	Blood group, Rh-factor
b) Microbiological analyses	Hepatitis, venereal diseases
c) Genetic analyses	Karyotyping, biochemical tests (if indicated)
d) Semen analyses	See Table 3.

from Rh-positive men. Also, semen of A- or B-donors should not be given to recipients with blood group O if possible.

2. *Screening tests for hepatitis and venereal diseases.* A variety of microorganisms have been isolated from human semen, including: mycoplasmas (DeLourois et al., 1974), cytomegalovirus CMV (Lang and Kummer, 1975), herpes simplex virus (DeTure et al., 1975), hepatitis antigen B (Heathecote, et al., 1974) and gonococcus (Sherman and Rosenfeld, 1975; Fiumara, 1972). Not all of these however, require screening. The possible role of semen contaminated with CMV in the genesis of intrauterine infection, for example, need further exploration (Lang, 1978).

Three diseases are known to be transmissible via artificial insemination: hepatitis, syphilis and gonorrhea. Hepatitis can be screened in blood samples or in semen cultures for hepatitis antigen and antibody. Screening for venereal disease consists of a serum test for syphilis and a semen culture on Thayer-Martin medium for gonorrhea. The risks of transferring gonococcal infections via AID are

considerable as most donors are in the age group of 20 to 24 years, which show the greatest incidence of gonorrhea (Nolan and Osborne, 1973; Panikabutra, 1973; Jennings et al., 1977).

The following guidelines should be regarded when screening for gonorrhea. a) Each ejaculate coming from every donor considered for AID should be screened. b) Continuous testing of all specimens is essential since gonorrhea is sometimes discovered in asymptomatic donors, whose test has previously been negative (Feldschuh, 1978). c) There is no reliable rapid test as yet for the detection of gonococci. Therefore, the culture method, requiring a minimum of 24 hours, is still the method of choice (Shermann and Rosenfeld, 1975). It seems desirable to screen every specimen for any kind of contamination (Bartlett, 1978). However, the size of a given sample restricts the extent of microbiological testing, as 0.2–0.4 ml of semen is used per microbial isolation for a total of 1.2 ml per sample. In the future, there may be methods such as sensitive radioimmunoassays that minimize the amount of semen required for the various isolations (Noguchi et al., 1978).

3. *Genetic screening*. With proper screening, the risk of genetic disease transmission by donor semen is far less than with natural mating in the general population. Minimal genetic screening should consist of a three-generation family history giving special attention to any type of birth defects, unexplained deaths before the age of 30, habitual abortions, or fertility problems. A recent study of current AID practice in the U.S. revealed that the screening for genetic diseases is inadequate. There should be a list of genetic traits to be used routinely when taking a family history. Likewise, screening should be conducted by professionals trained in evaluating genetic traits (Curie-Cohen et al., 1979).

Regarding the low frequency of congenital abnormalities and spontaneous abortions resulting from artificial insemination, the value of expensive cytogenetic analyses remains questionable (the average cost of karyotyping is about \$ 200).

4. *Semen analyses*. As semen qualities are highly variable, three semen samples of every potential donor should be initially examined, including the following parameters:

a) Volume of ejaculate. A volume of less than 1 ml does not guarantee a sufficient buffering effect on the vaginal fluid of the recipient; consequently, a minimum of 2.5 ml is mandatory.

b) Coagulation and liquefaction time. Disorders in coagulation and liquefaction are indicators of reduced fertility (Amelar, 1962; Moon and Bunge, 1968; Bunge, 1970). There are no pharmacological agents that can improve poor liquefaction without affecting other important parameters of semen quality.

c) Sperm motility. Although sperm motility is considered one of the most important aspects of fertility, a suitable definition for the measurement of this parameter is still lacking, and all ranking systems are subjective. Several photographic techniques and sperm velocity tests have been introduced but the advantage of objectivity faces the disadvantage of being time consuming (Bartak, 1971; Atherton, 1977).

d) Sperm morphology. Human semen is characterized by morphologic heterogeneity and a rather high percentage of abnormal spermatozoa, but more than 50% of abnormal spermatozoa indicates reduced fertility (Zaneveld and Polakoski, 1977; Hafez, 1976). The consensus opinion is that 70% or more of sperm should show normal morphological structure for the semen to be potentially fertile (Sherman, 1978).

e) Sperm count. Only a few studies have critically investigated the amount of human spermatozoa required for conception. Fertility of donor semen is not particularly well related to sperm density. A minimum of 25 million actively motile spermatozoa, accurately timed to pre-ovulation, is necessary to achieve an acceptable frequency of conception (Matthews et al., 1979; Kerin, 1980). Considering the problems involved with the exact timing of ovulation for AID, the sperm counts of a semen sample for insemination should not be below those anticipated in an average fresh ejaculate, i.e. 40 million/ml. More than 130 million/ml are required for frozen semen. After allowing for dilution factors, freezing losses, etc. at each insemination, only approximately 10 million motile spermatozoa/ml would be introduced (Richardson, 1980). The paucity of data regarding the physiology of human fertilization makes it difficult to formulate recommendations concerning standards for donor semen

Table 3. Standards for acceptable donor semen.

	Parameters	Minimum requirements
Ejaculate	Volume	2.5 ml
	Viscosity	Length of semen thread 3–5 cm
	Coagulum	Present in fresh semen
	Liquefaction time of coagulum	5–20 min
	pH	7.2–7.8
Spermatozoa	Sperm count	60×10^6/ml (fresh semen)
		130×10^6/ml (frozen semen)
	Sperm viability	50%
	Sperm motility	60%
	Sperm progression	4 (Eliasson scale)
	Sperm morphology	70%

Table 4. The evaluation of semen during cryo-preservation and storage.

Assessment	Stage	Abbreviation
1.	Motility of untreated semen prior to freezing	PFM (Pre-Freeze Motility)
2.	Motility following dilution with cryo-protective medium	PDM (Post-Dilution Motility)
3.	Motility after being frozen for 1 day	PTM (Post-Thaw Motility)
4.	Motility after being frozen, and stored for 7 days	PTM (Post-Thaw Motility)
5.	Motility immediately before insemination	PIM (Pre-Insemination Motility)

Authorized table from: Richardson D (1980) In Richardson, Joyce and Symonds eds. Frozen human semen, p 49. The Hague: Martinus Nijhoff.

upon proven factual evidence. Semen specimens can apparently be accepted for AID when the main parameters are within the range indicated in Table 3. These minimal standards may appear rather high, usually eliminating two thirds of the potential donors (Beck, 1977).

f) Microbiological tests. Screening for bacteria and white blood cells should be part of every semen analysis as infections of male accessory organs are often asymptomatic (Nikkanen et al., 1979). At significant concentrations, bacteria (especially *E. coli*) cause a decrease in sperm motility by at least 50% and induce sperm agglutination, resulting in a reduced chance of conception (Derrick, 1977). Each semen sample for freeze storage must be cultured for gonorrhea because the gonococcus is not as fragile as once assumed and will survive freezing and storage (Feldschuh, 1978).

g) Assessment of freezability. Despite availability of adequante techniques for frozen storage of human semen, subsequent fertilizability of a specimen is never guaranteed, and semen samples of normal quality may lose their fertilizability during cryopreservation. When human semen is frozen and stored, approximately one third of the initial motility is lost in the cryopreservation process, regardless of the cryoprotective medium (Richardson, 1980). According to results of repeated freeze-thawing, the extent of adverse effect during freeze-preservation appears to be in direct relationship to the quality of a specimen. The cryo-survival is calculated from the

$$\text{formula cryosurvival} = \frac{\text{post-thaw motility}}{\text{pre-freeze motility}} \times 100.$$

Table 5. Criteria for rejection of a donor.

Type of investigation	Parameters	
Personal history	Age above 30 to 35 years	
	Consanguinity with the recipient	
	Increased risk of radiation or chemical exposure	
	Cytostasis therapy	
	Alcohol abuse	
	Drug abuse	
	Diabeter (in the donor himself or in his family)	
Physical investigation	Venereal disease	
	General infection	
	Genital infection	
Genetic history	Possible hereditary illness of the donor	
	Birth defect	of any
	Unexplored death below the age of 30	family
	Habitual abortions	member
	Fertility problems	
Genetic analysis	Chromosome abnormality	
	Biochemical disorders	
Semen analysis	Lack of liquefaction	
	Total sperm count below 40×10^6	
	Percent motile sperm	
	$<50\%$ 1 h after ejaculation	
	$<40\%$ 3 h after ejaculation	
	Percent abnormal sperm forms $>50\%$	
	Positive gonorrhea culture	

Semen showing less than 40% of motile sperm has a compromised fertility potential (Beck and Silverstein, 1975). Post-thaw motility recovery rate of cryopreserved semen has a direct correlation with the pre-freeze quality of the sample (Ansari, 1980). Consequently, potential donor semen should have minimal initial motility of 60%. A sperm progression rating of 4 or higher should be seen (Eliasson, 1971). A cryo-survival rate of 50% is considered the minimal standard (Sherman, 1978).

At specific stages during cryopreservation, the ability to undergo freezing and thawing of a specimen is monitored by five motility determinations (Table 4). Post-thaw motility alone is a poor guide to fertility of any individual specimen. Whether the quality of motility is more definitive in predicting fertilizing ability of spermatozoa is not known in the absence of a reliable objective assessment for this semen parameter (Read, 1980).

Other factors such as prolonged interval between collection of specimen and freezing and prolonged duration of cryopreservation may also influence post-frozen-storage fecundity unfavorably (Ansari, 1980). The inclusion of a cervical mucus penetration test (Kremer and Jager, 1976) would assess whether the migration rate and/or velocity of spermatozoa has been significantly affected by freezing and thawing. This penetration test requires further refinement with regard to establishing minimal standards for frozen thawed spermatozoa.

1.3. Rejection

Most clinicians rely on sperm banks and their standards of donor screening; however, the variation in the criteria for rejection is rather widespread (Table 5). A definite reason for excluding a semen sample is the detection of gonorrhea since the addition of penicillin to the ejaculate is of questionable clinical prudence due to allergic reactions (Sherman and Rosenfeld, 1975). A questionable concern with genetic screening is whether to use donors whose background indicates an unusual tendency towards multiple pregnancies (Finegold, 1964).

1.4. Matching

The couple should be consulted in this final step of donor selection. The extent of matching the donor to the infertile husband, differs with various authors. Most physicians only match the phenotype regarding racial background, body build, hair and eye color, and complexion (Taymor, 1973; Beck, 1976). It is usually the wish of the couple to make the progeny physically appear as the natural child of the husband (Curie-Cohen et al., 1979). This practice reduces the dangers inherent in positive eugenics (Roberts, 1964) by limiting the number of characteristics that can be selected by the inseminating physicians and their clients. Some andrologists usually match blood type and Rh-factor of donor and husband (Beck 1976, Friedman, 1977; Pollock, 1967). It is more reasonable to match both ABO and Rh-type of donor and recipient to rule out any chance of blood incompatibility.

Results from in vitro sperm penetration tests in cervical mucus are beneficial to the individual selection of the most suitable semen samples for a recipient. The velocity and depth of penetration, the number and survival time of donor's spermatozoa in recipient's cervical mucus correlate best with the conception rate (Jaszczak and Hafez, 1977). Spot checks of semen quality and compatibility can be made 15–20 min after insemination by microscopic examination of the cervical mucus (Goss, 1975).

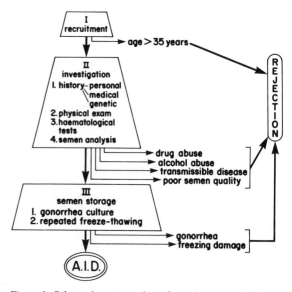

Figure 1. Schematic presentation of step-by-step evaluation of donors for AID.

1.5. Change of donor

There are two main reasons for replacing the donor:

1. Generally, human insemination demands a limitation of the number of conceptions from any single donor to avoid inadvertent consanguinity. To minimize eugenic problems, semen from the same donor should not be used after successful insemination of more than five (Weller, 1977), or a maximum of 15 women (Hansen et al., 1979).

2. For any couple, the donor should be changed after two or three unsuccessful inseminating cycles (Beck, 1976; Friedman, 1977) to choose a semen with proven fertility.

2. THE RECIPIENT

2.1. Selection

There is no agreement as yet of the criteria for selecting recipients suitable for undergoing AID. Regarding the material and personal expense involved with AID, the selection of recipients should include more than counselling of the couple, thereby not leaving the decision to them as to whether or not the woman is suitable for artificial insemination. Selection of the recipient requires the following: 1) proof of infertility in the male partner (azoospermia or gross oligozoospermia), by accurate semen analysis and/or by several failures of AIH, provided they were not due to the female partner, and 2) exclusion of identified pathology interfering with the recipient's fertility.

1. *Counselling interview.* As the psychological aspect of AID is obvious, it is essential that the couple be completely at ease with the procedure. During a counseling interview, the AID procedure, including the associated legal, psychological, and religious problems, is explained (Bromwich et al., 1978; Quinlivan, 1979; Pennington and Naik, 1977). It might be ideal to include a medical social worker in the consultation to help the couple clarify any problems or questions concerning AID (Ledward et al., 1976; Bromwich et al., 1978). During the initial interview, the couple — once willing to undergo AID — are advised to be prepared for six months of insemination while

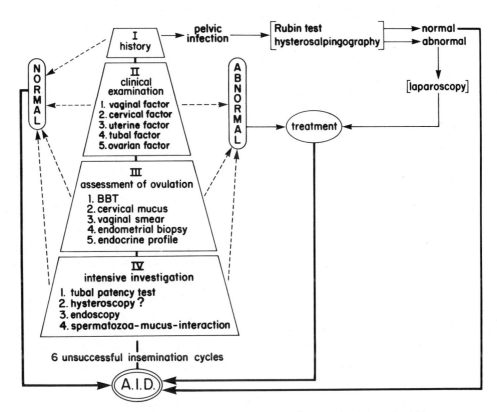

Figure 2. Schematic presentation of step-by-step evaluation of recipients for AID.

realizing that the majority of AID conceptions can be expected during this period, and that a major cause of AID failure is discontinuation from the program.

2. *Assessment of AID indication.* In order to assess the indication for most AID requests, the infertility of the male partner has to be determined. Apparent male infertility can cover many grades from subfertility to absolute sterility (Parkes 1973). The result of a single sperm analysis is an unreliable indicator of fertility (Edwards, 1973). Several semen analyses are required as severe oligozoospermia represents a gray zone, and borderline counts may respond to urologic therapy or may be an indication for AIH instead of AID.

Rh-incompatibility as a reason for AID is assessed either by a history of fetal hemoblastosis or by blood grouping of both partners. Severe hereditary diseases requiring AID are proven either by a history of genetic malformation or by chromosome analysis.

3. *Blood grouping and Rh-typing of the recipient.* Knowing the recipient's blood group and Rh-type is necessary for the selection of a suitable donor, but there is no need to perform blood grouping of the male partner.

4. *Recording the physical characteristics of both partners.* Knowledge of the physical characteristics (i.e. race, height, stature, complexion, color of eyes and hair) is a supposition for matching a potential donor to the male partner of the recipient.

2.2. Investigation

To date, there are no agreed criteria for selecting recipients suitable for AID. The extent of investigative procedures differs among various centers. The recipient should generally be in good physical and psychological condition, thus allowing her to carry a child through pregnancy and adequately raise thereafter. However, thoroughness of the fertility work-up is controversial. One group of authors may start AID when the woman appears to be fertile, whereas another group may perform hysterosalpingography routinely during the pre-insemination investigation. The following reasons justify an in-depth investigation of the recipient:

1. In 95% of cases, AID is achieved because of male infertility; however, the finding of a male

factor in an infertile couple does not rule out the possibility of fertility problems in the female partner. Reproductive abnormalities and irregular ovulatory patterns in the woman are the second most common cause of failure in AID programs (Quinlivan, 1979).

2. Comparison of AID results before and after careful female fertility evaluation shows that prior investigation improves the success rate and reduces the number of treatment cycles required (Rajan and John 1978). Pregnancy rates of AID drop from about 35–45% to 20% when an associated female subfertility factor is involved and may reach 67% after elimination of those women with associated causes of subfertility (Friedman, 1977). The pregnancy rate is also higher in women with demonstrated fertility (Dixon and Buttram, 1976).

3. The often large amount of money, time, physical and psychological energy of both physician and client should not be wasted on "hopeless cases".

For these reasons, the extent of thoroughness in the investigation of the woman's fertility should not only depend on the fertility work-up of her partner. It cannot be enough to "assume" the fertility of a woman just because her partner is infertile. However, comparing complication rate and informational value of some diagnostic methods necessary to achieve a complete fertility work-up, the aim must be to adopt a middle course. There seems to be two types of investigational procedures: a) investigation prior to AID, and b) investigation concomitant with AID.

2.3. Investigation prior to AID

1. History

a) Age of the recipient. Although there seems to be a trend towards diminished fertility with increasing age, a relationship between age and pregnancy rate in AID has not been noted (Dixon and Buttram, 1976; Pennington and Naik, 1977; Chong and Taymor, 1975). It does not seem necessary to create an age limit for recipients comparable to the 35 year limit for donors. The inseminating physician should give full information about the declined pregnancy rate with advancing age and about the increased incidence of mongolism after the age of 35, but AID cannot be refused if the patient is willing to accept the risk.

b) Gynecological and obstetrical history. Answers to the following questions will determine the extent of explorations necessary to prove the recipient's fertility: pregnancy or abortion? fertility treatment? gynecological investigation? (i.e. hysterosalpingography, laparoscopy etc.) gynecological surgery? pelvic or genital infection (especially tuberculosis)?

2. *Physical investigation.* During the gynecological examination, special attention has to be placed on the four critical anatomical points of possible fertility defects: cervical factor (cervical stenosis, polyps, erosions), uterine factor (congenital defects, tumors, retroflexio uteri), tubal factor (peritubal adhesions, pyosalpinx), and ovarian factor (tumors, periovarian adhesions). These disorders, which eventually influence the chance of fertilization, need further investigation.

Women with a known factor of infertility must not necessarily be excluded from the AID program since recipients with known pathology including cervical polyps, ovarian cysts and endometriosis may conceive (Symonds, 1980). Some factors respond to treatment: Uterine or ovarian tumors and peritubal or periovarian adhesions can be treated surgically. However, the overall success rate of correcting cervical disorders by estrogen therapy, midcycle sounding or cryosurgery is rather poor (Davajan, 1977).

3. *Microbiological analysis.* Acute vaginal and endocervical infections (viral, bacterial, monilial or trichomonal) affect sperm transport in various ways. Cervicitis reduces the penetration of spermatozoa in cervical mucus (Horne et al., 1974; Patton and Taymor, 1975). Furthermore, infections may potentiate the immune response against spermatozoa (Katshi et al., 1968). Therefore, any genital infection requires bacteriological evaluation and specific therapy.

4. *Assessment of ovulation.* The reliable confirmation of the recipient's reproductive ability is an inevitable step before starting AID procedure. The following tests detect ovulation: a) recording of basal body temperature (BBT), b) investigation of cervical mucus, c) vaginal smear, d) premenstrual endometrial biopsy, and e) endocrine profile.

a) Recording of the BBT. A BBT chart sup-

posedly indicates ovulation when it shows a biphasic change in temperature with a sustained rise of more than 0.5° for 14 days following ovulation (Newton, 1977). The rise in body temperature is a helpful but not at all infallible hint that the egg has been shed, as the cyclic thermogenesis may be influenced by emotion, activity, and ovarian hormones (McLaren, 1973).

A monophasic BBT is not invariably associated with anovulation, but can and does occur during ovulatory cycles (Jones, 1975; Moghissi, 1976). This indicates that there are both false-negative and false-positive results.

b) Investigation of cervical mucus. Most clinicians prefer to examine the cervical mucus to detect ovulation. The clinical condition of the cervix is assessed by a cervical score method of four parameters, namely, volume of mucus, degree of ferning, length of spinnbarkeit, and cervical dilatation (Insler and Melmed, 1972). Each parameter is ascribed a score of 0 to 3, the maximal possible cumulative score being 12. The advantage of this method is that the subjective clinical parameters of the cervical score give a reliable objective prediction in terms of the total score, and that there is no need for technical or biochemical facilities (Kerin, 1980).

An "ovutime tackiness rheometer" has been designed to identify the mid-cycle fertile period through changes in the biophysical characteristics of cervical mucus (Kopito and Kosasky, 1979). The pre-ovulatory decrease of some enzymes, such as alkaline phosphatase (Moghissi, 1976), amylase (Skerlavay et al., 1968) and muramidase (Schumacher, 1969), may faciliate the detection of ovulation after developing a simple colorimetric assay.

c) Vaginal smear. Vaginal smears serially collected by a standardized technique and stained using the Papanicolaou method, may indicate ovulation. The vagina responds to the increasing pre-ovulatory estrogen level by hyperplasia of the basal epithelium. Prior to ovulation, exfoliated karyopycnotic and eosinophilic cells are characteristic; after ovulation, there is predominance of exfoliated intermediate cells. The detection of this shift in cell type in a vaginal smear is an indicator for ovulation.

d) Premenstrual endometrial biopsy. If ovulation has occurred, an endometrial biopsy sample taken 2–3 days before menstruation shows the typical secretory phase. Non-ovulation is proven by persistance of the proliferative phase of the endometrial pattern (Konicks et al., 1977); however, this painful procedure is not recommended.

e) Preovulatory endocrine profile. By correlating the secretion pattern of progesterone and the endometrial biopsy dating, the time of the cycle can be determined (Newton, 1977). If plasma progesterone levels are not available, its urinary metabolite pregnandiol can be measured; values greater than 5 ng/l usually indicate ovulation (Klopper and Billewicz, 1963).

A single clinical or laboratory test is unsatisfactory, and the combination of several indirect techniques provides a better chance of ovulation detection, but is not conclusive. The only absolute proof of ovulation is the finding of a ruptured Graafian follicle with recovery of the egg. However, ultrasonic examination of ovaries (Hackeloer et al., 1978; Ylostalo et al., 1978) is still on the experimental level, and laparoscopy is no practical procedure for every day investigation (Newton, 1977).

In practice, a combination of the BBT with cervical mucus quality is taken as an indicator for ovulation. As the postovulatory characteristics of cervical mucus are due to the presence of progesterone and usually coincide with a rise in BBT, a combination of these three parameters is considered most reliable for detection of ovulation.

2.4. Investigation concomitant to AID

The majority of candidates do not need a complete sterility survey which is published by the American Society for the Study of Sterility. If the woman has a normal BBT chart indicating ovulation, no history suggestive of tubal or uterine infection, and appears healthy after physical examination, AID can be performed without initiating further testing (Guttmacher, 1960).

About 90% of AID pregnancies occur during the first six inseminating cycles, if careful pre-insemination investigation of the recipient is provided. In case of failure during this period, further investigations have to be performed. Patients over age 30 may especially benefit from these extensive investigations to exclude any treatable factors that might

otherwise delay pregnancy (Sulewski et al., 1978).

1. *Tubal patency tests.* Since the incidence of tubal factors as a cause of infertility is about 20–40% (Moghissi and Sim, 1975), tubal patency is of special interest for AID. However, the necessity of routine patency tests is as controversial as is the question of the most reliable method.

a) Uterotubal insufflation test (Rubin test). Only a few authors perform a carbon dioxide insufflation test to establish tubal patency (Rajan and John, 1978; Friedman, 1977). This test is associated with a high incidence of false-positive and -negative results (Whitelaw et al., 1970). Because of greater familiarity with other diagnostic tests (hysterosalpingography, culdoscopy and laparoscopy), the Rubin test tends to be outmoded (Parsons and Sommers, 1978).

b) Hysterosalpingography (HSG). Hysterosalpingography as part of the AID evaluation program remains controversial. Some 75% of U.S. clinicians obtain HSG routinely before starting AID. Others employ HSG only in case of historical or physical findings suggestive of pelvic pathology, or after several unsuccessful AID cycles (Nash et al., 1979; Chong and Taymor, 1975; Goldenberg and White, 1977; Warner, 1974). Two questions have to be considered when judging HSG prior to AID:

1) What is the prospective incidence of tubal patency disturbance in patients undergoing AID, and what are the results of routine HSG in preliminary AID evaluations so far? and

2) Can HSG be considered as a screening device for tubal patency?

As previously mentioned, the incidence of tubal factors as a cause in infertility is about 30%, referring to the infertile woman, not to candidates for AID with a negative history of PID. There are no conclusive data about the percentage of pathological salpingograms in AID candidates, although many publications name HSG as a routine method of pre-insemination procedures (Goss, 1975; Macourt and Jones, 1977; Sulewski et al., 1978; Pennington and Naik, 1977; Nash et al., 1979; Quinlivan, 1979). There are some severe arguments against using HSG as part of the routine pre-AID evaluation, because it does not fulfill all the demands for a screening procedure such as simple technique, significant results and low risk: i) Rigid adherence to technical details in performing HSG is necessary to make the interpretation meaningful (Sweeney, 1962). Retrospective analysis of HSGs often show a less than optimal technique in the studies categorized as abnormal (Nash et al., 1979), denoting that the procedure is not as easy as usually assumed. ii) The incidence of significantly abnormal HSG is low (Nash et al., 1979), particularly with respect to patency and motility of the tubes. Information of HSG is not precise enough to justify an operative correction without laparoscopy (Parsons and Sommers, 1978). When carefully performed and correctly interpreted, the results of HSG and laparoscopy disagree in about 40% of cases (Gomel, 1977; Maathuis et al., 1972; Swolin and Rosencrantz, 1972; Keirse and Vandervellen, 1973; Moghissi and Sim, 1975). iii) Results of HSG do not necessarily correlate with pregnancy outcome. There is no significant difference in the conception rates between women with normal and slightly pathological HSG who underwent AID (Nash et al., 1979). iv) The procedure of HSG is not without risk. The introduction or exacerbation of PID, uterine perforation, and remarkable radiation exposure have been noted (Warner, 1974; Shirley, 1971).

The following guideline for use of HSG has been recommended (Nash et al., 1979): a) pre-insemination HSG in case of any history suggesting tubal occlusion, and b) post-insemination HSG after six unsuccessful AID cycles. Insemination is undertaken when bilateral tubal patency is evident, or when the uterus is normal and one of the tubes shows normal filling and spilling. If HSG is normal after the first AID cycles, laparoscopy should be postponed for an additional 3 to 6 months of AID (Goldenberg and White, 1977).

2. *Endoscopy*. Endoscopic techniques by culdoscopy or laparoscopy allow direct visualization of the pelvic organ and positive diagnosis of tubal patency, when combined with hydrotubation using a colored dye. Routine laparoscopy is not advisable, as women with impaired fertility have ovulatory difficulties rather than tubal problems which are not visible during pelvic inspection (Read, 1980; Symonds, 1980). Endoscopy is recommended to the patient if:

a) Initial history, physical examination or BBT pattern suggest a possible abnormality such as endometriosis, tubal affection, or disorders of ovulation.

b) HSG studies, after six unsuccessful AID cycles, are without significant results. Laparoscopy can detect unsuspected lesions such as peritubal adhesions and endometriosis causing infertility in about 50% of the cases with so-called "unexplained infertility" in the apparently normal woman (Peterson and Behrman, 1979; Drake et al., 1977). Both lesions may not be detected by HSG and are associated with greatly reduced conception rates.

c) HSG results are abnormal. Even if HSG indicates the existence of a tubal block, corrective surgical procedures should await the results of laparoscopy which provide direct visualization. This particularly applies to blockage at the cornual ends of the tubes. Laparoscopy must be performed as a two-puncture technique with elevation of uterus and adnexes. Corrective therapy of severe pelvic abnormalities may be possible, especially in case of endometriosis, which is a common cause of AID failure. If a surgically correctable factor can be identified and treated, an additional 20% of AID failures may be expected to become pregnant (Collman and Stoller, 1962; Sulewski et al., 1978).

3. *Hysteroscopy*. The diagnostic value of hysteroscopy is still uncertain. Some recommend the technique for direct visualization of the uterine tubal opening (Edstrom and Fernstrom, 1979; Lindeman, 1972; Cohen and Dmowski, 1973). However, hysteroscopy does not show any advantage over HSG in the study of tubal patency and uterine cavity.

4. *Spermatozoa–mucus interaction*. One reason for AID failure may be that the recipient's mucus is hostile to spermatozoa (Quinlivan, 1979). The incidence of sperm agglutinating activity is 5% in women with unknown infertility and 80% in women with no demonstrable organic cause of infertility (Franklin and Dukes, 1964; Dukes and Franklin, 1968). If the post-insemination test is satisfactory (more than 6 spermatozoa per high-power field, progressing in clear mucus within 16 hours after insemination) it is unlikely that there are pathological anti-sperm antibodies in the woman. If the post-insemination test is unsatisfactory, a sperm–cervical mucus test for "cervical hostility" must be performed (Hendry et al., 1978).

An interaction between spermatozoa and cervical

mucus may be evaluated either by: a) in vitro sperm penetration in cervical mucus, carried out as slide or capillary tube test (Miller and Kurzrock, 1932; Kremer, 1965; Jaszczak and Hafez, 1977) or b) spermatozoa cervical mucus contact test or SCMC-test (Kremer and Jager, 1976).

The SCMC test is a simple screening method for detecting anti-sperm-antibodies in the recipient. A strongly positive SCMC test means that sperm agglutinins are present in the blood serum and in the genital secretions of the woman. A negative SCMC test may sometimes be accompanied by sperm agglutinins in the blood serum, but very seldom by sperm agglutinins in the genital secretions (Kremer et al., 1977).

2.5. Rejection of a recipient.

The reasons for rejecting a candidate for AID vary among different centers and involve a mixture of medical and ethical criteria.

1. *Ambivalent attitude towards AID.* Mixed feelings towards the procedure in one or both of the partners may be a reason for rejection because of the dubious legal situation and the future parents–child interaction.

2. *Alcoholism or drug abuse.* Alcoholism and drug abuse of the recipient may interfere with the stability of the marriage and the education of the child; therefore, AID is not advised in this situation.

3. *Medical contraindications.* The only absolute contraindications for AID are diseases that may affect the life of the mother or have any negative influence on the pregnancy outcome such as: a) acute infection of the genital area, b) acute infection with possible fetal loss or malformation (rubella, cytomegalovirus disease etc.), c) hereditary disease, d) severe diseases that may not allow child bearing, such as tuberculosis, severe diabetes mellitus and carcinoma, and e) exposure to therapeutic radiation or cytostatic therapy. Another medical reason for rejection is the diagnosis of bilateral tubal occlusion.

3. CONCLUDING REMARKS

There is a remarkable lack of standardization of criteria for the selection of both, donor and recipient for instrumental insemination (AID). Criteria for donor selection include: personal, physical and genetic history, physical examination, laboratory tests for venereal diseases and hepatitis, and three semen samples. The characteristics of somatotype will facilitate matching the donor with the husband's phenotype. Blood grouping and Rh-typing is necessary to avoid blood incompatibility between the prospective mother and the progeny. Before freeze-storage, semen samples are cultured for gonorrhea and tested for post-thawing fertilizing ability. Only excellent quality semen should be subjected to cryopreservation, with resultant adequate post-thaw characteristics in terms of good progressive motility and high sperm survival rates. The number of pregnancies produced by a single donor should be limited to avoid the possibility of consanguineous matings.

Before adopting an AID program, the couple should undergo a counselling interview to discuss the AID procedure including the associated legal, religious, and psychological problems. The large number of dropouts after a few cycles of AID suggests a need for intensive and continuous psychological support. Since the male and/or female partner may have one or more components of infertility, both should be initially examined. The partner of a potential recipient requires a recent and detailed medical history, complete hormone profile, analysis of at least two semen samples, and a chromosome analysis, if indicated.

The necessity of an in-depth evaluation of the recipient is emphasized, as the finding of a male factor does not rule out the possibility of infertility in the female partner. Reproductive abnormalities are a major cause of unsuccessful AID. Improved pregnancy rate and decrease in the total number of inseminating cycles required are related to thorough investigation of female fertility before AID. The woman's fertility potential should be optimal in terms of spontaneous ovulation, a normal functional and patient genital tract, and an age of less than 35 years. The initial evaluation of the recipient includes history, physical examination and assessment of ovulation. Hysterosalpingography (HSG), or other means to prove tubal patency as part of the pre-insemination evaluation, are controversial. Pre-insemination HSG should be performed only in case of any history suggesting tubal occlusion, as the procedure is not without risk. Since most AID pregnancies occur during the first 6 cycles of insemination, post-insemination testing, immunologic testing for sperm antibodies, and more intensive investigations such as tubal patency tests and endoscopy methods should be limited to those women who fail to conceive within 6 properly-timed AID cycles. Careful pre-insemination assessment provides an average 70–80% pregnancy rate in most AID programs. Some women, however, will fail to conceive despite normal female fertility, and standardized selection of donors.

REFERENCES

Amelar RD (1962) Coagulation, liquefaction and viscosity of human semen. J Urol 87: 187.

Ansari AH (1980) Repeated freeze-thawing for assessment of semen freezability. In Emperaire JC, Audebert A, Hafez ESE, eds. Homologous artificial insemination (AIH). Clinics in Andrology, Vol I, pp 177–186. The Hague: Martinus Nijhoff.

Atherton RW (1977) Evaluation of sperm motility. In Hafez ESE, ed Techniques of human andrology, pp 173–189. Amsterdam Elsevier/North Holland Biomedical Press.

Bartak V (1971) Sperm velocity test in clinical practice. Int J Fertil 16: 107.

Bartlett DE (1978) Microbial contaminants in frozen semen. In: The integrity of frozen spermatozoa, pp 173–180. The National Research Council ed. Washington, DC. National Academy of Sciences.

Beck WW (1976) A critical look at the legal, ethical and technical aspects of artificial insemination. Fertil Steril 27: 1.

Beck WW (1977) Artificial insemination. In Hafez ESE, ed. Techniques of human andrology, Biomedical Press. Amsterdam: Elsevier/North-Holland pp 421–431.

Beck WW, Silverstein J (1975) Variable motility recovery of spermatozoa following freeze preservation. Fertil Steril 26: 863–867.

Blank CE (1960) Apert's syndrome (a type of acroencephalosyndactyly). Observations on a British series of 39 cases. Ann Hum Genet 24:151.

Bromwich P, Kilpatrick M, Newton J (1978) Artificial insemination with frozen stored donor semen. Br J Obstet Gynaecol 85: 641.

Bunge RG (1970) Some observations on the male ejaculate. Fertil Steril 21: 639.

Chong AP, Taymor ML (1975) Sixteen years' experience with therapeutic donor insemination. Fertil Steril 26: 791.

Cohen MR, Dmowski WP (1973) Modern hysteroscopy, diagnostic and therapeutic potential. Fertil Steril 24: 905.

Collman RD, Stoller A (1962) A survey of mongoloid births in Victoria, Australia 1942–1975. Am J Publ Health 52: 813.

Curie-Cohen M, Luttrell L, Shapiro S (1979).Current practice of artificial insemination by donor in the United States. N Engl J Med 300:585.

Davajan V (1977) In vivo postcoital test. In Hafez ESE, ed. Techniques of human andrology, pp 373–379. Amsterdam: Elsevier/North-Holland Biomedical Press.

DeLourois J, Blades M, Harrison RF et al. (1974) Frequency of mycoplasma in fertile and infertile couples. Lancet 1: 1073.

Derrick FC (1977) Bacteriological examination of ejaculate. In Hafez ESE, ed. Techniques of human andrology, pp 311–321. Amsterdam: Elsevier/North-Holland Biomedical Press.

DeTure FA, Drylie DM, Kaufman H, Centifanto Y (1975) Human male reproductive organs harbor herpes simplex virus type 2. Summary of a presentation at the Southeast Section of the American Urological Association, as reported in: Infectious diseases, Vol 1.

Dixon RE, Buttram VC (1976) Artificial insemination using donor semen; a review of 171 cases. Fertil Steril 27: 130.

Drake T, Tredway D, Buchanan G, Takaki N (1977) Unexplained infertility, reappraisal. Obstet Gynec 50: 644.

Dukes CD, Franklin RR (1968) Sperm agglutinins and human infertility: female. Fertil Steril 19: 263.

Edstrom K, Fernstrom I (1979) The diagnostic possibilities of a modified hysteroscopic technique. Acta Obstet Gynec Scand 49: 327.

Edwards RG (1973) Biological aspect of AID. In: Law and ethics of AID and embryo transfer, pp 3–11. Ciba Foundation Symposium 17. Amsterdam: Excerpta Medica, Elsevier/North-Holland.

Eliasson R (1971) Standards for investigation of human semen. Andrologie 3: 49.

Erickson D, Cohen MM (1974) A study of parental effects on the occurrence of fresh maturations for the Apert syndrome. Ann Hum Genet 38: 89.

Feldschuh J (1978) Artificial insemination in clinical practice. In: The integrity of frozen spermatozoa, pp 212–214. The National Research Council, ed. Washington, DC: National Academy of Sciences.

Feldschuh J (1978) Current clinical applications of sperm banking. In: The integrity of frozen spermatozoa, tp 212–219. The National Research Council, ed. Washington, DC: National Academy of Sciences.

Finegold WJ (1964) Artificial insemination. Springfield, Ill: CC Thomas.

Fiumara NJ (1972) Transmission of gonorrhea by artificial insemination. Br J Vener Dis 48: 308.

Franklin RR, Dukes CD (1964) Antispermatozoal antibody and unexplained infertility. Am J Obstet Gynecol 89: 6

Friedman S (1977) Artificial donor insemination with frozen human semen. Fertil Steril 28: 1230.

Godden JO (1973) International symposium on gonorrhea. Can Med Assoc J 109: 1043.

Goldenberg RL, White R (1977) Artificial insemination. J Reprod Med 18: 149.

Gomel V (1977) Laparoscopy prior to reconstructive tubal surgery for infertility. J Reprod Med 18: 251.

Goss DA (1975) Current status of artificial insemination with donor semen. Am J Obstet Gynecol 22: 246.

Guerrero RI (1975) Spontaneous abortion and aging of human ova and spermatozoa. New Eng J Med 293: 573.

Guttmacher AF (1960) The role of artificial insemination in the treatment of sterility. Obstet Gynecol Surv 15: 767.

Hackeloer BJ, Fleming R, Robinson HP, Adam AH, Coutts JRT (1978) Ultrasound assessment of follicular growth. A new technique for observation of ovarian development. Int Symp on the Functional Morphology of the Human Ovary, Glasgow, Scotland.

Hafez ESE (1976) The human semen and fertility regulation in the male. International Conference in Andrology. J Reprod Med 16: 91.

Hansen KB, Nielson NC, Rebbe H (1979) Artificial insemination in Denmark by frozen donor semen supplied from a central bank. Br J Obstet gynecol 86: 284.

Heathecote J, Cameron CH, Dane DS (1974) Hepatitis-B antigen in saliva and semen. Lancet 1: 71.

Hendry WF, Morgan H, Stedronska J, Scammell G, Chamberlain CVP (1978) The clinical significance of antisperm antibodies in male subfertility: crossed hostility testing and prednisolone treatment. In Cohen J, Hendry WF ed. Spermatozoa, antibodies and infertility, pp 129–139. Oxford: Blackwell Scientific Publications.

Herrman J (1966) Der Einfluss des Zeugungsalters auf die Mutationen zu Haemophilie A. Humangenetik 3: 1.

Horne HW, Kundsin RB, Kosasa TS (1974) The role of mycoplasma infection in human reproductive failure. Fertil Steril 25: 380.

Hutton EM, Thompson MW (1970) Parental age and mutation rate in Duchenne muscular dystrophy. Am J Hum Genet 22: 26a.

Insler VH, Melmed I (1972) The cervical score. Int J Gyn Obst 10: 223.

Jaszczak S, Hafez ESE (1977) In vitro sperm penetration in cervical mucus. In Hafez ESE, ed. Techniques of human andrology, pp 379–399. Amsterdam: Elsevier/North-Holland Biomedical Press.

Jennings RT, Dixon RE, Neetles JB (1977) The risks and prevention of Neisseria gonorrhoeae transfer in fresh ejaculate donor insemination. Fertil Steril 28: 554.

Jones G (1975) Luteal phase defects. In Behrman SJ, Kistner RW, eds. Progress in infertility 2 nd edn, pp 299–324. Boston: Little, Brown.

Joyce DN (1979) Artificial insemination by donor. IPPE Medical Bulletin. Vol 13, p 1.

Katshi S, Aguirre A, Katshi G (1968) Inactivation of sperm antigens by sera and tissues of the female reproductive tract. Fertil Steril 19: 740.

Keirse MJ, Vandervellen R (1973) A comparison of hysterosalpingography and laparoscopy in the investigation of infertility. Obstet Gynecol 14: 685.

Kerin J (1980) Determination of the optimal timing of insemination in women. In Richardson DW, Joyce D, Symonds EM, eds. Frozen human semen, pp 105–129. The Hague: Martinus Nijhoff.

Klopper A, Billewics W (1963) Urinary excretion of oestriol and pregnanediol during normal pregnancy. J Obstet Gynaec Brit Cwlth 70: 1024.

Konicks PR, Goddeeris PG, Lauweryns JM, Hertog HC, Brosens IA (1977) Accuracy of endometrial biopsy dating in relation to the midcycle luteinizing hormone peak. Fertil Steril 28: 443.

Kopito LE, Kosasky HJ (1979) The tackiness rheometer determination of the viscoelasticity of cervical mucus. In Hafez ESE, ed. Human ovulation, pp 351–365. Amsterdam: Elsevier/North Holland.

Kremer J (1965) A simple sperm penetration test. Int J Fertil 10: 201.

Kremer J, Jager S (1976) The sperm–cervical mucus contact test. A preliminary report. Fertil Steril 27: 335.

Kremer J, Jager S, Kuiken J (1977) The clinical significance of antibodies to spermatozoa. In: Immunological influence on human fertility, pp 47–66. Proceedings of the workshop in fertility in human reproduction. Department of Biological Science, University of New Castle, Australia. Sydney: Academic Press.

Lang DJ, Kummer JT (1975) Cytomegalovirus in semen; observations in selected populations. J Infect Dis 132: 472.

Lang DJ (1978) Viruses in human semen. In: The integrity of frozen spermatozoa, pp 237–249. The National Research Council, ed. Washington DC: National Academy of Sciences.

Ledward RS, Crich J, Sharp P, Cotton RE, Symonds EM (1976) The establishment of a programme of artificial insemination by donor semen within the national health service. Br J Obstet Gyn 83: 917.

Lindeman H (1972) The use of CO_2 in the uterine cavity for hysteroscopy. Int J Fertil 17: 221.

Lynas MA (1958) Marfan's syndrome in Northern Ireland. An account of 13 families. Ann Hum Genet 22: 289.

Maathuis JB, Horbach JG, Mall HEV van (1972) A comparison of the results of hysterosalpingography and laparoscopy in the diagnosis of Fallopian tube dysfunction. Fertil Steril 23: 428.

Macourt DC, Jones GR (1977) Artificial insemination with donor semen. Med J Aust 1: 693.

Matthews CD, Broom TJ, Crawshaw KM, Hopkins RE, Kerin JF, Svigos JM (1979) The influence of inseminating timing and semen characteristics on the efficiency of a donor insemination program. Fertil Steril 31: 45.

McLaren A (1973) Biological Aspects of AID In: Law and ethics of AID and embryo transfer, pp 3–11. Ciba Foundation Symposium 17 Amsterdam: Elsevier/North-Holland.

Miller EG, Kurzrock R (1932) Biochemical studies of human semen: factors affecting migration of sperm through cervix. Am J Obstet gynecol 24: 19.

Moghissi KS (1976) Accuracy of basal body temperature for ovulation detection. Fertil Steril 27: 1415.

Moghissi KS, Sim GS (1975) Correlation between hysterosalpingography and pelvic endoscopy for the evaluation of tubal factor. Fertil Steril 26: 1178.

Moon KH, Bunge RG (1968) Observations on the biochemistry of human semen. II. Alkalin phosphatase. Fertil Steril 19: 766.

Murdoch JL, Walker AA, Hall JG, Abbey H, Smith KS, McKusick VA (1970) Achondroplasia: a genetic and statistical survey. Ann Hum Genet 35: 227.

Nash D, Haning RV, Shapiro SS (1979) The value of hysterosalpingography prior to donor artificial insemination. Fertil Steril 31: 378.

Newton JR (1977) The investigation of the infertile couple. A critique of the currently available diagnostic tests. In Diczfalusy E, ed. Regulation of human fertility pp 111–135. Proceedings of WHO symposium on advances in fertility regulation, Moscow. Copenhagen: Scriptor.

Nikkanen V, Groenroos M, Suominen J (1979) Silent infection in male accessory genital organs and male infertility. Andrologia 11: 236.

Noguchi PD, Kiss JE, Petricciani JC (1978) Microbial contamination of human semen. In: The integrity of frozen spermatozoa, pp 216–226. The National Research Council, ed. Washington, DC: National Academy of Sciences.

Nolan GH, Osborne N (1973) Gonococcal infections in the female. Obstet Gynecol 42: 156.

Panikabutra K (1973) Clinical aspects of uncomplicated gonorrhoea in the female. Br J Vener Dis 49: 213.

Parkes A (1973) Discussion: biological aspects. In: Law and ethics of AID and embryo transfer, pp 3–11. Ciba Foundation Symposium 17. Amsterdam: Elsevier/North-Holland.

Parsons L, Sommers SC (1978) Gynecology, 2nd edn, Vol I p 412. Philadelphia: WD Saunders.

Patton WC, Taymor ML (1975) An investigation of the relationship between cervical mycoplasma infection, the postcoital test and infertility. Fertil Steril 26: 211.

Pennington GW, Naik S (1977) Donor insemination: report of a two-year study. Br Med J 1: 1327.

Penrose LS, Camb FRS (1955) Parental age and mutation. Lancet II: 312.

Peterson EP, Behrman SJ (1970) Laparoscopy of the infertile patient. Obstet Gynecol 35: 363.

Peterson RN, Freund M (1976) Metabolism of human spermatozoa. In: Hafez ESE, ed. Human semen and fertility regulation in men, pp 176–186. Saint Louis: Mosby CV.

Pollock M (1967) Sex and its problems. VIII Artificial insemination. Practitioner 199: 244.

Portnoy J, Mendelson J, Clecner B, Heisler L (1974) Asymptomatic gonorrhea in the male. Can Med J 110: 169.

Quinlivan WL (1979) Therapeutic donor insemination. Results and causes of nonfertilization. Fertil Steril 32: 157.

Rajan R, John R (1978) Some aspects of artificial insemination using donor semen. J Obstet Gynecol India 28: 1076.

Read MD (1980) The relationship between methods of freezing human semen and successful AID. In Richardson DW, Joyce D, Symonds EM, eds. Frozen human semen, pp 89–103. The Hague: Martinus Nijhoff.

Richardson DW (1980) Factors influencing the fertility of frozen semen. In Richardson DW, Joyce D, Symonds EM, eds. Frozen human semen, pp 35–55. The Hague Martinus Nijhoff.

Roberts G (1964) Some reflections on positive eugenics. Perspect Biol Med 7: 297.

Schoysman R (1975) Problems of selecting donors for artificial insemination. J Med Ethics 1: 34.

Schumacher GFB (1969) Cyclic changes of muramidase in cervical mucus. J Reprod Med 3: 171.

Sherman JK (1978) Banks for frozen human semen. Current status and prospects. In: The integrity of frozen spermatozoa, pp 78–91. The National Research Council, ed. Washington, DC: National Academy of Sciences.

Sherman JK (1978) Proposed stadards for cryobanking of human spermatozoa. Am Assoc Tissue Banks; 1st Am Meeting 136.

Sherman JK, Rosenfeld JJ (1975) Importance of frozen-stored human semen in the spread of gonorrhea. Fertil Steril 26: 1043.

Shirley RL (1971) Ovarian radiation dosage during hysterosalpingography. Fertil Steril 22: 83.

Skerlavay M, Epstein JA, Sobrero AJ (1968) Cervical mucus amylase level in normal menstrual cycles. Fertil Steril 19: 726.

Smith CAB (1972) Note on the estimation of parental age effects. Ann Hum Genet 35: 227.

Sulewski JM, Eisenberg F, Stenger VG (1978) A longitudinal analysis of artificial insemination with donor semen. Fertil Steril 29: 527.

Sweeney WJ (1962) Pitfalls in present day methods of evaluating tubal function. II. Hysterosalpingography. Fertil Steril 13: 124.

Swolin K, Rosencrantz N (1972) Laparoscopy vs hysterosalpingography in sterility investigations; a comparative study. Fertil Steril 23: 270.

Symonds EM (1980) Factors influencing successful AID with frozen semen. In: Richardson DW, Joyce D, Symonds EM, eds. Frozen human semen, pp 133–155. The Hague: Martinus Nijhoff.

Taymor ML (1973) Induction of ovulation with gonadotropins, Clin Obstet Gynecol 16: 201.

Tunte W, Becker PE, Von Knorre G (1967) Zur Genetik der Myositis ossificans progressiva Humangenetik 4: 320.

Tunte W (1972) Human mutations and paternal age. Humangenetik 16: 77.

Warner MP (1974) Artificial insemination. Review after 32 years of experience. MY State J Med 74: 2358.

Weller J (1977) First results and experiences with artificial donor insemination AID in the treatment of sterile and infertile couples. Zentrabl Gynaekol 99: 264.

Whitelaw MJ, Foster T, Graham WH (1970) Hysterosalpingography and insufflation: a 35 year clinical study. J Reprod Med 4: 41.

Witherington R, Black JB, Karow AM (1977) Semen cyropreservation: an update. J Urol 118: 510.

Ylostalo P, Ronnberg L, Jouppila P (1978) Simultaneous monitoring of the growth of the ovarian follicle with ultrasound and oestrogen assays during ovulation induction. 3rd Reinier De Graaf Symp, Maastricht, The Netherlands.

Zaneveld LJ, Polakoski KL (1977) Collection and physical examination of the ejaculate. In Hafez ESE ed. Techniques of human andrology, pp 147–173. Amsterdam: Elsevier/North-Holland Biomedical Press.

Author's address:
Dr U. Hermanns
Städtische Frauenklinik Osnabrück
Osnabrück, FRG

15. A SIMPLE TECHNIQUE FOR RAPID SPERM COUNT AND DATA DOCUMENTATION

F. Maleika, B. Angerer and C. Lauritzen

In clinical routine work, a single hemocytometer count is widely used to determine whether a patient's sperm concentration is normal or pathological. This procedure of diagnosis presents a complete overestimation of the method. There are two major variations when measuring sperm concentrations: 1) Biological variations which mainly depend on time of sexual abstinence (Schirren, 1972) and general health condition; 2) Variations due to the employed technique and the executing technician. Regarding biological variations, a single sperm count results in a confidence interval between 0.5 n and 2.3 n, i.e. For a measured concentration of 10 million spermatozoa/ml, the confidence interval varies between 5 million/ml (oligozoospermia) and 23 million/ml (normozoospermia) (Schwartz, 1974). Considering the analysis itself, a variation of 20% is due to the technique and 25% is due to the technician (Freund and Carol, 1964). The two major sources of technical errors in the hemocytometer technique are inadequate mixing of the fresh sample and the necessary dilution with a spermicidal solution.

The standard dilution is 1:20 (Zaneveld and Polakoski, 1977) but dilutions of 1:50, 1:100 or 1:200 are also employed (Eliasson, 1971). Therefore, errors in mixing and pipetting are subsequently magnified.

A time-consuming factor of the 100 μm thick hemocytometer preparation is the lapse of 1 hour in order to allow spermatozoa to settle motionless in one focal plane. The dilution and handling of the hemocytometer's technique is time-consuming and increases inaccuracy. An advanced 10 μm chamber has been designed (Makler, 1978a, b) and recently improved (Makler, 1980), which makes it possible to count native semen after mixing. With this technique, microphotographs are used in order to avoid immobilization of spermatozoa by heat and to enable the procedure of counting and motility analysis in a single preparation (Makler et al., 1979a, b).

In order to expedite time and efficiency, a Polaroid system has been adapted to provide an instant and permanent visual documentation of sperm count (Maleika et al., 1980). Repeated measurements are thus easy to obtain and analysis of data can be made after any lapse of time. Also, the sperm count can be submitted to a quality control.

1. MICROPHOTOGRAPH TECHNIQUE

1.1. Method

Polaroid microphotographic sperm count was taken using the Makler chamber. Although the present study only deals with sperm count, the same single preparation is also used for motility examination. Therefore, the glass sperm collector, the pipettes and the Makler counting chamber should maintain a temperature of 37° C throughout the entire analysis (Atherton, 1977).

After ejaculation, the graduated glass sperm collector containing the specimen is placed in a waterbath at 37° C in order to allow a suitable time for liquefaction. The entire specimen is then gently mixed for 5 min. A drop of native semen is inserted into the warmed Makler counting chamber. Using an Olympus BH phase contrast microscope with a 100 W halogen light source and an Olympus Polaroid microphotograph camera (Fig. 1), three prints on Polaroid Type 667 Land Film are exposed in 1/250 second under a × 200 magnification. A uniform distribution of spermatozoa indicates adequate mixing. Sperm heads are counted by staining them with red ink to avoid error.

Hafez ESE & Semm K (Eds) Instrumental insemination.

118

1.2. Validation of the method

A total of 50 randomized ejaculates, ranging from 0 to 371 × 10⁶ spermatozoa/ml were evaluated. Three-fold measurements were executed within a coefficient of variation of 6.14%. There is no important variation of CV related to different spermatozoal concentrations. The coefficients of variation from individual counts are distributed in a normal fashion around the middle CV. These results confirm the accuracy of Makler's counting chamber.

2. EVALUATION

Polaroid microphotographs of the Makler counting chamber simply the procedure for daily routine work. In comparison to the hemocytometer meth-

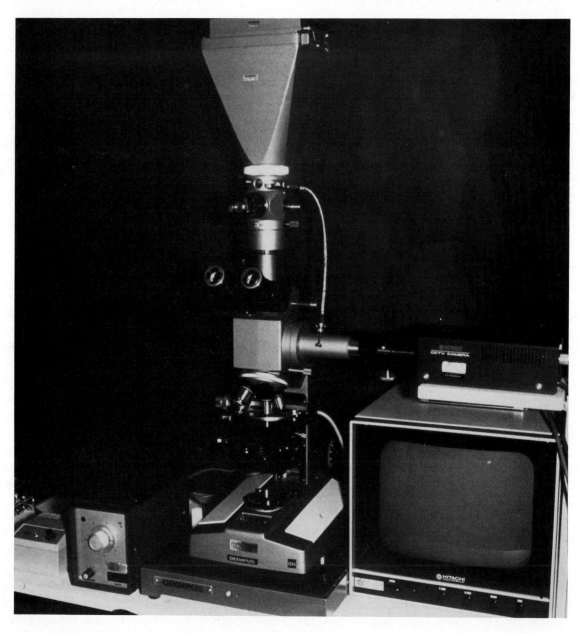

Figure 1. The Polaroid microphotographic system for instant sperm count and visual documentation: a phase contrast microscope topped by a Polaroid camera. The microscope is fitted with an incorporated warming stage and a separate one on the left side for motility analysis.

od, it results in increased accuracy. The simple handling should encourage its use by private gynecologists performing inseminations. Split ejaculate inseminations can be rapidly quantified.

For specialized laboratories the Polaroid microphotograph sperm count will provide, at a low price, a permanent documentation and enable them to proceed to a quality control.

Because of the biological variations and the possible technical errors it is unwise to pronounce a diagnosis based on only a single sperm count. In normal amounts two specimens are evaluated with an interval of around 8 weeks. When low spermatozoal concentrations are found a minimum of three specimens should be analyzed before a pathological diagnosis can be pronounced. When optimal mixing is established, three-fold counts of one pipetting from a native specimen should be sufficient. When the hemocytometer technique is used, two pipettings from one diluted sample are necessary to prove the accuracy of the dilution.

The entire analyses should be repeated if the coefficient of variation out of three counts passes beyond 10%. Therefore, it is unnecessary to discuss whether preparations containing agglutinated spermatozoa should be remade. If agglutinations are scrutinized, it is better not to mix at all, since the mixing procedure disrupts agglutinations (Dahlberg, 1978). The hemocytometer method becomes even more inaccurate in severe oligozoospermia (below 5 million spermatozoa/ml) and sperm dilutions should be completely avoided (Zaneveld and Polakoski, 1977). For the Makler chamber, sixfold measurements should be executed in counts below 20 million/ml, because the coefficient of variation has depassed 10% in the related study. The polyzoospermic specimen count does not present any problem because they can always be counted in their own undiluted medium. Using the Makler chamber, difficulties can be encountered in identification of leukocytes, because only a 200-fold magnification can be used (Eliasson and Maleika, 1980).

Motility analysis has to be performed at 37° C. The pattern of movement as well as the speed of spermatozoa are impaired at 20° C (Jondet, 1976). Polaroid multiexposures were adopted to the Makler method for precise and instant motility analysis and the first promising results were obtained. Avoiding time-consuming development of negatives and possible errors of coordination, a Polaroid procedure should achieve widespread use for objective motility analyses in private offices. The major difficulty arises from the enormous intensity of light needed for stroboscopic multiexposures on Polaroid films, the camera back being very distant from the objective and the Makler chamber appearing to be too light absorbing for this purpose. The quality of prints are therefore still unsatisfactory. Only very powerful electronic stroboscopic flashes should be used. Mechanical stroboscopes are not suitable for Polaroid but are good for negative films.

REFERENCES

Atherton RW (1977) Evaluation of sperm motility. In Hafez ESE ed. Techniques of human andrology, p 173–187. Elsevier/North-Holland Biomedical Press.

Dahlberg B (1978) Infection of the male reproductive tract. Prog. Reprod Biol vol 3, pp 46–59. Basel: Karger.

Eliasson R (1971) Standards for investigation of human semen. Andrologie 3: 49.

Eliasson R, Maleika F Discussion at Xth World Congress on Fertility and Sterility, Madrid, 5–11 July 1980.

Freund M, Carol B (1964) Factors affecting hemocytometer counts of sperm concentration in human semen. J Reprod Fertil 8: 149.

Jondet M (1976) Congelation du sperme. Bull Acad Vet France 49: 373.

Makler A (1978a) A new chamber for rapid sperm count and motility estimation. Fertil Steril 30: 313.

Makler A (1978b) A new multiple exposure photography method for objective human spermatozoal motility determination. Fertil Steril 30: 192.

Makler A, Zaidise I, Paldi E, Brandes JM (1979a) Factors affecting sperm motility. I. In vitro change in motility with time after ejaculation. Fertil Steril 31: 147.

Makler A, Itskovitz J, Brandes JM, Paldi E (1979b) Sperm velocity and percentage of motility in 100 normospermic specimens analyzed by the multiple exposure photography MEP method. Fertil Steril 31: 155.

Makler A (1980) The improved ten-micrometer chamber for rapid sperm count and motility evaluation. Fertil Steril 33: 337.

Maleika F, Schäffer E, Lauritzen Ch (1980) A simple technique for objective measurement and evaluation of sperm motility and concentration (abstract) Arch Androl 5: 6. Paper presented at World Conference for instrumental insemination, in vitro fertilization and embryo transfer. Kiel, West Germany, 24–27 September 1980.

Schirren C (1972) Practical andrology. Berlin: Hartmann.

120

Schwartz D (1974) Spermiogramme et fertilité du couple. Contraception Fertilité Sexualité 6: 767.

Zaneveld LJD, Polakoski KL (1977) Collection and physical examination of the ejaculate. In Hafez ESE ed. Techniques of human andrology, pp 147–172. Elsevier/North-Holland Biomedical Press.

Author's address:
Dr B Maleika
Department of Obstetrics and Gynecology
University of Ulm
Prittwitzstrasse 43
7900 Ulm/Donau, FRG.

16. PREOVULATION: VARIABILITY, PREDICTION AND FERTILITY POTENTIAL

C.D. Matthews, T.J. Broom, J.F. Kerin and L.W. Cox

1. DETECTION OF HUMAN PREOVULATION

1.1. Physical signs and symptoms

The time of ovulation may be associated with such subjective physical symptoms as mid-cycle abdominal pain, increased awareness of cervical mucus and minor vaginal blood loss.

Mid-cycle pain has been traditionally considered to be due to the rupture of the follicular contents into the peritoneal cavity. Recently (O'Herlihy et al., 1980; Kerin et al., 1981), it has been recognized that the majority of women who complain of pain, have thin-walled, unruptured follicles at laparoscopy. In addition, such preovular follicles are distorted by distended bladder associated with ultrasound examination. This has suggested that 'tension' inside the follicle is not the cause of the pain and a role for prostaglandin F2α has been postulated (O'Herlihy et al., 1980). Many women can be taught to appreciate the ovarian discomfort associated with the preovular follicle and can successfully localize the side of imminent ovulation. This simple clinical finding may have more usefulness than has been previously ascribed.

The physical changes which occur in preovular cervical mucus have been well reviewed (Hafez, 1980), are easily recognizable and quantified. A cervical score (Insler et al., 1972) generally correlates well between different observers and maximal cervical scores are associated with Day −1 and Day 0 (Day 0 being the day of peak serum luteinizing hormonal values) (Kerin et al., 1976).

Cervical scores in the same individual can vary from cycle to cycle, presumably due to changes in follicular maturation and steroid production. In addition, poor scores may be associated with clomiphene therapy. Clomiphene appears to optimize cervical function when prescribed for conditions where pre-existing follicular development has been poor (mostly anovular conditions), but is consistently associated with poorer cervical responses when prescribed at high dosage in consecutive but apparently ovular cycles. Several explanations may be possible, including a direct effect on the cervical receptor of the biologically weak oestrogenic action of clomiphene, or perhaps the small rises (0.5–1 ng/ml) of serum progesterone seen frequently in the follicular phases of about 50% of clomiphene-treated cycles (Matthews et al., 1981b).

Many women are able to recognize changes in cervical function and thereby roughly predict the time of ovulation. The self-recognition of changes in cervical function is currently the best simple method of recognizing the preovular time.

Finally, it is important to realize that poor cervical function may be associated with conceptional cycles. About 9% of conceptions on AID. programs are associated with a less than 50% optimal cervical score, even when all periovular days have been assessed (Matthews, 1980).

1.2. Basal body temperature (BBT)

The recognition and documentation of changes in BBT has provided more objectivity in localizing preovulation and the combination of symptothermal methods (Billings, 1972) is now being used extensively for natural family planning. The nadir of BBT possibly relates to the oestrogen zenith prior to ovulation, and the elevation of body temperature to the secretion of thermogenic progestagens from the early corpus luteum.

The recording of BBT changes during the cycle, whilst inexpensive and easily performed, documents only a single point every 24 hours and it is not surprising to find when either the nadir of BBT or the initial significant upward shift is related to the

Hafez ESE & Semm K (Eds) Instrumental insemination.

endocrinological events, that there is a scatter of days around Day 0 (Matthews, 1981a). The accuracy of basal temperature recordings to localize ovulation has also been questioned by Lenton et al. (1977).

1.3. Endocrinological markers of preovulation

With the increasing demand for the precise localisation of human ovulation for AID, more sophisticated endocrinological and physical methods have been tried.

1.3.1. Preovular estrogens. The dominant follicle is responsible for the major portion of the preovular estrogen surge seen in the plasma (Baird, 1974). Though estradiol, estrone and estriol are secreted by the maturing follicle, the ratio of estradiol to estrone increases progressively towards ovulation (Guerrero et al., 1976), and the measurement of estradiol is a good indicator of follicular development and maturity (Thornycroft et al., 1974). Estrogen production peaks 64 to 22 hours (mean 34 hours) prior to ovulation (see Descomps et al., 1980, for review) and though considerable fluctuation is apparent when plasma oestradiol is measured prior to ovulation (Guerrero et al., 1976; Broom et al., 1979), the estrogen rise precedes, the LH rise when adequate sampling has been undertaken. Once-daily sampling may provide an unclear picture. When the data from daily plasma sampling was analyzed, Broom et al. (1979), found that the maximum mean estradiol levels occurred in plasma on Day -1 in 19 (67%) of 28 cycles analyzed. In the remaining cycles, estradiol appears to peak coincident with maximal LH values. In addition, more than a single peak of estradiol appeared to occur prior to ovulation in 12 of the 28 cycles. Neither was the fall of plasma estradiol prior to the LH peak precise enough to use to recognize preovulation; only 18 (64.3%) showed a 25% estradiol fall at ovulation.

Thus plasma LH monitoring is a superior method of determining preovulation in the human than the measurement of estradiol. More frequent sampling may provide a more distinct and predictable picture; indeed, the greater the frequency of sampling and measurement of any chosen parameter, the greater the reliability and usefulness which can

be placed on the results. Rapid radioimmunoassay (RIA) techniques for plasma estrogen, using specific or near specific antibodies, are perfectly feasible, but blood sampling does impose practical clinical limitations and inconvenience.

Estrogens in the blood are excreted by the kidney as glucuronides and the measurement of the native steroids, estrone, estradiol and estriol, requires preliminary hydrolysis and extraction. The pattern of estrogen conjugates in urine is marked by a low constant output during the early follicular phase, which rises to a maximum between Day -2 and Day 0.

Whilst intra-subject variation of urinary glucuronides may be wide, the proportion of individual glucuronides to the total conjugates appears to be steady for any particular individual. The major estrogen metabolites in urine include estriol 3 glucuronide (E3-3-g), estrone 3 glucuronide (E1-3-g), estriol 16α glucuronide (E3-16α-g), estradiol 3 glucuronide (E2-3-g), and estradiol 17β glucuronide (E2-17β-g). Almost certainly, other estrogen metabolites remain to be identified in urine. The direct measurement of estrogen conjugates by RIA has been achieved, and the usefulness of the findings explored to determine the optimal metabolite to detect preovulation in the human. Using a significant rise in excretion of the metabolite (a measured value exceeding calculated baseline values by two standard deviations), Baker et al. (1980) demonstrated that the greatest increase occurred with estradiol 17β glucuronide (3.4 $\pm$ 0.8 times); unfortunately, the low absolute levels of this metabolite made it unsuitable for routine study.

More satisfactory for the recognition of preovulation was the measurement of estrone 3 glucuronide (2.8 $\pm$ 1.1 times). The results obtained are similar to those calculated by Adlercreutz et al. (1980) who used similar methodology but employed different mathematical criteria (either a cusum method, using the day of 3rd consecutive increase as a marker for impending ovulation, or the 50% increase over basal values). These workers also included the measurement of urinary estradiol and estrone, and confirmed these steroids to be excellent preovulatory markers, in addition to the estrone 3 glucuronide metabolite.

The excretion of the metabolite of progesterone 5β pregnanediol 3α glucuronide in urine, has also been shown to be a valuable adjunct to the determination of preovulation. Employing precise measurements of both estrone 3 glucuronide and pregnanediol 3α glucuronide throughout the cycle, Baker et al. (1980), were able to demonstrate a significant increase in the ratio detected 120–48 hours prior to maximum LH values. A major advantage of the use of this ratio was that it was independent of the concentration and rate of excretion of the metabolites, and could be applied to non-24 hour urinary collections.

The direct measurements of estrogen and progesterone metabolites in urine by RIA would seem, therefore, to herald the next generation of determinants of preovulation, at least for populations with access to sophisticated laboratory technology. The adaptation of such methods to simpler subject-orientated markers is yet a further possible step forward for the future.

1.3.2. L.H. The most striking endocrinological change prior to ovulation is the plasma surge of LH. The detail of the physiological effects of LH on the maturing follicle and egg are still somewhat uncertain, but are clearly linked with the change in steroid profile from the maturing follicle to the early corpus luteum, and are coincident with maturing changes in the egg itself. The temporal relationship between the LH surge and ovulation has been explored (cf. Descomps et al., 1980, for review). There is a 24 hour lag period prior to ovulation, from the start of the LH surge to egg release, and about a 9 hour period between maximum plasma LH levels and ovulation. Although there appears to be precision in the temporal relationship between the action of LH and ovulation, many aspects need further exploration, including the variation in timing between subjects, the pulsatile nature of LH, and the fact that the process of ovulation itself appears to be spread over a period of time.

The use of a marker so close to egg release places considerable demands even on a sophisticated laboratory. Normally, plasma LH assays require 3 to 4 days to obtain the level of sensitivity normally demanded clinically; however, given the considerable difference between basal levels and peak LH values, most LH assays can be modified to recognize Day 0, given some sacrifice of accuracy of the lower basal values. Several methods (Vekemans and Robyn, 1971; Schmidt-Gollweitzer et al., 1977; Matthews et al., 1979) have been advocated for the rapid detection of plasma LH. Both radioimmuno- and radioreceptor procedures have been described, the latter offering the greatest theoretical potential, but having had the more limited development to date. The modification of routine RIAs of LH by reducing the incubation time (by use of higher temperatures), and employing rapid separation and counting techniques, allow a practical procedure and results to be available within 4–8 hours. The recognition of Day 0 when rapid and conventional assay technology is compared can be 100% (Broom et al., 1979).

A question not yet clarified accurately is whether a delay exists between the level of LH in the plasma and its excretion into urine. Using a 12-hourly collection system, Roget et al. (1980) found the only positive correlation to be between the plasma levels 36 hours prior to the end of urine collection. Our own studies, Kerin et al. (1981), and those of others (Lopata et al., 1980; Trounsen, 1980), suggest little delay. It remains an interesting question whether the signal to ovulation is the rise from baseline levels, the timing of the maximum secretion of LH, or perhaps the exposure of the follicle to a quantum of LH.

The other possibilities for LH secretion to be used for the detection of preovulation, not as yet well explored, may be the combination of LH and other preovular markers. LH and estradiol have been postulated (Roget et al., 1980) to be useful. These authors showed that if LH and estradiol are both elevated, ovulation is close, and even closer if LH remains elevated in the presence of a falling level of plasma estradiol. Unexplored to date is the LH/progesterone relationship, which may provide an even more critical measurement of the time of pre-ovulation.

1.3.3. 17-Hydroxyprogesterone and progesterone. The rise of serum 17-hydroxyprogesterone and progesterone, is reported as one of the earliest results of the luteinizing action of LH on the follicle. A mid-cycle rise in these two steroids, coincident with the LH peak (Ross et al., 1970; Thornycroft et al., 1971), and before the LH peak (Aedo et al., 1976), has been demonstrated. Thornycroft et al. (1974) also showed that some variability existed in the rise of these steroids during individual cycles. Whilst specific antisera are available to allow the direct RIA measurement of these steroids, the quality of the methodology is demanding because of the low absolute levels of these steroids at mid-cycle. A minimal detection limit of 0.25–0.5 ng per ml is needed to detect the earlier stages of progesterone rise from follicular levels. Our own data (Matthews et al., 1981b), derived from the daily sampling of 115 ovulatory cycles, indicate that the rise from baseline of progesterone (or 17-hydroxyprogesterone) occurred at Day 0, and median values increase on Days +1 and +2. The 95% confidence limits of the data, however, can overlap each day. The stability of secretion of the steroid hormones is one major advantage when compared with the measurements of protein hormones in the serum.

The urinary metabolic product of progesterone, namely 5β pregnanediol 3α glucuronide, has already been referred to as being, perhaps, the most useful marker of preovulation when used in the form of a ratio with estrone 3 glucuronide.

1.4. Ultrasound

The application of ultrasonic techniques to determine follicular growth and ovulation, has already made a major contribution to the understanding of ovarian physiology. The increased sophistication of modern ultrasound scanners has confirmed the early experience from Germany (Hackeloer et al., 1978) which detailed the earliest information of the ovulatory process. Several studies (Queenan et al., 1980; Kerin et al., 1981) are now in general agreement that there is a rise in diameter of the dominant follicle destined to ovulate, from 9.8 mm ± 1.9 at Day -5, to 21.1 mm ± 3.5 at Day 0. The wide range in the diameter of the preovular follicle precludes its use alone as an index of ovulation. Clear, too, is the spectrum of findings of follicular growth, regression, and re-emergence possible, together with their variable temporal relationship with the menstrual cycle. Several ultrasonic appearances appear to be consistent with ovulation, and at least four types of ultrasonic appearance of corpus lutea can be distinguished (Queenan et al., 1980). Ovulation, as judged by the ultrasonic approach, appears to occur between 12 and 37 hours after the first significant increase in the concentration of urinary LH. Ultrasound techniques demand considerable skill and application, and are not free from technical errors and misinterpretation. A further problem not resolvable by ultrasound is the detection of luteinized, yet apparently non-ovular follicles (Edwards and Steptoe, 1975). In spite of some limitations, ultrasound has become an important noninvasive technique which has added considerable precision to other parameters of determing preovulation.

2. APPLICATION OF TECHNIQUES OF DETERMINING PREOVULATION

Whilst it is clear that current in vitro fertilization programs using natural cycles demand the sophisticated techniques of LH and ultrasonic monitoring, the application of such methods to programs of AID (Matthews et al., 1980), and intercourse timing (Edmonds et al., 1979), have not demonstrated major benefits when compared with the simpler methods. The general efficiency of AID does not appear to hinge on the very accurate localization of ovulation, although it is clear that the highest conception rates occur when insemination is performed at Day 0 or Day -1 (Matthews et al., 1979; Propping et al., 1980).

3. VARIATION OF THE NORMAL MENSTRUAL CYCLE

When apparently normal ovular menstrual cycles are monitored, one striking finding is the variation in the time of the LH peak and ovulation, even for cycles of an overall standard length. Using a spectrum of 293 ovulatory cycles of varying length (23 to 34 days), McIntosh et al. (1980) have calculated 95% confidence limits on the expected day of the LH peak. Even for subjects with a mean 28 $\pm$ 0.5 standard deviation cycle, the occurrence of the LH surge can extend from Day 12 to Day 16 of the 28 day cycle.

The endocrinological factors underlying cycles of varying lengths and the subsequent fertility potential of such cycles has been explored by Broom et al. (1981). When the follicular phases of 51 cycles were divided into short (less than 12 days), normal

(12–16 days), and long (greater than 16 days), and mid-cycle steroids and LH analyzed, no significant differences were observed between the groups when the quantitative aspects of the LH surge or the plasma progesterone levels associated with the early corpus luteum were considered. Plasma androstenedione and oestradiol levels were found to be significantly lower in the short cycles when compared with cycles with normal or long length follicular phases, thereby supporting a role for both these steroids in LH modulation. When the prior 265 cycles of 92 consecutive patients who had conceived with AID were analyzed, statistical analysis failed to reveal significant differences in fertility potential of cycles with follicular phases varying from 9 to 25 days.

REFERENCES

Adlercreutz H, Lehtinen T, Kairento AL (1980) Prediction of ovulation by urinary estrogen assays. J Steroid Biochem 12: 395.

Aedio AR, Nuez M, Landgren BM, Cekan Z, Diczfalusy E (1977) Studies on the pattern of circulating steroids in the normal menstrual cycle. Acta Endocr 84: 320.

Baird DT, Fraser IS (1974) Blood production and ovarian secretion rates of estradiol-17β and estrone in women through the menstrual cycle. J Clin Endocr Metab 38: 1009.

Baker TS, Jennison K, Kellie AE (1980) A possible method for the detection of ovulation and the determination of the duration of the fertile period. J Steroid Biochem 12: 411.

Billings EL, Billings JJ, Brown JB (1972) Symptoms and hormonal changes accompanying ovulation. Lancet 1: 282.

Broom TJ, Matthews CD, Cooke ID, Ralph MM, Seamark RF, Cox LW (1981) Endocrine profiles and fertility status of human menstrual cycles of varying length. Submitted for publication Fertil Steril.

Broom TJ, Matthews CD, Crawshaw KM (1979) A comparison of plasma oestradiol and luteinising hormone as endocrinological markers of preovulation. Infertility 2: 29.

Descomps B, Nicolas JC, Chikhaoui Y, Crastes Y, De Paulet A (1980) Prediction and detection of ovulation by hormonal measurements: contribution of a new enzymic method. J Steroid Biochem 12: 385.

Edmonds DK, Matthews CD, Crocker J, Broom TJ, Morris DG (1979) Accurate coital timing. Failure to obtain useful results in normal infertile couples. Infertility 2: 201.

Edwards RG, Steptoe PC (1975) Induction of follicular growth, ovulation and luteinization in the human overy. J Reprod Fert Suppl 82: 121.

Guerrero RT, Aso T, Brenner PF, Cekan Z, Landgren BM, Hagenfeld K, Diczfaluzy (1976) Studies on the pattern of circulating steroids in the normal menstrual cycle. Acta Endocr Copenh 81: 133.

Hackeloer BJ, Robinson HP (1978) Ultraschalldarstellung des wacksedon Follikels und Corpus Luteum in normalen physiologischen. Geburtshilfe Frauenheilkd 30: 163.

Hafez ESE (1980) Prediction and detection of ovualtion: physiological and clinical parameters. In Emperaire JC, Audebert A, Hafez ESE, eds. Homologous artificial insemination (AIH). Clinics in andrology, vol 1, pp 38–54.

Insler V, Melmed H, Eichenbrenner I, Serr D, Lunenfeld B (1972) The cervical score. Int J Gynaec Obstet 10: 223.

Kerin JF, Edmons DK, Warnes GM, Cox LW, Seamark RF, Matthews CD, Young GB, Baird DT (1981) Morphological and functional relationships of Graafian follicle growth in ovulating women using ultrasonic, laparoscopic and biochemical measurements. Br Commonwealth J Obstet Gynaec (in press).

Kerin JF, Matthews CD, Svigos JM, Makin AE, Symons RG, Smeaton TC (1976) Linear and quantitative migration of stored semen through cervical mucus during the periovular period. Fertil Steril 27: 1054.

Lenton EA, Weston GA, Cooke ID (1977) Problems in using basal body temperature recordings in an infertility clinic. Br Med J 1: 803.

Lopata A, Johnston IWH, Hoult IJ, Speirs AI (1980) Pregnancy following intrauterine implantation of an embryo obtained by in vitro fertilisation of a preovular egg. Fertil Steril 33: 117.

Matthews CD (1980) The technique and outcome of AID. In Wood C, Leeton J, Kovacs G, eds. Artificial insemination by donor (1980). Melbourne: Brown Prior Anderson.

Matthews CD, Broom TJ, Black T, Tansing J (1981a) Optimal features of basal body temperature. Recordings associated with conceptional cycles. Int J Fertil. (in press).

Matthews CD, Broom TJ, Crawshaw KM, Hopkins RE, Kerin JFP, Svigos JM (1979) The influence of insemination timing and semen characteristics on the efficiency of a donor insemination programme. Fertil Steril 31: 45.

Matthews CD, Broom TJ, Ralph MM, Kerin JFP (1981b) Unpublished observations.

McIntosh JEA, Matthews CD, Crocker JM, Broom TJ, Cox LW (1980) Predicting the luteinising hormone surge: relationship between the duration of the follicular and luteal phases and the length of the human menstrual cycle. Fertil Steril 34: 125.

O'Herlihy C, Robinson HP, DeCrespigny LJ (1980) Mittleschmerz is a preovular symptom. BMJ 5 April. 280 986.

Propping D, Katzorke T, Tauber PF, Ludwig H (1980) Value of BBT chart in choice of insemination day. Arch Androl 5: 17.

Queenan JT, O'Brien GD, Bains LM, Simpson J, Collins WP, Campbell S (1980) Ultrasound scanning of ovaries to detect ovulation in women. Fertil Steril 34: 99–000.

Roget M, Grenier J, Houlbert C, Castanier M, Feinstein MC, Scholler R (1980) Rapid radioimmunoassays of plasma LH and estradiol-17β for the prediction of ovulation. J Steroid Biochem 12: 403–000.

Ross GT, Cargille CM, Lipsett MB, Rayford PL, Marshall JR, Strott CA, Rodbard D (1970) Pituitary and gonadal hormones in women during spontaneous and induced ovulatory cycles. Recent Prog Horm Res 26: 1.

Schmidt-Gollwitzer K, Schmidt-Gollwitzer M, Sackman U, Eiletz J (1977) Ovulation timing by a radioreceptor assay for human luteinizing hormone. Int J Fertil 22: 232.

Thorneycroft IH, Mishell DR, Stone SC, Kharma KM, Nakamura RM (1971) The relation of serum 17-hydroxy-progesterone and estradiol-17β levels during the human menstrual cycle. Am J Obstet Gynaec 111: 947.

Thorneycroft IH, Sribyatta B, Tom WK, Nakamura RM, Mishell DR (1974) Measurement of serum LH, FSH, proges-

126

terone, 17-hydroxyprogesterone and estradiol-17β levels at 4
hour intervals during the pre-ovulatory phase of the menstrual
cycle. J Clin Endocr Metab 39: 754.

Trounsen A (1980) Personal communication.

Vekemans M, Robyn C (1971) A four hour radioimmunoassay
for human luteinizing hormone (h^{LH}) in plasma using double
antibody technique. Acta Endocr Kbh Suppl 155–158.

Author's address:
Dr C.D. Matthews
Department of Obstetrics and Gynaecology
The University of Adelaide
The Queen Elizabeth Hospital
Woodville, South Australia, 5011

17. PREDICTION AND DETECTION OF OVULATION FOR INSEMINATION: CORRELATION OF ULTRASONIC, CLINICAL AND ENDOCRINOLOGIC RESULTS

P. SAINT-POL, P. GOEUSSE, J.P. GASNAULT, A. POTIER and M. DELECOUR

Ovulation is estimated by currently accepted methods using both cervical mucus changes and basal body temperature for women who receive artificial insemination either by husband (AIH) or by donor (AID). This clinical management benefits from the knowledge of exact stage of follicular growth. An exciting new development is the application of diagnostic ultrasound to the monitoring of follicular development on spontaneous cycles (Hackeloer et al., 1979; Hall et al., 1979) and during induction of ovulation (Hackeloer et al., 1979; Ylostalo et al., 1979). This non-invasive technique causes no potential harm to an early conceptus and, results are immediate. This chapter compares ultrasonic, clinical and endocrinologic evaluation of follicular growth in women receiving artificial insemination.

1. ULTRASONIC SCANNING OF THE OVARY

Using the full bladder technique (Hackeloer et al., 1977, 1978), serial longitudinal and transverse scanning of the pelvis are performed. The follicle is recognized as a small cystic structure surrounded by tissue (ovarian) of relatively low amplitude echo and is surrounded by the more dense echoes of posterior and lateral pelvis walls and the inferior surface of the bladder (Fig. 1). The maximum diameters of the follicle may be measured in both longitudinal and transverse planes. The average of these measurements are used for the purpose of this analysis. Measurements are not normally made until the follicle is over 10 mm in diameter since smaller structures could be confused with artefact echo-free areas. The ALOKA scanner B (type 60 c) with a gray scale (type ERG 2 AHS) ultrasonic apparatus is used together with a 3 MHz-transducer. Follicles are found in only one ovary in any

given cycles and with few exceptions only a single follicle is identified.

2. HORMONAL ASSAYS

FSH, LH, estradiol and progesterone are measured by specific, precise and sensitive radioimmunoassays (EAC kits). Blood samples are obtained by

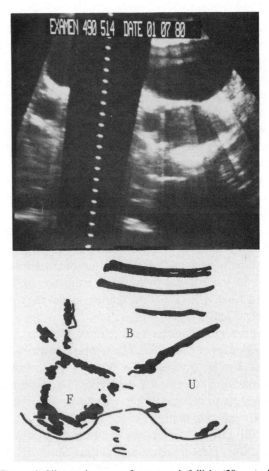

Figure 1. Ultrasonic scan of a normal follicle (20 mm). B: bladder, F: follicle, U: uterus.

Hafez ESE & Semm K (Eds) Instrumental insemination.

128

puncturing the antecubital vein. The plasma is separated and stored at $-20°$ C until assay is made.

3. BASAL BODY TEMPERATURE (BBT)

Women are instructed to record oral, vaginal or rectal temperature with a basal thermometer every morning upon awakening prior to getting out of bed or any physical activity. The temperature record shows a typical biphasic pattern during ovulatory cycles; the "presumed day of ovulation" is defined as being the lowest point prior to a sustained rise of $0.2°$ C. The BBT record does not predict the day of ovulation but rather provides evidence of ovulation after it has occurred (Moghissi et al., 1972).

4. PHYSICAL PROPERTIES OF CERVICAL MUCUS

Secretion of cervical mucus is regulated by ovarian hormones. Estrogen stimulates the production of large amounts of thin, watery alkaline acellular cervical mucus with intense ferning spinnbarkeit and sperm receptivity. Progesterone inhibits the secretory activity of cervical epithelium and produces scanty, viscous, cellular mucus with low spinnbarkeit and absence of ferning which is impenetrable by spermatozoa.

Insler et al. (1972) have devised a cervical score to monitor ovulation time. In this system, the quantity, spinnbarkeit and ferning capacity of cervical mucus and the appearance of the external os are clinically assessed. A 4 point score (0 to 3) is given to all parameters with the exception of the appearance of the external os which is estimated by a 3 point score. The sum of the score provides the total cervical score.

Patients: 30 patients were selected after six well timed cycles of I.A. without conception, in an effort to determine the usefulness of a daily ultrasonic examination during a five day periovulatory period according to previous BBT. On retrospective analysis, the population was divided into two groups: Group 1 comprises 15 normal cycles with ultrasonic measurements and plasma hormone estimations correlated with clinical data before, dur-

ing and after the midcycle. Group 2 comprises 15 cycles which were determined "abnormal" when they were explored either at or after the LH peak.

5. OVULATORY CYCLES

Five out of 15 patients had a clomiphene induction treatment during the protocol. Nine more cycles were monitorized by clinical and ultrasonic evaluations without hormonal assays.

5.1. *Ultrasonic measurements*

The follicular diameter measurements are summarized in Fig. 2 and Table 1 (N = 24 cycles). Days prior to follicle shrinking are denoted negative; range, means and S.D. are indicated for each day in the induction treatment group (N = 7) and in the spontaneously ovulatory group (N = 14). The average values with and without treatment may be compared by a Mann and Whitney "non-parametrical test". F.D. at J-3 is statistically higher (U = 2) in the induction therapy group. By using all sucessful measurements, the linear regression was calculated between follicular diameter and estradiol

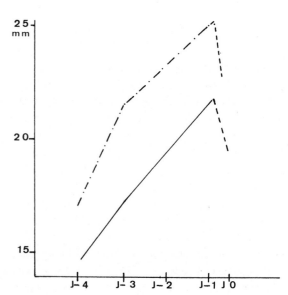

Figure 2. Ultrasonic measurements. Mean follicular diameters relative to the days before follicle shrinking (Day 0) in the induction treatment group (interrupted line) and in 14 spontaneous ovulatory cycles (solid line).

Table 1. Ultrasonic measurements.

	Range	Mean ± S.D.
Without treatment	13–19	15 ± 2.5
	16–20	18 ± 1.7
	15–24	20 ± 2.5
	19–30	22 ± 3.3
With induction	14–19	17 ± 2.9
	20-23	22 ± 1.1
	20–31	23 ± 5.2
	20–30	25 ± 4.8

serum values using a Spearman test, r:0.6953. At least 95% of the circulating estradiol emanates from the growing follicle (Baird and Fraser, 1974). The positive correlation coefficient between peripheral plasma estradiol estimation and ultrasonic follicular diameter measurements on paired data 0.6953 is very closed to the 0.711 correlation coefficient.

5.2. Hormonal findings

The midcycle FSH peak is always measured at the same time as the LH peak. The LH peak value which is more than twice the value the day before and day after, is preceded either by estradiol peak value 11 times (73%), or both LH and estradiol are evaluated at the same time (27%). Progesterone increases as follows: 33% the day after, 60% two days after and 7% three days after. The results for FSH, LH, estradiol and progesterone plasma levels from group 1 cycles are shown in Fig. 3. Days are designated relatively to the day of the LH peak. Days prior to the peak are designated negative while those after are denoted positive. The Mann and Whitney "non-parametrical test" allows comparison between average values of the assays with and without induction therapy. LH at J-1 is statistically higher in the induction group (U = 7)

The shrinking of the follicle is observed when the LH peak value is evaluated in 20% cases on the same day, 67% cases the day after, 13% cases two days after. Progesterone level as high as 3 ng/ml is evaluated the day of the shrinking of the follicle in 33% cases, the next day in 47% cases and two days after in 20% cases.

5.3. Clinical observations

The best cervical score is always obtained on the

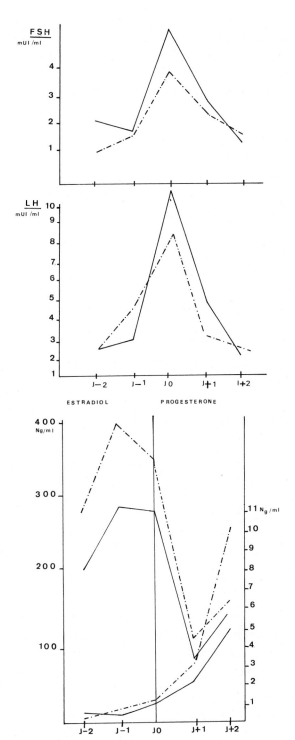

Figure 3. Hormonal profiles.
J 0: day of the LH peak

	J−1	J 0	J+1	J+2
Peak of estradiol	73%	27%		
Shrinking of the follicle		20%	67%	13%

same day that the LH peak value is measured, and is drastically lower when progesterone equals 2 ng/ml or more. J.O. is the lowest point on the BBT chart prior to a rise of at least 0.2° C. The shrinking of the follicle, i.e. ultrasonic appreciation of ovulation, occurs the same day for 33% of the cycles, the day after for 42%, two days after for 21%, and three days after for 4% of the cycles; while progesterone levels reach 3 ng/ml on J.O. 7% cases, the day after 47% cases, two days after 33% cases and three days after 10% cases (Table 2). These findings are almost identical to previously published data (Renaud et al., 1979, 1980).

6. ATYPICAL CYCLES

Fifteen patients had atypical cycles while following the protocol study. Some cycles may therefore differ from others for the same woman, mostly when psychological factors interfere with planned examinations.

6.1. Variability of cycles

In seven cycles, the ultrasonic monitoring was started at or after the LH peak as indicated by plasma progesterone levels. No follicle was detectable and the corpora lutea were recognized four times. Two of the patients were under induction treatment. Ovulation occurred 2 or 3 days before the usual timing (according to BBT).

6.2. Short luteal phase

Four cycles had a short luteal phase whereas the maximum follicular diameter measured never exceeded 15 mm or else was not detectable. LH and FSH peaks were not well defined; progesterone

reached 3 ng/ml. Accumulation of follicular fluid is an essential component of follicular development (Henderson, 1979). Furthermore, follicular dimensions based on the volume of aspirated fluid correlates well with the ultrasound measurements (O'Herlihy et al., 1979). In group 2, short luteal phase (defined as less than 10 days between the lowest point prior to a sustained rise and the onset of the next menstrual period) was preceded by no follicular growth. Only the bad cervical mucus score clinically suggested the eventuality of an abnormal cycle as in anovulatory cycles.

6.3. Anovulatory cycles

In two anovulatory cycles, the low hormonal levels and poor cervical mucus correlate with the lack of follicle observation. BBT recordings confirm the anovulation.

6.4. Abnormal cycles

For the same patient with clomiphene therapy, the follicular diameter reached 44 mm and three more follicles were seen of 17 mm each. No gonadotropin peak was measured. The BBT chart was irregular and hormonal levels were low.

7. CONCLUDING REMARKS

In ovulatory cycles, a regular follicular growth of a least 2 mm/day is noted until a maximum value is reached. In five cases, the follicular diameter was equal during two days before shrinking. The ultrasonic follicular diameter measurements in the induction therapy group are statistically different from those of spontaneous cycles only three days before follicle shrinking.

The midcycle surges of LH and FSH are always simultaneous (Dhont et al., 1974; Dupon et al., 1973; Mishell et al., 1971). A peak of estradiol occurred in every subject. Progesterone never reaches 3 ng/ml which is considered as ovulatory (Israel et al., 1972), before the day after the peak of LH. In normal ovulatory response to clomiphene, the peak of serum estradiol are neither higher than those in spontaneous cycle, nor average progesterone values opposite of Dodson et al. series

Table 2. Sequence of clinical, hormonal, ultrasonic results.

JO, lowest point of temperature	J 0	J+1	J+2	J+3
Shrinking of the follicle	33%	42%	21%	4%
P 3 ng/ml	7%	47%	33%	10%
J 0 = shrinking of follicle day				
P 3 ng/ml	33%	47%	20%	

(1975). LH value is statistically higher in the induction group the day before the peak value.

The sequence of clinical hormonal ultrasonic results is presented in Table 2. The follicle shrinking, i.e. ultrasonic ovulation assessment, can occur up to three days after the lowest point of BBT, i.e. day of presumed ovulation. Progesterone plasma level equals 3 ng/ml as late as two days after follicle shrinking and three days after the presumed ovulation day, according to the BBT chart. This finding correlates with the observation of Ross et al. (1970) which states that the BBT is extremely sensitive to small amounts of progesterone and is consistent with an early luteinization. Yet, it is difficult to evaluate the exact timing of ovulation, i.e. ovum extrusion, even by a daily examination, leaving a 24 hour period between each evaluation. Should artificial insemination be continued while the BBT rises, even if the cervical mucus score lowers? A regular follicular growth up to 17 mm guarantees a normal ovulatory cycle and an ovulation, which ultrasonically occurs in the next 48 hours. Artificial insemination can be started when those conditions are fulfilled. The efficiency of this new technique has to be appreciated in terms of pregnancy rate in which more cycles should be evaluated. When a cervical mucus study is unreliable due to a cervical pathology, cases can be managed with ultrasonic exploration.

ACKNOWLEDGMENTS

With acknowledgments to Dr A. Racadot for hormonal assays (Laboratory of Biochemistry U.S.N.A C.H.R., Lille Cedex).

REFERENCES

Baird DT, Fraser IS (1974) Blood production and ovarian secretion rates of estradiol and estrone in women throughout the menstrual cycle. J Clin Endocr Metab 38: 1009.

Dhont M, Vandekerckhove D, Vermeulen A, Vandeweghe M (1974) Daily concentrations of plasma LH-FSH estradiol estrone and progesterone throughout the menstrual cycle. Eur J Obstet Gynec Repr Biol 4 suppl 1 S 153.

Dodson KS, Macnaughton ML, Coutts Jr T (1975) Infertility in women with apparently ovulatory cycles: II the effects of clomiphene treatment on the profiles of gonadotrophin, and sex steroid hormones in peripheral plasma. Br J Obstet Gynaecol 82: 625.

Dupon C, Hosseinia A, Kim MH (1973) Simultaneous determination of plasma estrogens, androgens and progesterone during the human menstrual cycle. Steroids 22: 47.

Hackeloer BJ, Nitschke S, Daume E, Sturm G, Buchholz R. Ultraschalldarstellung von Ovarveranderungen. Geburtshilfe Frauenkerlkd 37: 185.

Hackeloer BJ, Robinson HP (1978) Ultraschalldarstellung des wachsenden Follikels und Corpus luteum in normalen physiologischen Zyklus. Geburtschilfe Frauenheilkd 38: 163.

Hackeloer BJ, Fleming R, Robinson HP, Adam A, Coutts JR (1979) Correlation of ultrasonic and endocrinologic assessment of human follicular development. Am J Obstet Gynec 135: 122.

Hall DA, Harn LE, Ferrucci Jr JT, Black EB, Braitman BS, Browly WIFI, Nikrui N, Kelley JA (1979) Sonographie morphology of the normal menstrual cycle. Radiology 133: 185.

Insler V, Mac Lamed H, Eichenbrenner I, Seer DH, Lunenfeld B (1972) The cervical score, a simple semiquantitative method for monitoring of the menstrual cycle. Int J Fertil 10: 223.

Israel R, Mischell DR, Stone SC, Thorneycroft IH, Moyer DL (1972) Single luteal phase progesterone assay as an index of ovulation. Am J Obstet Gynec 112: 104, 3.

Mischell DJ, Nakaruma RM, Grasignani P, Stone S, Kharma K, Nagata Y, Thorneycroft IH. Serum gonadotropin and steroid patterns during the normal menstrual cycle. Am J Obstet Gynec 111: 60.

Moghissi KS, Syner FV, Evans TN (1972) A composite picture of the menstrual cycle. Am J Obstet Gynecol 114: 405.

O'Herlihy C, De Crespigny L, Lopata A, Johnston I, Hoult I, Robinson H (1980) Preovulatory follicular size: a comparison of ultrasound and laparoscopic measurements. Fert Steril 34: 14.

Ylostalo P, Ronnberg L, Jouppila P (1979) Measurement of the ovarian follicle by ultrasound in ovulation induction. Fert Steril 31: 651.

Renaud R, Macler J, Dervain I, Ehret C, Aron C, Plasroser S, Spira A (1980) Echographic study of follicular maturation and ovulation during the normal menstrual cycle. Obst Gyn Survey 35: 7 451.

Ross GT, Cargille CM, Bipsett MG, Rayford PL, Marshaff Jr, Shott CA, Rodbard D. Pituitary and gonadal hormones in women during spontaneous and induced ovulatory cycle. Recent Prog Horm Res 26: 1.

Author's address:
Dr P. Saint-Pol
Laboratory of Histology, Faculty of Medicine
Place de Verdun, 59045 Lille Cedex, France.

18. IRREGULAR MENSTRUAL CYCLES DURING AID: USE OF SYNTHETIC LH-RH AND ITS ANALOGS FOR TIMING OF OVULATION

TH. KATZORKE

1. DEVELOPMENT OF IRREGULAR OR ANOVULATORY CYCLES DURING AID

There are remarkable psychological effects of AID on the menstrual cycle. Approximately 80% of women undergoing AID have normal, biphasic ovulatory BBT charts with constant cycle lengths of 28 ± 2 days at the beginning of treatment. However, during AID almost half of the women have disturbed menstrual cycles which lead to a low pregnancy rate (Katzorke et al., 1980d; McBain, 1980). The other 20% of women exhibit primary irregular fluctuations before AID of more than ± 3 days for the day on which the BBT dips, or show anovulatory cycles, the latter requiring induction of ovulation (Fig. 1). When all women are grouped together, the overall pregnancy rate is approximately 40%, requiring an average of 5 cycles to achieve a pregnancy (Table 1). Of the women undergoing AID treatment who originally have normal cycles, slightly more than one third are pregnant after 6 consecutive insemination cycles. An equal number of women develop irregular cycles, and the remaining 26% are without any obvious disturbance, but not pregnant. Timing of insemination which is solely based on the analysis of previous BBT records therefore fails frequently.

It has further been determined whether a correlation exists between the type of irregularity which develops and the outcome of AID (Katzorke et al., 1979). During the first 6 insemination cycles, 61% of regularly ovulating patients develop delayed ovulation, or, less frequently, early ovulation. During the 6th to 12th insemination cycles, the number of delayed ovulators is equal to the number of early ovulators. The success of AID is correlated with the type of irregular ovulation: in the case of early ovulation, more pregnancies occur (72%) than in the case of delayed ovulation (28%). Regarding the first 6 insemination cycles, disturbances occur most

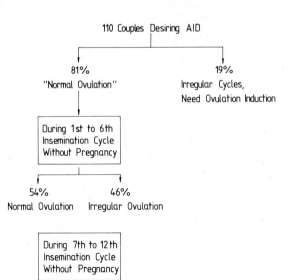

Figure 1. AID — incidence of normal and irregular ovulations (fluctuations of the ovulation day of more than ± 3 days, including anovulation) during AID-treatment.

Table 1. AID: Overall pregnancy and abortion rates in non-treated women.

(N = 110)	Regular ovulation	Irregular ovulation	Overall pregnancy rate	Abortion rate
Before AID	81%	19%		
During insemination cycle 1–6	54%	46%	36%	12%
During insemination cycle 7–12	43%	57%	42%	15%

(Katzorke et al., 1980d)

Hafez ESE & Semm K (Eds) Instrumental insemination.

frequently during the 3rd and 4th cycles (45%), which probably leads to the lower pregnancy rate observed during these insemination cycles. The occurrence of irregular cycles is more often associated with older patients and couples with longer duration of infertility (Katzorke et al., 1979).

The question of whether analysis of BBT charts before AID treatment can predict the future success of this treatment has also been addressed (Katzorke et al., 1980d). In other words, is there a connection between the occurrence of irregular cycles previous to AID and its future success? A comparison was made of the two extreme ovulation days in 3 cycles before the beginning of AID, and the cycles in which a pregnancy occurred. No significant difference was present between the two groups (Table 2). The occurrence of irregular ovulation previous to AID is therefore not a contraindication for beginning treatment. There is no correlation between ovulation characteristics preceding AID treatment and the time required for a pregnancy. It should be emphasized, however, that the existence of deviations is an important factor and should be noted and corrected early.

In our experience, a high pregnancy rate is present during the 1st and 2nd cycles and a lower pregnancy rate during the 3rd and 4th cycles, probably due to the increased number of irregular ovulators during these cycles (Table 3). Because the occurrence of irregular ovulations prior to AID treatment does not allow prediction of subsequent success, and to prevent further occurrence of ovulation irregularity, we have proposed the early application of "ovulation timing" and/or "pinpointing" substances.

Table 2. AID: Does analysis of BBT-charts before AID-treatment predict future success?

N = 110	Variation of the ovulation day before AID				
	0 to 1 day	2 days	3 days	4–5 days	≥6 days	An-ovulation
Pregnant after 6 insemination cycles	21	13	8	7	4	0
Not pregnant after 6 insemination cycles	20	14	13	4	3	3

2. THE PROBLEMS OF PINPOINTING OVULATION

Delays in ovulation and subsequent shift in BBT patterns have been observed in patients undergoing AID (Czyba et al., 1978; Katzorke et al., 1980d; McBain, 1980). Therefore, if one bases the timing of ovulation only on data obtained from previous BBT records (i.e. predictive information), treatment may often fail. Daily examination of cervical mucus ferning and Spinnbarkeit at midcycle is time-consuming, subjective, and increase the emotional and financial burden for the patient (Klay, 1976). Due to the episodic secretion of LH, the LH-peak cannot be identified with certainty unless frequent serial assays are performed. If the LH-peak can be identified, however, it is the day with the highest fertility rate (Matthews et al., 1978). There seems to be no correlation between the day of BBT rise and the LH-peak day, however (Morris et al., 1976; Matthews, 1980).

In order to improve pregnancy rates it is essential to perform AID as close as possible to the time of ovulation. For a positive and very recent indication that ovulation has occurred (ovulation pinpointing), daily examination for cervix scoring and a rapid LH-radioimmunoassay (RIA) (Hosseinian and Kim, 1976) or radioreceptorassay (RRA) (Schmidt-Gollwitzer et al., 1978) are useful, but unfortunately not practical for a variety of reasons including costs and the long distance required for some patients to reach insemination centers. For these reasons and the fact that AID treatment is only offered by a relatively small number of facilities, it would be advantageous to see patients only once or twice during one cycle, and to perform the insemination on the day(s) during which the probability of ovulation would be the greatest, providing better success rates. In order to follow this schedule, however, either the insemination service must be available 7 days a week, or ovulation must be timed (medically induced).

3. TIMED INDUCTION OF OVULATION

3.1. Previous reports

Ovulation timing in normally ovulating women

Table 3. Artificial insemination donor: analysis of results related to the AID-cycle.

Insemination-cycle	No. of cases	No. of "drop-outs" at the end of cycle	No. of pregnancies	Monthly pregnancy-rate (%)	% of total pregnancies	Cumulative pregnancy rate (%)
1	415	43	76	18	36	36
2	296	34	51	17	24	61
3	211	33	23	11	11	72
4	155	20	12	8	6	78
5	123	18	17	14	8	85
6	88	15	13	15	6	92
7	60	10	5	8	2	94
8	45	12	3	8	1	95
9	30	2	1	3	1	96
10	27	0	4	15	2	98
>10	23	18	5	22	2	100

(Katzorke et al., 1980b)

(causing ovulation to occur on a specific, predetermined day) has been accomplished successfully with clomiphene citrate (Klay, 1976) and hMG-hCG (Berger and Taymor, 1971; Edwards and Steptoe, 1975). LH-RH can be administered on a specific day of the cycle for timed ovulation (and therefore also pinpointing of ovulation) and, on the other hand, as one possible method of contraception (Schally et al., 1972).

Clinical trials with LH-RH for timing of ovulation have been performed previously in association with AID/AIH (Gigon et al., 1973; Grimes et al., 1975; Taymor and Jittivanih, 1978). Triggering of ovulation in the late follicular phase of the menstrual cycle appears to be possible if the follicle has reached an advanced stage of maturation, indicated by high preovulatory serum estradiol (Gigon et al., 1973; Grimes et al., 1975). However, it is difficult to evaluate the efficacy of treatment in normally ovulating women since spontaneous ovulations can always occur. In randomized studies, the results obtained after single injections of LH-RH (100–500 μg) did not differ from those obtained after placebo treatment (Nillius and Wide, 1976; Reyes et al., 1977). Multiple LH-RH administration by the practical intranasal route may be more effective (Nillius and Wide, 1976). However, the optimal therapeutic regimen for timing of ovulation by LH-RH remains to be established.

Several stimulating LH-RH analogs have been synthesized and evaluated (cf. Schally et al., 1976). Long acting stimulatory LH-RH analogs should be more successful than LH-RH itself (which has effects on gonadotropin secretion of relatively short duration) because their administration leads to a prolonged elevation of plasma LH and FSH. Programmed ovulation has been attempted with a potent, long acting LH-RH analog, D-Leu[6]-des-Gly[10]-LH-RH-ethylamide (Zanartu et al., 1975). When a single injection of the potent analog (500–1000 μg) was given on day 13 of the cycle of ten women pretreated with ethinylestradiol, signs of recent ovulation were observed on day 15 in seven, and on day 16 in two cases. Neither ethinylestradiol given alone on days 9 to 11, LH-RH alone, nor the more potent LH-RH analog given alone on day 13 induced ovulation.

3.2. Use of LH-RH and HOE 766

The low pregnancy rate in patients undergoing AID, together with the uncertainty regarding the possibility of medically induced, timed ovulation, lead to the following question. Is it possible to improve the pregnancy rate, compared to an untreated control group, in patients undergoing AID therapy 1) by oral application of high doses of synthetic LH-Releasing Hormone (LH-RH), or 2) by nasal application of a potent stimulatory LH-RH analog (HOE 766) (Katzorke et al., 1978, 1980c)?

3.2.1. Patient group. One hundred and thirty-two women between 20 and 40 years of age (mean age = 28.3 years) with a period of infertility between 1 and 10 years due to male partner factors were examined. Before AID was begun, each woman underwent a gynecologic examination, serum hormone work-up (LH, FSH, estradiol, progesterone, prolactin), hysterosalpingography, and in special cases diagnostic laparoscopy for evaluation of possible tubal factor.

Fresh donor semen (0.5–1.0 ml) was administered intracervically. When the first two cycles of insemination did not result in a pregnancy, ovulation timing was begun during the third insemination cycle.

3.2.2. Administration of LH-RH or HOE 766. Ovulation timing was attempted either by administration of high doses of synthetic LH-RH or a potent, long acting stimulatory analog, D-Ser-(TBU)[6]-ethylamide[10]-LH (HOE 766, Hoechst Co., Frankfurt/Main, West Germany) (Fig. 2). HOE 766 is an analog which stimulates the release of LH and FSH and has, compared to the natural decapeptide LH-RH, 20 to 170 times greater the stimulus on secretion of LH, FSH and 17-β-estradiol in normally ovulating women (Dericks-Tan et al., 1977) and in women having secondary amenorrhea (Katzorke et al., 1980a). An intravenous bolus injection of LH-RH (500 or 1000 μg) or intranasal spray application of the analog HOE 766 (100 or 200 μg, supposed resorption quotient 1–4%) was administered one or two days before the earliest expected BBT rise, as determined by the analysis of control cycles in the normally cyclic women prior to initiation of therapy.

3.2.3. Ovulation and corpus luteum function. To document ovulation and to check corpus luteum function, BBT measurement and serum levels of LH, FSH and progesterone were monitored. Treatment was considered successful only for those cycles in which ovulation occurred within 48 hours after application of the ovulation triggering substance (indicated by hyperthermia $>0.5°$ C and/or serum progesterone concentrations >1.5 ng/ml) (Laborde et al., 1976), and which exhibited normal corpus luteum function (at least 12 days of hyperthermia and progesterone levels >4.0 ng/ml) (Table 4). Serum gonadotropin and progesterone levels >4.0 ng/ml) (Table 4). Serum gonadotropin and progesterone levels were measured by commercially available radioimmunoassay.

3.2.4. Effect of LH-RH and HOE 766 on ovulation, pregnancy and abortion rates. Tables 5 and 6 show the ovulation and pregnancy data, respectively, for untreated women and women treated with an ovulation timing agent. The pregnancy rate increased from 34% in the untreated group to 65% by nasal application of 200 μg LH-RH analog. The overall pregnancy rate achieved during use of either LH-RH or the analog HOE 766 was 51% after 2 untreated and one timed cycle, compared to a 34%

Table 4. Criteria for successful timing of ovulation.

Result	Criteria
Successful ovulation timing	Progesterone greater than 1.5 ng/ml within 48 hours after drug administration Temperature rise greater than 0.5° C within 48 hours after drug administration At least 12 days of hyperthermia
Short or insufficient luteal phase	Serum progesterone less than 4.0 ng/ml, but greater than 1.5 ng/ml Hyperthermia shorter than 12 days

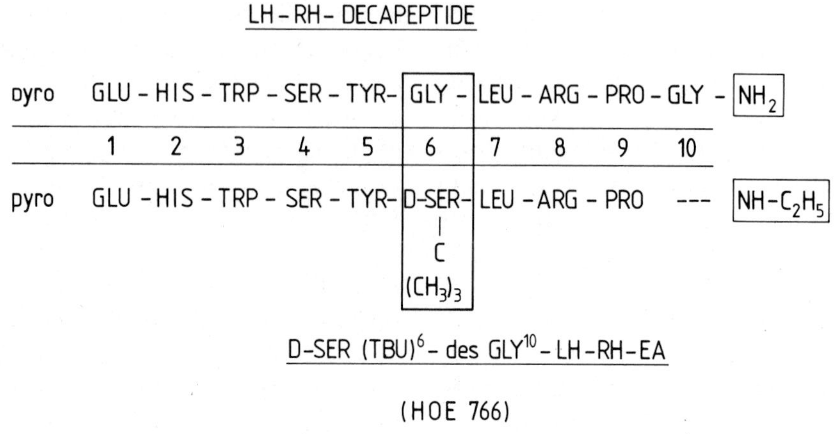

LH – RH – DECAPEPTIDE

Figure 2. Formula for LH-RH and HOE 766.

Table 5. AID: Ovulation characteristics during the use of different drugs for "ovulation timing".

Substance	Patients (N)	Successful ovulation timing	No. of short luteal phases	Unsuccessful ovulation timing
500 µg LH-Rh (I.V.)	20	11	2	7
1000 µg LH-RH (I.V.)	20	15	1	4
100 µg HOE 766 (intranasal)	20	15	1	4
200 µg HOE 766 (intranasal)	20	17	0	3
Total treated	80	58	5	17
Untreated	52	(30)*	8	–

* Spontaneous ovulations
(Katzorke et al., 1980c)

Table 6. AID: Results of AID during use of different agents for "ovulation timing".

Substance	Patients (N)	No. of pregnancies	% of ovulations resulting in pregnancies	No. of abortions (% of pregnancies)
500 µg LH-RH (i.v.)	20	8	73%	2
1000 µg LH-RH (i.v.)	20	9	60%	1
100 µg HOE 766 (intranasal)	20	11	74%	2
200 µg HOE 766 (intranasal)	20	13	77%	2
Total treated	80	41 (51%)	71%	7 (17%)
Untreated	52	18 (34%)	60%	3 (17%)

(Katzorke et al., 1980c)

pregnancy rate after 3 untreated consecutive cycles. The spontaneous abortion rate was influenced by neither of the drugs.

Of the 80 treated women, 58 showed successful ovulations (73%), whereas in the 52 untreated women 30 spontaneous ovulations occurred (58%), and with a higher number of luteal defects. The pregnancy rate for treated women increased to 51% after 6 cycles, compared to a pregnancy rate of 34% in untreated women. In other words, 71% of the ovulations were resulting in a pregnancy in treated cases and 60% in untreated cases.

Two other ovulation inducing or timing agents (clomiphene citrate and hMG-hCG) were studied. The overall pregnancy rate could be increased from 34% to 42% (insemination cycles 1 to 6) and from 39% to 50% (insemination cycles 7 to 12) by

application of these agents. The use of these agents decreased the time required for pregnancy so that in fewer consecutive cycles more pregnancies occurred (Table 7).

The single application of high doses of synthetic

Table 7. AID: pregnancy rate in 6 consecutive AID-cycles: results of an untreated and a regulated group.

	Insemination cycle					
	1	2	3	4	5	6
Clomiphene, hMG/hCG or LH-RH/analogue regulated (N = 55)	25	13	11	3	2	1
	45%	23%	20%	6%	4%	2%
Untreated (N = 30)	9	8	3	4	3	3
	30%	27%	10%	13%	10%	10%

LH-RH or of the analog HOE 766 leads to an increased number of ovulations and to a higher pregnancy rate. With the LH-RH analog, it was advantageous to use single, higher doses rather than midcyclic application for 2 or 3 days, which can lead to suppression of ovulation (Katzorke et al., 1978). Definitive statements regarding the use of synthetic LH-RH and its analogs for timing of ovulation are difficult to make since spontaneous ovulations cannot be excluded. The pregnancy rate can definitely be improved, however, by treatment with these agents (Table 8).

4. CONCLUDING REMARKS

Increasing irregularity of the menstrual cycle during

Table 8. Administration of ovulation inducing substances during artificial insemination by donor (AID).

Advantages	Disadvantages
Scheduled insemination	Expensive and not economic
Higher pregnancy rate in shorter time	Masking or loss of spontaneous ovulations
Less ovulation disorders	Risk of multiple pregnancy
Less emotional stress	

AID, especially persistent late ovulation, explains the low pregnancy rate after more than six unsuccessful insemination cycles, and is probably an expression of the number of psychically labile women which increases constantly during AID. The psychological conflicts exert a negative effect on the hypothalamic LH-releasing center, and influence the pituitary–ovarian axis (Schally et al., 1972). The psychological problems, which include the frustration generated by unsuccessful AID, therefore complicate the process of conception. Since the pregnancy rate after AID is highest in the first insemination cycles (Dixon and Buttram, 1976; Katzorke et al., 1980b), it is proposed that ovulation timing, without previous expanded hormone analysis which only delays the treatment, should be started after two unsuccessful insemination cycles to eliminate possible stress-induced conception failures. High doses of LH-RH and one of its stimulating analogs are helpful.

ACKNOWLEDGEMENT

Thanks are due to Dr. J. C. Goodpasture for valuable help and discussion in preparing the manuscript. (D-Ser(TBU)[6]-LH-RH 1–9 EA (HOE 766, burserelin) was generously supplied by Dr. M. von der Ohe, Hoechst AG, Frankfurt/Main, West Germany.

REFERENCES

Berger WJ, Taymor ML (1971) Combined human menopausal gonadotropin therapy and donor insemination. Fertil Steril 22: 787.

Czyba JC, Cottinet D, Souchier C (1978) Perturbations de l'ovulation consécutives à l'insémination artificielle avec donneurs (AID). J Gyn Obst Biol Repr 7: 499.

Dericks-Tan JSE, Hammer E, Taubert HD (1977) The effect of D-Ser (TBU)[6]-LH-RH-EA[10] upon gonadotropin release in normally cyclic women. J Clin EndocrinoL Metab 45: 597.

Dixon RE, Buttram VC (1976) Artificial insemination using donor semen: a review of 171 cases. Fertil Steril 27: 130.

Edwards RG, Steptoe PC (1975) Induction of follicular growth, ovulation and luteinization in the human ovary. J Reprod Fert Suppl 22: 121.

Gigon U, Stamm O, Werder H (1973) Induction of ovulation timing with HCG or synthetic LH-RH in cases of sterility (Die Bedeutung der getimten Ovulationsinduktion mittels HCG oder synthetischem LH-RH in der Sterilitätsbehandlung). Geburtsh Frauenheilk 33: 567.

Grimes EM, Taymor ML, Thompson IE (1975) Induction of timed ovulation with synthetic luteinizing hormone-releasing hormone in women undergoing insemination therapy. I. Effect of a single parenteral administration at midcycle. Fertil Steril 26: 277.

Hosseinian AH, Kim MH (1976) Predetermination of ovulation timing by luteinizing hormone assay. Fertil Steril 27: 369.

Katzorke Th, Propping D, Tauber PF, Ludwig H (1978) Programming of ovulation with a new LH-RH analogue (HOE 766; D-Ser-(TBU)[6]-EA[10]-LH-RH) for artificial insemination. V Europ Congr Ster Fert Venice Italy.

Katzorke TH, Propping D, Tauber PF (1980) Méthodes et résultats de la régulation de l'ovulation. Methods and results for regulated ovulation during artificial insemination. Symposium international sur l'insémination artificielle et la conservation du sperme. Paris France 1979. In David G, Price WS, eds, Human artificial insemination and semen preservation, pp 361–370. New York: Plenum.

Katzorke Th, Propping D, Ohe M vd, Tauber PF (1980a) Clinical evaluation of the effects of a new long-acting super-active luteinizing hormone-releasing hormone (LH-RH) analog, D-Ser-(TBU)[6]-des-Gly-10-Ethylamide-LH-RH, in women with secondary amenorrhea. Fertil Steril 33: 35.

Katzorke Th, Propping D, Tauber PF, Ludwig H (1980b) Artificial insemination with donor semen (AID), 144 pregnancies in 290 couples (Artifizielle Insemination mit Spendersamen (AID); 144 Schwangerschaften bei 290 Ehepaaren). Der Frauenarzt 21: 405.

Katzorke Th, Tauber PF, Propping D, Ludwig H (1980c) Timing of ovulation: use of synthetic LH-RH and its stimulatory analogs. Arch Androl 5: 19.

Katzorke Th, Propping D, Tauber PF, Ludwig H (1980d) Analysis of cycle changes following AID. Arch Androl 5: 48.

Klay LJ (1976) Clomiphene — regulated ovulation for donor artificial insemination. Fertil Steril 27: 383.

Laborde N, Carril M, Cheviakoff S, Croxatto HD, Pedroza E, Rosner JM (1976) The secretion of progesterone during the periovulatory period in women with certified ovulation. J Clin Endocrin Metab 43: 1157.

Matthews CD, Kerin LFP, Hopkins R, Wheatley BP, Makin M Svigos JM (1978) The characterization of thawed semen, and the timing and route of insemination associated with conception in the human. Int J Fertil 23: 158.

Matthews CD (1980) The technique and outcome of AID In: Wood C, Leeton J, Kovacs G eds. Artificial insemination by donor, pp 63–80. Melbourne: Brown Prior Anderson.

McBain JC (1980) The timing of ovulation for AID. In: Wood C, Leeton J, Kovacs G, eds. Artificial insemination by donor, pp 50–62. Melbourne: Brown Prior Anderson.

Morris NM, Underwood LE, Easterling W (1976) Temporal relationship between basal temperature and luteinizing hormone surge in normal women. Fertil Steril 27: 780.

Nillius SJ, Wide L (1976) Luteinizing hormone-releasing hormone for induction of follicular maturation and ovulation in women. In: Charro-Salgado AL, Fernandez-Durango R, Lopez del Campo JG, eds. Basic applications and clinical uses of hypothalamic hormones, p 291. Amsterdam: Excerpta Medica.

Reyes FI, Winter JSD, Rochefort JG, Faiman CH (1977) Luteinizing hormone-releasing hormone as an ovulation trigger in regularly ovulation women: problems in assessment of efficacy. Fertil Steril 28: 1175.

Schally AV, Kastin AJ, Arimura A (1972) The hypothalamus and reproduction. Am J Obstet Gyn 114: 423.

Schally AV, Kastin AJ, Coy DH (1976) LH- releasing hormone and its analogues: recent basic and clinical investigation. Int J Fertil 21: 1.

Schmidt-Gollwitzer K, Eiletz J, Schmidt-Gollwitzer M (1978) Radioreceptor assay for human LH: detection of ovulation for artificial insemination. In Emperaire JC, Audebert A, eds. Proc 1st Int Symp on Artificial Insemination: Homologous and Male Subfertility, p 16. Bordeaux.

Taymor ML, Jittivanih B (1978) Ovulation regulation with HMG for artificial insemination. In Emperaire JC, Audebert A, eds. Proc 1st Int Symp on Artificial Insemination: Homologous and Male Subfertility, p 26.

Zanartu J, Rosner JM, Guiloff E, Ibarra-Polo AA, Croxatto HD, Croxatto HB, Aguilera E, Coy HD, Schally AV (1975) Attempts to programme ovulation with exogenous oestrogens and LH-RH analogue. Br Med J 2: 527.

Author's address:
Dr Thomas Katzorke
Fertility Institute
Kettwiger Strasse 2-10
43 Essen, FRG

19. ADDITION OF PHARMACOLOGICAL AGENTS TO THE EJACULATE

J.D. Paulson, R. Harrison, W.B. Schill and J. Barkay

A total understanding of human spermatozoal metabolism is yet to be achieved. The natural activators of the metabolic systems in spermatozoa still remain to be identified. Much knowledge has been applied from experimental animal data, which does not always apply to men. Therefore, the site of action of the interaction between motility and capacitation are not as yet completely understood. There are many factors involved in and affecting the process of spermatozoal motility; because of this, an ejaculate with spermatozoa having abnormal motility but with other normal parameters may well benefit from the addition of some pharmacological agent to it in order to increase motility. This beneficial effect may increase the chance of pregnancy after insemination.

Knowledge of the anatomical mechanisms of motility of the spermatozoa has increased rapidly. Electron microscopic studies have shown that the motility of human spermatozoa is produced in the axial spiral complex of the tail (Pedersen, 1970) by a sliding mechanism of axonemal microtubules with respect to one another under the gripping action of the outer and inner dynein arms (Huxley, 1969). Contractions and relaxations in the tail are produced, propelling the spermatozoon in a quasi-purposeful manner, a self-propulsion that must suffice if it is to achieve contact with the released ovum after the impetus given by the contraction of elements of the male reproductive system and the possible copulatory motor activity of the genital tract of the female.

Immature spermatozoa are incapable of self-propulsion and while this property, like fertilization capacity (Cooper and Orgebin-Crist, 1975), is acquired in the epididymis (Gadden, 1968), they only become truly motile upon ejaculation. Motility is affected adversely by the age of the man (MacLeod, 1951), certain spermatozoal shapes (Mitchell et al.,

1976), the part of the ejaculate in which the spermatozoon is extruded (Eliasson and Lindholmer, 1972), and the morphology and length of time after ejaculation (Bartak, 1971). External influences, such as temperature (Zaneveld and Polakoski, 1977), light (Van Duijn and Van Lierop, 1966), pH (Kroeks and Kremer, 1977), sources of irradiation (Norman et al., 1962), and the presence of antibodies (Fjallbrant, 1968), may also affect motility. In addition, abnormalities in the seminal plasma (Polakoski and Zaneveld, 1977) and cervical mucus (Wolf et al., 1977) can be related to motility of the spermatozoa. There is also a correlation between sperm metabolism and concentration of zinc (Huacuja et al., 1973) and spermine (Fair et al., 1972).

1. PHARMACOLOGICAL AGENTS

Several pharmacological agents have been utilized to increase motility in semen specimens which had poor motility: 1) methylxanthines, 2) kinins, 3) caffeine and kinin 4) prostaglandins, and 5) L-arginine.

1.1. Methylxanthines

Methylxanthines — caffeine, theophylline, and aminophylline — are inhibitors of phosphodiesterase. Addition of these substances in proper dosages may increase the concentration of cyclic AMP and cyclic GMP in spermatozoa (Fig. 1). Cyclic AMP stimulates human sperm motility (Hicks et al., 1972a) and ATP is converted to cyclic AMP under the influence of adenylcyclase. Because of buildup of cyclic AMP, addition of a methylxanthine to the ejaculate increases energy production by accelerating glycolysis and stimulating

Hafez ESE & Semm K (Eds) Instrumental insemination.

motility. Metabolic activity of both epididymal (Drevius, 1971) and ejaculated (Garbers et al., 1971) bull spermatozoa was shown to be stimulated by methylxanthines such as caffeine (1, 3, 7-trimethyl-2, 6-dioxopurine). The stimulatory affect is greater on the precapacitated specimens although motility is only progressive if seminal plasma is also present (Hoskins and Casillas, 1975).

The addition of caffeine to human semen in a final concentration of approximately 6 mmol not only stimulates a greater number of spermatozoa to become motile but also increases the rate of motility and forward progression of the spermotozoa (Bunge, 1973; Haesungcharern and Chulavatnatol, 1973; Schoenfield et al., 1973, 1975). The addition of caffeine to specimens that are cryopreserved stimulates motility (Paulson et al., 1981). Harrison (1978) noted significant stimulation of spermatozoal motility in 34 patients, 14 of whom had semen analyses within normal limits, using the same dosage regimen as previously described. These specimens were artificially inseminated with no pregnancies after the addition of caffeine. Scanning

electron microscopy (Harrison et al., 1980) demonstrated that incubation of caffeine may have a detrimental effect on human spermatozoa and this may be an explanation as to why there are poor pregnancy results.

1.2. Kinins

Kinins are polypeptides produced through an enzymatic breakdown of a precursor substrate kininogen, by a kininogenase (kallikrein), a proteolytic enzyme present in tissues. Kinins are potent pharmacologically and, in very low doses, have the ability to cause vasodilatation leading to a lowering of blood pressure. They also increase capillary permeability, produce edema and pain and contract or relax different smooth muscles, including the uterus and small bowel. Factors involved in the formation and destruction of the kallikrein–kinin system are similar in form to those of coagulation, fibrolysis, and the complement system (Fig. 1). The components of this mechanism are all present in the male and female genital secretions (Palm et al., 1976; Schill

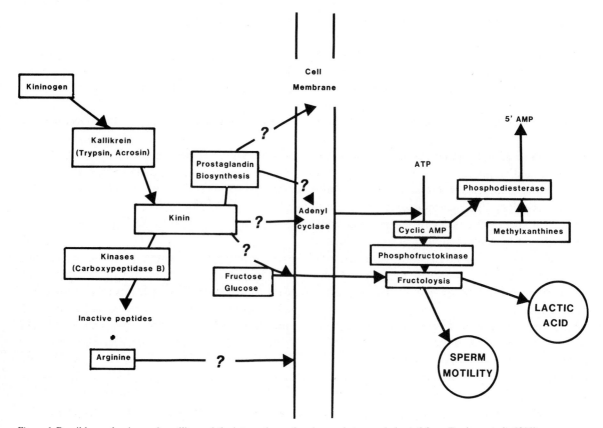

Figure 1. Possible mechanisms of motility and the interactions of various substances (adapted from Paulson et al., 1980).

and Preissler, 1977) and continuous production and destruction of these elements occur as long as kininogen, kinin-liberating proteinases (kallikrein) and kinin-inactivating enzymes are present. Acrosin, as well as trypsin and kininogenase from the prostate, has the ability to liberate kinins from kininogen (Palm and Fritz, 1975). This proteolytic enzyme, which allows penetration of the zona pellucida of the ovum, is in the acrosome of the spermatozoa and is in an enzyme-inhibitor complex and zymogen form in the seminal plasma (Fritz et al., 1975; Polakoski et al., 1977). As spermatozoa penetrate the cervical mucus, acrosin could be released, thereby liberating kinins and increasing and potentiating motility.

The addition of hog pancreatic kallikrein to human samples with decreased sperm motility can cause an increase in sperm motility, not only in the total number of motile spermatozoa, but also in the number of progressively moving spermatozoa (Schill et al., 1974; Leidl et al., 1975; Schirren, 1975; Wallner et al., 1975; Steiner et al., 1977; Schill and Haberland, 1974a). There is an increase in the mean velocity (Steiner et al., 1977) and a small improvement in the viability (Leidl et al., 1975) of these samples. The metabolic state is increased as demonstrated by an increase in fructolysis (Schill 1975a), increased oxygen consumption (Leidl et al., 1975), increased lactic acid and CO_2 production (Leidl et al., 1975; Schill et al., 1975) and increased intracellular cyclic AMP levels (Schill and Preissler, 1977). This effect on semen samples that were 24 hours old by the addition of kallikrein was also noted (Schill, 1975b), as was this effect on samples that were cryopreserved (Schill et al., 1976; Schill and Pritsch, 1976; Schill, 1977). Inactivation by acid denaturation or inhibition by the trypsin-kallikrein inhibitor from bovine organs (Trasylol® [Bayer A.G.]) demonstrates that the increase in spermatozoal motility seen by the addition of kallikrein can be attributed to its enzymatic properties as a kinin-releasing proteinase (Schill, 1975d). There is a shorter duration of increased spermatozoal motility by kinins in comparison to kallikrein. The direct stimulatory effect of motility by the addition of bradykinin and kallidin lasts between one and two hours (Schill, 1975b). This is probably a direct effect of the kinases on the kinins in the seminal plasma, in comparison to the longer effect of

increased motility with the addition of kallikrein due to continuous liberation of kinins from kininogen for long time intervals. The addition of a potent kinase, carboxypeptidase-B decreases motility of the spermatozoa in the ejaculates with good semen quality (Schill and Haberland, 1974b). The kallikrein–kinin system may, therefore, contribute to the regulation and stimulation of spermatozoal motility.

A significant correlation exists with in vitro cervical mucus penetration and conception indices and fertilizing ability (Ulstein, 1972, 1973). In vitro cervical mucus penetration can be improved by the addition of pancreatic kallikrein (Wallner et al., 1975; Schill et al., 1975, 1976; Schill and Preissler, 1977). This increased cervical mucus penetration depth by the addition of kallikrein was negated when a kallikrein inhibitor (Trasylol) was added. The effect of bradykinin (a kinin) was similar to that of kallikrein in its ability to stimulate oligospermic semen specimens with increased cervical mucus penetration.

1.3. Caffeine and kinin

There are different changes in sperm motility when comparing caffeine and kallikrein to the same ejaculate (Schill, 1975c). There is an immediate increase in sperm motility after the addition of caffeine and this effect remains relatively constant during the first several hours; however, by 24 hours, the caffeine-treated samples demonstrate the same motility as untreated controls. Kallikrein's effect is delayed with a maximum stimulation at 2 hours. The addition of both caffeine and kallikrein simultaneously to a sample further increases the motility of the spermatozoa significantly over that produced by either alone.

The addition of caffeine and kallikrein in final concentrations of 5 mmol and 5 KU/ml (KU = kallikrein unit) respectively to cryopreserved samples which have thawed, demonstrate a significant improvement over the post-thaw total motility by an increase of 81% with caffeine and 73% with kallikrein after one hour of incubation (Schill et al., 1979). A similar pattern of 80% increase with caffeine and 54% increase in the presence of kallikrein is observed after incubating for 4 hours. The simultaneous addition of both substances demon-

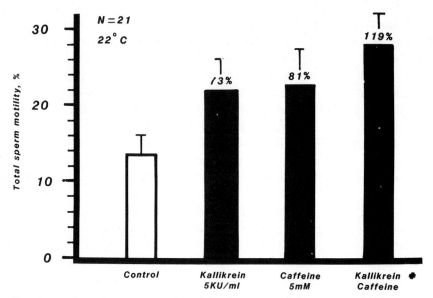

Figure 2. The motility after one hour of cryopreserved thawed ejaculates after the addition of kallikrein, caffeine and both (adapted from Paulson et al., 1980).

strate significantly better motility than either agent alone with an average increase of 119 % after one hour and 114% after 4 hours (Fig. 2). The forward progressive motility of the spermatozoa are also improved by the addition of both caffeine and kallikrein. As with the total motility, the best stimulation of the forward progressive motility is obtained by the simultaneous addition of both substances to the cryopreserved thawed specimens (Fig. 3). There is a significant increase in fructolysis after 4 hours of incubation in the presence of caffeine. Kallikrein, however, shows a statistically significant increase in fructose utilization only after 24 hours (Schill et al., 1978). Cervical mucus penetration depth by sperm is improved by the addition of either caffeine or kallikrein initially. However, no difference to the controls could be noted after a 2 hour time period (Schill et al., 1978). Significantly increased penetration is also observed by the simultaneous addition of both substances. In a study involving 57 ejaculates containing hypokinetic spermatozoa (Fig. 4), the addition of caffeine and kallikrein demonstrated that in 40% there was no response to either caffeine or kallikrein; 39% showed stimulation with either caffeine or kallikrein; 12% demonstrated an increase only with caffeine; and 9% only with kallikrein (Schill, 1978).

1.4. Prostaglandins

Prostaglandins are 20-carbon fatty acids containing

a 5-membered ring. They are vasodepressors and have smooth muscle contracting properties. They constitute one of the most biologically active types of compounds discovered with 5 groups of naturally occurring prostaglandins existing. Individual prostaglandins vary widely in potency and in their activities.

Prostaglandin-E levels are decreased in infertile males (Bygdeman et al., 1970; Hawkins, 1967; Collier et al., 1975). Prostaglandin F2α added to semen specimens in concentrations 100 times greater than found in normal semen results in significant

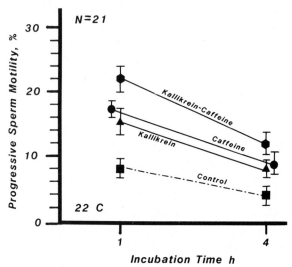

Figure 3. Forward progressive motility of cryopreserved ejaculates after thawing after the addition of pharmacological agents (adapted from Paulson et al., 1980).

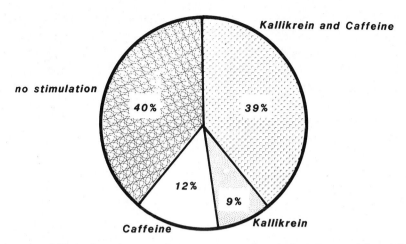

Figure 4. The percentage of 57 ejaculates demonstrating a response to pharmacological agents (adapted from Schill, 1978).

inhibition of spermatozoal motility (Cohen et al. 1977). In contrast, the addition of physiologic levels of prostaglandin F2α to spermatozoa increases in vitro penetration depth into cervical mucus (Eskin et al., 1973). The time required for spermatozoal penetration of cervical mucus is greatly diminished by the addition of small doses of prostaglandin F1α or F2α (Hunt and Zaneveld, 1975). The addition of prostaglandin-E is less effective.

1.5. L-arginine

L-arginine is a nonessential amino acid found in seminal plasma. Acrosin, the proteolytic enzyme at the head of the sperm, preferentially catalyzes the hydrolysis of arginine substrates (Paulson et al., 1979). Kinases cleave the carboxy-terminal arginine from kinins yielding arginine and inactive peptides. A clinical report of pregnancy success with oligozoospermic individuals given oral arginine (Schachter et al., 1973) spurred an interest in this amino acid as a possible therapeutic modality in treatment of oligozoospermia; others, however, were not able to reproduce these results (Jungling and Bunge, 1976). In vitro testing performed by the addition of L-arginine in a final concentration of 4 mmol demonstrated an average increase of forward motility was 82% in comparison to controls (Keller and Polakoski, 1975). Other amino acids, both similar in structure and arginine analogs (D-arginine, L-nitroarginine, L-homoarginine, L-lysine, and L-ornithine) are not effective in stimulation.

2. MODE OF ACTION

Human spermatozoa have an absolute requirement for hexoses from exogenous sources to drive glycolysis; however, the final energy driving motility is chiefly provided internally, with the plasma membrane helping to control and modulate the effects from the differing external environments. This energy source is ATP situated on the mitochondria adjacent to the axial spiral complex. Ca^{2+} plus Mg^{2+} mediate the appropriate ATPase activity metabolism (enzymatic hydrolysis) of the 150 moles of ATP present in each spermatozoon and this initiates the tail motion (Petersen and Freund, 1973). Other organic phosphates present act as reserves (Newton and Rothschild, 1961). Oxidative metabolism occurs (Petersen and Freund, 1973), and this involves the cyclic AMP system (Hicks et al., 1972b). Endogenous respiratory activity, possibly a derivative of the oxidation of intracellular phospholipids (Mann, 1964; Poulos and White, 1973), can support motility (Nevo 1966). Motility ceases within a few hours at ATP levels soon become depleted unless fructose helps in the regeneration of ATP (Petersen and Freund, 1970). The chiefly gycolytic metabolism has minimal oxygen consumption, and most of the sugars (hexoses) that the human spermatozoa consume appear to be broken down into the suspending medium as lactic acid, whether or not there has been oxygen present (MacLeod and Freund, 1958).

The pathway in man appears to be under the

influence of nucleotide phosphodiesterase enzymes (Hicks et al., 1972a), the release of which is inhibited by high ATP levels. Therefore, as the levels are used up, the enzymes are released which results in an increase in glycolysis (Atkinson and Walton 1967). A role for cyclic AMP related to capacitation has been seen in rabbits (Rosado et al., 1974), but the natural activators of this mechanism in the human remain to be identified. Cyclic AMP binds on the surface of the membrane of the spermatozoa (Rosado et al., 1976) and the amount present is directly related to spermatozoal activity (Tash and Mann, 1973). Higher levels of AMP increase enzymatic activation, which suggest that the amount present appears to be directly related to this spermatozoal activity of the cyclic nucleotides (cAMP and cGMP) which are intimately connected with sperm metabolism.

The mode of action of increased motility in the ejaculate is different after the addition of caffeine and kallikrein in fresh (Schill, 1975c) and cryopreserved thawed specimens (Schill et al., 1979). The simultaneous addition of both substances led to improvement of spermatozoal motility over and above the addition of either alone (Schill, 1975; Schill et al., 1978). Although there is an increase in intracellular cyclic AMP levels after stimulation by the kinins (Schill and Preissler, 1977), the amount is small. Therefore, it is doubtful that the kinins increase sperm motility in the same physiological way that the methylxanthines do (Fig. 1). The mode of increase of the motility by kinins has still not been elucidated. A prostaglandin synthesis effect by kinins has been suggested (Damas and Deby, 1974; Ferreira et al., 1974). When mefenamate, a prostaglandin synthesis inhibitor (in vitro) was added to an ejaculate, the kallikrein–kinin effect on sperm motility and oxygen consumption was inhibited (Gryglewski, 1974). The additions of prostaglandins to the ejaculate containing mefenamate and kallikrein however, restores and increases the motility. Kinins may also help facilitate transport of hexoses into the cell. Prostaglandins, in addition to their relationship with the kinin system interact with other systems. Although caffeine stimulates spermatozoal motility due to its action as a phosphodiesterase inhibitor with subsequent buildup of cyclic AMP, it will inhibit prostaglandin-15-dehydrogenase (Marrazzi and Matschinsky, 1972), an important enzyme in the degregation process of prostaglandins. Prostaglandins can produce their actions as part of an interaction with the cyclic AMP system (Ramwell and Shaw, 1971), and in most systems, prostaglandin-E is a strong simulus for the accumulation of cyclic AMP (Marsh and LeMaire, 1974).

The stimulatory mechanism for increased spermatozoal motility by the addition in vitro of L-arginine remains unresolved. L-arginine is a nonessential amino acid. Therefore, there should be no shortage of this element in vitro; however, the concentration of arginine in men with normal sperm counts is higher than that in oligozoospermic and azoospermic individuals (Krampitz and Doepfmer 1962). The terminal guanidine group as well as the chain length of the amino acid may be important for its actions in vitro (Keller and Polakoski, 1975).

3. CONCLUDING REMARKS

Unfortunately, in vitro addition of caffeine and subsequent inseminations fail to improve pregnancy rates. The effects of methylxanthines and kinins are not uniform in all semen specimens. Especially where semen samples are already poor, these substances may not really make samples as "normal" as they apparently become. There may, however, be other reasons for such results. The addition of caffeine to "normal" specimens prior to cryopreservation has produced no adverse affects on fertility rates, although such semen is obviously impeccable in quality from the beginning. The results of the addition of kallikrein to hypokinetic specimens with an increased pregnancy rate of 39% is encouraging and the addition of pharmacological agents to the ejaculate may be beneficial in certain instances to improve fertility.

REFERENCES

Atkinson EE, Walton GE (1967) Adenosine triphosphate concentration in metabolic regulation. J Biol Chem 242: 3239.

Barkay J, Zuckerman H Paper presented at the 1st International Symposium on AIH and male subfertility. Bordeaux, 1978.

Bartak V (1971) Sperm velocity test in clinical practice. Int J Fertil 16: 107.

Bunge RG (1973) Caffeine stimulation of ejaculated human spermatozoa. Urology 1: 371.

Bygdeman M, Fredericsson B, Svanborg K, Samuelsson B (1970) The relation between fertility and prostaglandin content of seminal fluid in man. Fertil Steril 21: 622.

Cohen MS, Colin MJ, Golimbu M, Hotchkiss RS (1977) The effects of prostaglandins on sperm motility. Fertil Steril 28: 78.

Collier JG, Flower RJ, Stanton SL (1975) Seminal prostaglandins in infertile men. Fertil Steril 26: 868.

Cooper TG, Orgebin-Crist MD (1975) The effect of epididymal and testicular fluid on the fertilizing capacity of testicular and epididymal spermatozoa. Andrologia 7: 85.

Damas J, Deby C (1974) Libération de prostaglandines par la bradykinine chez le rat. C R Soc Biol 168: 375.

Drevius LO (1971) The sperm rise test. J Reprod Fert 24: 427.

Duijn C van, Lierop JH van (1966) Effect of temperature on photosensitivity of spermatozoa. Nature 201: 5055.

Eliasson R, Lindholmer C (1972) Distribution and properties of spermatozoa in different fractions of split ejaculates. Fertil Steril 23: 252.

Eskin BA, Azarbal S, Sepic R, Slate WG (1973) In vitro responses of the spermatozoa-cervical mucus system treated with prostaglandin-F2x. Obstet Gynecol 41: 436.

Fair W, Clarke R, Wehner N (1972) A correlation of seminal polyamine levels and semen analysis in the human. Fertil Steril 23: 38.

Ferreira SH, Moncada S, Vane JR (1974) Prostaglandins and signs and symptoms of inflammation. In Robinson HJ, Vane JR, eds. Prostaglandin synthetase inhibitors, p 175. New York: Raven.

Fjallbrant B (1968) Interrelation between high levels of sperm antibodies, reduced penetration of cervical mucus by spermatozoa and sterility in men. Acta Obstet Gynecol Scand 47: 102.

Fritz H, Schiessler H, Schill WB, Tscheache H, Heimburger N, Wallner O (1975) Low molecular weight proteinase (acrosin) inhibitors from human and boar seminal plasma and spermatozoa and human cervical mucus: isolation, properties, and biological aspects. In Reich E, Rifkin DB, Shaw E, eds. Proteases and biological control; Cold Spring Harbor Laboratory.

Gadden P (1968) Sperm maturation in the male reproductive tract: development of motility. Anat Rec 161: 471.

Garbers DL, First NL, Sullivan JT, Lardy HA (1971) Stimulation and maintenance of ejaculated bovine spermatozoa respiration and motility by caffeine. Biol Reprod 5: 336.

Gryglewski RJ (1974) Structure–activity relationships of some prostaglandin synthetase inhibitors. In Robinson HJ, Vane JR, eds. Prostaglandin synthetase inhibitors, p 33. New York: Raven.

Haesungcharern A, Chulavatnatol M (1973) Stimulation of human spermatozoal motility by caffeine. Fertil Steril 27: 662.

Harrison RF (1978) Insemination of husband's semen with and without addition of caffeine. Fertil Steril 29: 532.

Harrison RF, Sheppard BL, Kaliszer M (1980) Observations on the motility, ultrastructure and elemental composition of human spermatozoa incubated with caffeine. Andrologia 12: 34.

Hawkins DF (1967) In Ramwell PW, Shaw JE, eds) Symposium of the Worcester foundation for experimental biology, p 1. New York: Interscience.

Hicks JJ, Pedron N, Martinez-Manautoi J, Rosado A (1972a) Metabolic changes in human spermatozoa related to capacitation. Fertil Steril 23: 172.

Hicks JJ, Pedron N, Rosado A (1972b) Modifications of human spermatozoa glycolysis by cyclic adenosine monophosphate (cAMP), estrogens and follicular fluid. Fertil Steril 23: 886.

Hoskins DD, Casillas ER (1975) Function of cyclic nucleotides in mammalian spermatozoa. In Greepro L, Astwood EB, eds. Handbook of physiology, vol 5, sect 7: Endocrinology of the reproductive system: male. Washington DC: American Physiological Society.

Huacuja L, Sosa A, Delgrado NM, Rosado A (1973) Kinetic study of the participation of zinc in human spermatozoa metabolism. Life Sci 13: 1383.

Hunt WL, Zaneveld LJD: Prostaglandin effects on sperm penetration of cervical mucus. Presented at the International Conference of Andrology, Detroit, 1975.

Huxley HE (1969) Mechanism of muscular contraction. Science 164: 1356.

Jungling ML, Bunge RG (1976) The treatment of spermatogenic arrest with arginine. Fertil Steril 27: 282.

Keller DW, Polakoski KL (1975) L-arginine stimulation of human sperm motility in vitro. Biol Reprod 13: 154.

Krampitz G, Doepfmer R (1962) Determination of free aminoacids in human ejaculate by ion exchange chromatography. Nature 194: 684.

Kroeks M, Kremer J (1977) The pH in the lower third of the genital tract. In Insler V, Bettendorf G, eds. The uterine cervix in reproduction, p 109. Stuttgart: Thieme.

Leidl W, Prinzen R, Schill W-B, Fritz H (1975) The effect of kallikrein on motility and metabolism of spermatozoa in vitro. In Haberland GL, Rohen JW, Schirren C, Huber P,eds. Kininogenases, kallikrein: 2nd symposium on physiological properties and pharmacological rationale, p 33. Stuttgart: Schattauer.

MacLeod J (1951) Semen quality in 1,000 men of known fertility and 800 of infertile marriages. Fertil Steril 2: 115.

MacLeod J, Freund M (1958) Influence of spermatozoa concentration and initial fructose level on fructolysis of human semen. J Appl Physiol 13: 501.

Mann T (1964) Biochemistry of semen and of the male reproductive tract; 2nd edn. New York: John Wiley.

Marrazzi MA, Matschinsky M (1972) Properties of 15-hydroxyprostaglandin dehydrogenase: structural requirements for binding prostaglandins 1: 373.

Marsh JM, LeMaire WJ (1974) Cyclic AMP accumulation and steroidogenesis in the human corpus luteum: effect of gonadotropins and prostaglandins. J Clin Endocrinol Metab 39: 99.

Mitchell J, Nelson L, Hafez ESE (1976) Motility of spermatozoa. In: Hafez ESE, ed. Human semen infertility regulation in men. St Louis: Mosby.

Nevo A (1966) Relations between motility and respiration in human spermatozoa. Rep Fert 16: 351.

Newton AA, Rothschild L (1961) Energy-rich phosphate compounds in bull semen: comparison of their metabolism with anaerobic heat production and impedance change frequency. Proc Royal Soc Lond (Biol) 155: 183.

Norman C, Goldberg E, Porterfield I (1962) The effect of visible radiation on the functional life span of mammalian and avian sperm. Exp Cell Res 28: 69.

Palm S, Fritz H (1975) Kinases in cervical mucus and seminal plasma. In Haberland GL, Rohen JW, Schirren C, Huber P, eds. Kininogenases, Kallikrein: second symposium on physiological properties and pharmacological rationale. Stuttgart: Schattauer.

Palm S, Schill W-B, Wallner O, Prinzen R, Fritz H (1976) Occurrence of components of the kallikrein–kinin system in human genital tract secretions and their possible function in stimulation of sperm motility and migration. In Sicuteri F, Back A, Haberland GL, eds. Kinins: pharmacodynamics and biological roles, p 271 New York: Plenum.

Paulson JD, Parrish RF, Polakoski KL (1979) Comparative synthetic substitute kinetics of porcine acrosin and porcine beta-trypsin. Int J Biochem 10: 247.

Paulson JD, Harrison R, Schill WB, Barkay J (1981) Addition of pharmacological substances to the ejaculate. In Emperaire JC, Audebert A, Hazez ESE, eds. Clinics of Andrology, vol 1, Homologous artificial insemination (AIH), p 71. The Hague: Martinus Nijhoff.

Pedersen H (1970) Observations of the axial filament complex of the human spermatozoon. J Ultrastructure 33: 451.

Petersen RN, Freund M (1970) ATP synthesis and oxidative metabolism in human spermatozoa. Biol Reprod 3: 47.

Petersen RN, Freund M (1973) Effects of H^+ and certain membrane-active drugs on glycolysis, motility and ATP. Biol Reprod 8: 350.

Polakoski K, Zaneveld L (1977) Biochemical examination of the human ejaculate. In: Hafez ESE, ed. Techniques of human andrology, p 265. Amsterdam: North-Holland, Biomedical Press.

Polakoski KL, Zahler WL, Paulson JD (1977) Demonstration of proacrosin and quantitation of acrosin in ejaculated human spermatozoa. Fertil Steril 28: 688.

Poulos A, White I (1973) Phospholipid composition of human spermatozoa and seminal plasma. J Reprod Fertil 35: 265.

Ramwell P, Shaw H (1970) The biological significance of the prostaglandins. Ann NY Acad Sci 180: 10.

Rosado A, Hicks JJ, Reyes A, Blanco J (1974) Capacitation in vitro of rabbit spermatozoa with cyclic adenosine monophosphate and human follicular fluid. Fertil Steril 25: 82.

Rosado A, Huacuja L, Delgardo N, Pancardo R (1976) Cyclic AMP receptors in the human spermatozoa membrane. Life Sci 17: 1707.

Schachter A, Goldman JA, Zuckerman Z (1973) Treatment of oligospermia with the amino acid arginine. J Urol 110: 311.

Schill, W-B (1975a) Increased fructolysis of kallikrein-stimulated human spermatozoa. Andrologia 7: 105.

Schill W-B (1975b) Stimulation of sperm motility by kinins in fresh and 24 hours aged human ejaculates. Andrologia 7: 135.

Schill W-B (1975c) Caffeine and kallikrein-induced stimulation of human sperm motility: a comparative study. Andrologia 7: 229.

Schill W-B (1975d) Influence of the kallikrein–kinin system on human sperm motility in vitro. In Haberland GL, Rohen JW, Schirren C, Huber P (eds.) Kininogenase, second symposium on physiological properties and pharmacological rationale: kallikrein. Stuttgart: Schattauer.

Schill W-B (1977) Kallikrein as a therapeutical means in the treatment of male infertility. In Haberland GL, Rohen JW, Suzuki T, eds. Kininogenases, 4th symposium on physiological properties and pharmacological rationale: kallikrein p 251. Stuttgart: Schattauer.

Schill W-B (1978) Effect of kallikrein on the motility of fresh and frozen human semen. Presented to the 1st International Symposium on AIH and male subfertility, Bordeaux.

Schill W-B, Haberland GL (1974a) Kinin-induced enhancement of sperm motility. Hoppe-Seyler's Z Physiol Chem 355: 299.

Schill W-B, Haberland GL (1974b) In vitro stimulation of human sperm motility by kallikrein. World Cong Fertil Steril 8: 153.

Schill W-B, Preissler G (1977) Improvement of cervical mucus spermatozoal penetration by kinins: a possible therapeutical approach in the treatment of male subfertility. In Insler V, Bettendorf G, eds. The uterine cervix in reproduction, p 134. Stuttgart: Georg Thieme.

Schill W-B, Pritsch W (1976) Kinin-induced enhancement of sperm motility in cryopreserved human spermatozoa. Proc Int Congress Animal Reprod Artif Insemination 8: 1071.

Schill W-B, Pritsch W, Preissler G (1979) Effect of caffeine and kallikrein on cryopreserved human spermatozoa. Int J Fertil 24: 27.

Schill W-B, Braun-Falco O, Haberland GL (1974) The possible role of kinins in sperm motilities. Int J Fertil 19: 163.

Schill W-B, Leidl W, Prinzen R, Wallner O (1975) Stimulation of sperm motility and sperm metabolism by kallikrein, a kinin-liberating proteinase. Proc European Sterility Congres 4: 375.

Schill W-B, Wallner O, Palm S, Fritz H (1976) Kinin stimulation of spermatozoa motility and migration in cervical mucus. In Hafez ESE, ed. Human semen and fertility regulation in men, p 442. St Louis: Mosby.

Schirren C (1975) Experimental studies on the influence of kallikrein on human sperm motility in vitro. In Haberland GL, Rohen JW, Schirren C, Huber P, eds. Kininoginases, kallikrein, 2nd symposium on physiological properties and pharmacological rationale, p 59. Stuttgart: Schattauer.

Schoenfeld C, Amelar RD, Dubin L (1973) Stimulation of ejaculated human spermatozoa by caffeine: a preliminary report. Fertil Steril 24: 772.

Schoenfeld C, Amelar RD, Dubin L (1975) Stimulation of ejaculated human spermatozoa by caffeine. Fertil Steril 26: 158.

Steiner R, Hofmann N, Hartmann R (1977) The influence of kallikrein on the velocity of human spermatozoa measured by Laser-Doppler spectroscopy In Haberland GL, Rohen JW, Suzuki T, eds. Kininogenases, kallikrein: 4th symposium on physiological properties and pharmacological rationale, p 229, Stuttgart: Schattauer.

Tash JA, Mann FRC (1973) Adenosine 3'5' cyclic monophosphate in relation to motility and senescence of spermatozoa. Proc Royal Soc Lond (Biol) 184: 109.

Ulstein M (1972) Sperm penetration of cervical mucus as a criterion of male fertility. Acta Obstet Gynecol Scand 51: 335.

Ulstein M (1973) Fertility of donors at heterologous insemination. Acta Obstet Gynecol Scand 52: 97.

Wallner O, Schill W-B, Brosser A, Fritz H (1975) Participation of the kallikrein–kinin system in sperm penetration through cervical mucus: in vitro studies. In Haberland GL, Rohen JW, Schirren C, Huber P, eds Kininogenases, kallikrein; 2nd symposium on physiological properties and pharmacological rationale, p. 63. Stuttgart: Schattauer.

Wolf P, Blasco L, Khan MA, Litt M (1977) Human cervical mucus II: changes in viscoelasticity during the ovulatory menstrual cycle. Fertil Steril 28: 48.

Zaneveld L, Polakoski K (1977) Collection and the physical examination of the ejaculate. In Hafez ESE, ed. Techniques in human andrology, p 159. Amsterdam: North-Holland Biomedical Press.

Author's address:
Dr J.D. Paulson
4801 Kenmore Avenue
Alexandria, VA 22304, USA

20. AIH IN OLIGOZOOSPERMIC MEN

K. USTAY

Biological and clinical aspects of the sperm–cervix interaction have been extensively studied (Davajan et al., 1970; Hafez, 1973; Hartman, 1963; Kurzrock and Miller, 1928; Marcus and Marcus, 1963, 1965, 1975; Moghissi et al., 1964; Moghissi and Neuhaus, 1966; Moghissi, 1972; Southam and Buxton, 1956, 1957; Schwimmer et al., 1967).

Artificial insemination is unsuccessful with oligozoospermic patients. As cervical mucus is an important factor in infertility, mixing semen with cervical mucus may increase the success of artificial insemination. Most infertile couples have more than one contributing factor causing their infertility. The cervical factor is one of the most common, yet least studied and sometimes even ignored by the physician.

In husbands with oligozoospermia, insemination can be successful, provided the wife does not have any cervical problems. To study cervical mucus in infertile couples requires extensive hormonal and immunological tests which are still restricted to only a few research centers around the world (Davajan et al., 1970; Hartman, 1963; Nakamura et al., 1973). In most cases the psychological stress of the recipient of insemination may cause failure. This psychological factor may alter the hormonal status of the women, prevent ovulation and may cause hormonal changes as well as alter the daily characteristics of the cervical mucus.

1. SEMEN ANALYSIS

Four grades of semen characteristics have been recognized: Grade I indicates the semen is good and the patient is fertile. The minimum requirements for these semen are: sperm count (above 40.10^6 ml), motility (above 70% in the first hour) morphology (about 70% normal sperm), pH ($7.7 - 8.1$), liquefaction (10-20 min), no sign of infection and no agglutination.

Grade II semen indicates that the patient is subfertile, yet still has an opportunity for treating fertility. Artificial insemination by husband (AIH) is not performed with this grade. The standards are: sperm count ($20 \times 10^6 - 40 \times 10^6$ per ml), motility (above 40% in the first hour), morphology (about 50% or more normal), and all other standards similar to grade I.

Grade III indicates a lesser chance for improved fertility. If treatment is unsuccessful, artificial insemination can then be performed. The standards are: sperm count (about $5 \times 10^6 - 20 \times 10^6$ per ml), motility (between 15% and 30%), morphology (about 50% or more normal), and all other standards similar to grade I.

Grade IV indicates azoospermia when there is no possibility of pregnancy even when insemination is attempted. Before any insemination is performed from grade III men, a complete evaluation of hormonal status, anatomical and pathophysiological condition is made. The following examinations are performed; a) No signs of infection are allowed. All normal semen contain 3, 4 leukocytes per each high power field (HPF) but leukocytes above 10 per HPF require further investigation of semen cultures. b) These patients undergo the following hormonal studies: FSH, LH, Testosterone, and Prolactin. Should treatment prove unsuccessful, the semen is then used for insemination.

Prior to insemination, the wife should be carefully examined for proven fertility using several tests. The ovulation status is determined either by endometrial biopsy, serial vaginal hormonal smears or weekly FSH and LH determinations.

Tubal patency is tested by hysterosalpingography or laparoscopy. The cervical mucus is examined. The day of ovulation is determined either by BBT

Hafez ESE & Semm K (Eds) Instrumental insemination.
© *1982 Martinus Nijhoff Publishers, The Hague/Boston/London. ISBN 90-247-2530-5. Printed in the Netherlands.*

150

or daily urinary LH in at least two consecutive cycles prior to insemination.

2. TYPES OF INSEMINATION

2.1. Six types of insemination are used:

1. *Intrauterine insemination* is very seldom performed. Without cervical mucus, there is little success for the insemination. This type can be used in cases of cervical amputation only. No more than 0.2 ml of semen is placed into the uterine cavity. Otherwise, the uterus will contract, expel the semen and the patient will have severe abdominal cramps, sometimes accompanied with nausea and vomiting. It is also possible to introduce an infection into the uterine cavity which may follow with fever or even more serious complications.

2. *Paracervical insemination* is used more often. About 0.3 to 0.4 ml of semen is slowly deposited through the cervical os.

3. *Intracervical insemination* is seldom used. Insemination is performed slowly and semen is injected (about 1.5 – 2 cm) inside the cervical canal.

4. *Intravaginal insemination* is performed into the posterior fornix of the vagina where 2 to 3 ml of semen is deposited. A seminal pool is formed in the posterior vaginal fornix and the cervical column dips into the pool while the patient is lying in lithotomy position.

5. *Cervical cap insemination:* About 2 to 3 ml of semen are placed into a cervical cap then tightly placed into the cervix.

6. *Cervical adapter insemination.* A special type of adapter is used. Once a vacuum is formed within the cervix, the adapter is tightly fitted and from a second tubing, semen is injected into the cervix. This adapter remains in place for 2 or 3 days, and insemination is repeated each day.

3. SEMEN CONCENTRATION

The entire ejaculate is collected and after liquefaction the container is spinned for 2 min at 200 rpm. The supernatant is discarded, a sperm count is made, the material is adjusted to 30.10^6 per ml with Man-Ringer solution, and used promptly for insemination.

3.1. Mixing cervical mucus with semen prior to insemination

Better results are obtained if the semen used for artificial insemination is mixed with the cervical mucus prior to insemination. On the day of insemination the cervix is first dry-cleaned then the cervical mucus is aspirated (as much as 700 mg on days of ovulation) with a plastic needle gauge 16, or the cover sheath of the cardiac catheter to 5 ml syringe. Immediately thereafter, about 0.3 ml of newly masturbated split or concentrated ejaculate is aspirated into the same syringe. Within 2 min a sufficient mixture is obtained and is then slowly injected into the paracervical cavity. The cervical cap or a diaphragm is placed in the cervix and the patient remains in lithotomy position for 20 min.

4. CERVICAL MUCUS EXCHANGE

A poor postcoital test may result in patients with oligozoospermia. Poor cervical mucus may result from anatomical and pathophysiological defects (Davajan et al., 1970). The quality of the mucus may alter in patients with cervicitis. The pathophysiological defects caused by glycoproteins, enzymes and immunoglobulins due to hormonal disturbances, infections and surgical interventions, may interfere with sperm penetration in cervical mucus. Exchange of cervical mucus from another woman may help lessen this problem.

This can be performed by fertile young women donors with the same blood group and Rh factor. Both menstrual cycles are manipulated by hormones to coincide so that ovulation occurs on the same day. On the day of ovulation, the cervical mucus is aspirated and discarded from the recipient whose post-coital test is poor. The donor's cervical mucus is then aspirated and mixed with the split ejaculate or concentrated semen which is then injected into the cervix of the recipient. Inseminations are performed on three successive days around ovulation time. The exchange of cervical mucus is a new technique, but results so far are promising.

5. CERVICAL MUCUS –
SEMEN MIXTURE INSEMINATIONS

A total of 618 couples with oligozoospermic husbands were screened for this study which lasted for six years. Only 80 couples were good candidates (Table 1). Post-coital tests were performed on the cervical mucus in vitro with a good donor specimen. The following results were obtained with mixed insemination (semen + cervical mucus).

1) Inseminations were continuously performed monthly. The average months necessary for conception to occur were as follows: one month for one patient, 2–4 months for 12, 5–8 months for 11, 9–10 months for 7, 11–12 months for 2, 15–16 months for 1 and no conception occurred in 46 of the patients.

Table 1. Patients studied and their reproductive potential.

Parameters		
Years of marriage	Years	Couples
	1	8
	2	12
	3–5	14
	5–8	23
	8–10	16
	10–14	7
Age of wives	Years	Women
	22–25	18
	25–30	46
	30–35	10
	35–40	6
Sperm count of husbands	per ml	Men
	$10.10^6 - 15.10^6$	28
	$5.10^6 - 10.10^6$	38
	$1.10^6 - 5.10^6$	12
Post-coital test		Women
	Satisfactory	78
	Poor	2

2) Ejaculate type: From the 36 patients who were able to conceive, 26 were by split ejaculate and 8 were by using concentrated sperm.

3) Out of the 80 inseminated patients, the split ejaculate technique was used on patients with sperm counts above 10 million per ml. Out of 38 men with sperm counts between 5 and 10 million per ml, 22 used the split ejaculate technique; while the remaining 16, along with 12 others with sperm counts below 5 million per ml, used concentrated semen for inseminations. Out of 50 patients inseminated by split ejaculate semen, 26 conceived; whereas, only 8 out of 28 patients inseminated with concentrated semen conceived. Two patients were lost to follow-up.

4) The control group consisted of 38 oligozoospermic infertile couples who were inseminated using either split ejaculate (20) or concentrated sperm (18) without mixing of semen with cervical mucus.

From the control group, it took 2–4 months of inseminations for one patient to conceive, 5–8 months for 4 patients, 9–10 months for one and 11–12 months for 2. A total of 30 patients did not conceive. From the 8 patients who did conceive, 6 were by the split ejaculate technique and 2 were by concentrated semen.

CONCLUDING REMARKS

A pregnancy rate of 52% was obtained by using the split ejaculate technique for AIH and 28% by using concentrated sperm mixture of cervical mucus and semen. By using ordinary insemination techniques, the pregnancy rate ranged from 11 to 30%. Results with cervical mucus exchange are promising and further studies are needed.

REFERENCES

Davajan V, Nakamura RM, Karma K (1970) Spermatozoan transport in cervical mucus. Obstet Gynec Survey 25: 1.

Grant A (1958) Cervical hostility. Fertil Steril 9: 321.

Hafez ESE (1973) Hystology and microstructure of the cervical epithelial secretory system. In Elstein M, Moghissi KS, Borth R, eds. Cervical mucus in human reproduction. World Health Organization Colloquium, Geneva 1972. Copenhagen: Skriptor.

Hartman CG (1963) Mechanisms concerned with conception. New York: Pergamon Press.

Kurzrock R, Miller EG Jr (1928) Biochemical studies of human semen and its relation to mucus of cervix uteri. Am J Obstet Gynec 15: 56.

Marcus CC, Marcus SL (1975) The cervical factor. In Behrman SJ, Kistner RW, eds. Progress in infertility. Boston: Little, Brown.

Marcus CC, Marcus SL (1965) The cervical factor in infertility. Clin Obstet and Gynec, 8: 15.

Marcus CC, Marcus SL (1963) Cervical mucus and its relation to infertility. Obstet Gynec Survey 18: 749.

Moghissi KS, Dabich D, Levine J, Neuhaus OW (1964) Mechanism of sperm migration. Fertil Steril 15: 15.

Moghissi KS, Neuhaus OW (1966) Cyclic changes of cervical mucus proteins. Am J Obstet Gynec 96: 91.

Moghissi KS (1973) Semen migration through the cervix. In Elstein M, Moghissi KS, Borth R, eds. Cervical mucus in human reproduction. World Health Organization Colloquium, Geneva 1972. Copenhagen: Skriptor.

Nakamura RM, Davajan V, Saga M, Allerton SE (1973) Salient biological properties of cervical mucus. In Elstein M, Moghissi KS, Borth R, eds. Cervical mucus in human reproduction. World Health Organization Colloquium, Geneva 1972. Copenhagen: Skriptor.

Southam AL, Buxton L (1956) Seventy postcoital tests made during the conception cycle. Fertil Steril 7: 133.

Southam A, Buxton CL (1957) Factors influencing reproductive potential. Fertil Steril 8: 25.

Schwimmer WB, Ustay KA, Behrman SJ (1967) An evaluation of immunological factors of infertility. Fertil Steril 18: 167.

Author's address:
Dr K. Ustay
Department of Obstetrics Gynecology
Hacettepe School of Medicine
Ankara, Turkey

21. AIH USING SPLIT EJACULATE AND CAP INSEMINATION

N.L. STAHL

1. INTRODUCTION

Characteristics of the split ejaculate have long been recognized. MacCloud and Hotchkiss described the characteristics of the split ejaculate for the first time in 1942. This have been repeated by others (McDonough, 1979). Characteristically, the split ejaculate contains most of the viable motile sperm in the first impulse. This has led to investigations into the possibility of improving sperm density by using the first impulse of the ejaculate for homologous insemination in infertile couples.

In 1965, the Mylex Company introduced the Mylex™ Insemination Cup to facilitate artificial insemination by providing a vehicle whereby the sperm could be introduced against the cervix without exposure to the hostile vaginal environment. This chapter describes the combination of these techniques in an effort to achieve pregnancy in infertile couples.

2. TECHNIQUES OF SPLIT EJACULATE COLLECTION

2.1. Methods for collection

For split ejaculate insemination, the couple is instructed to obtain a semen specimen approximately one hour prior to the appointment for insemination. A masturbatory semen collection is required and the wife is encouraged to participate in this attempt if appropriate in their relationship.

2.2. Adequacy of splitting

In judging the adequacy of splitting the specimen, there sould be at least a one of five volume differential in the two specimens. This is also

confirmed by finding most of the viable motile sperm in the first collection and few viable sperm in the second portion. It is also necessary to keep the semen specimens warm during the trip to the office.

2.3. Examination of specimens

Upon arrival, both containers are examined to determine sperm density in a rough manner. On rare occasions, the sperm are all present in the second impulse rather than the first. In those instances, a different method of splitting is recommended. By trial and error, the optimum splitting is determined to obtain concentration of the semen. In most instances this represents a 50–50 split to give all the concentrated motile sperm in the last portion of the sample. On rare occasions, there is no difference in the sperm density or motility in the two specimens. In these instances, there is no advantage to split ejaculate techniques.

3. THE INSEMINATION CUP

3.1. Method of insertion

The cup that is currently recommended for insemination is manufactured by Mylex and comes in various sizes. Instruction in patient removal is very simple and seems to present no problem, and techniques for insertion are simple. With the usual patient, depression of the perineum allows the rounded end of the cup to be easily inserted into the vagina. This is then advanced by digital pressure and in most instances, a tactile sensation that it has slipped over the cervix is obtained. The adequacy of the position is always checked by using a speculum to visualize the Mylex cup in position. This is assured by seeing the cervical os through the Mylex

Hafez ESE & Semm K (Eds) Instrumental insemination.

cup. Although some authors have recommended the teaching of self-capping techniques (Whitlow, 1979) so that the couples may do the insemination procedure at home, it is found that this is not as satisfactory as using physician placement. Even with much experience utilizing this technique, improper cup position will be found with the cup either anterior or posterior to the cervix.

Using the syringe provided, the appropriate specimen is inserted through the tube of the cup and the ball is seated at the end of the tube by the cup.

3.2. Instructions for patient removal

The patient is then, on the first insemination procedure, returned to the office in one hour for a post-insemination test and at this time, instructions are given to her for removal. The patient removes the cup under supervision to ascertain that she can complete the process. Removal is easily accomplished with slight downward traction on the stem with digital self-examination and breaking the suction by reaching over the rim of the cup, the cup can then be easily removed. The instruction section for removal is included for each of the insemination cups.

Once this technique has been taught, the patient then on subsequent inseminations can be allowed to remove the cup herself at home at her convenience. It is recommended that this be left in place for one or two hours, but the cup is comfortable and causes no problems if left in place for up to ten hours.

3.3. Care of the Insemination Cup

The cup is removed in subsequent cycles by the patient, cleaned with pure water — no detergents — and is reuseable by the same patient for a prolonged period of time.

4. INSEMINATION TECHNIQUES AND TIMING OF INSEMINATION

4.1. Methods for determination of ovulation

The patient, on the appropriate day of her cycle based upon either history or evaluation of the cervical mucus or basal body temperature charts, is inseminated every other day for two times. On rare occasions, it is helpful to inseminate three times when there is trouble determining the appropriate time in the cycle or the cycle is variable. The couple is instructed not to have intercourse the day prior to, or the day of, in semination on each occasion. In dealing with oligozoospermic males however, it seems better to lessen the number of ejaculates around the times that fertilization is atempted.

It is good practice to always do a post-insemination test the first time that a split ejaculate insemination is attempted. The procedure is truly indicated if you have a marked improvement in the post-coital test with a post-insemination test and seems to be superfluous if you do not have such improvement in the number of motile sperm in the mucus.

Prior to the insemination, no other female factors of infertility should have been identified. It is wise to check during the early portions of the semination program that the procedure itself has not caused anovulatory cycles. This is easily done by having the patient return in one week for a mid-luteal phase serum progesterone.

5. ADDING SURFACE TENSION LOWERING AGENTS

5.1. Benefits of using Alevaire[R]

One of the advantages of using the Mylex insemination cups is that one may use other agents to help sperm motility in the sperm concentration. It is very helpful to use a surface tension lowering agent along with the split specimens to improve sperm concentration in the mucus. Early in the utilization of this technique, the effectiveness of Alevaire in improving cervical mucus sperm penetration was apparent. In the first several patients using this technique, on alternate months the split ejaculate technique was used without Alevaire and with Alevaire. Subsequently, Alevaire has been used in each treatment cycle. It appears not to influence adversely the effectiveness of the technique and based upon observation of increased sperm density in the mucus, may be helpful. Alevaire is no longer manufactured however, and it will require further study to determine which of the other available surface tension lowering agents can be safely used without harm.

6. ALTERNATIVES TO CUP INSEMINATION

6.1. Patient vs physician insemination

There are those who advocate that this technique may be taught to couples so that the husbands can carry out the insemination procedure at home with the wife inserting the cup. The husband can then insert the sperm with the syringe containing his split ejaculate specimen. Although this is certainly less expensive for the couple, the safeguards of making sure of absolute positive placement are not obtained under these circumstances. However for those patients in whom office insemination is not economically or logistically feasible, this may be a reasonable alternative.

6.2. Coital techniques

The other alternative to the split ejaculate cup insemination is the technique of split ejaculate coitus which has been claimed to improve fertility potential. This was offered to patients on several occasions and it was found that the placement of the split ejaculate into the posterior fornix during intercourse in difficult. Most of the couples returned to the office requesting a return to the cup insemination method once they have attempted this coital technique.

7. PATIENT SELECTION

7.1 Indications for AIH

Patient selection is apparently the most controversial portion of this chapter. Many authors will take exception to the liberal indications suggested for this technique. Review of the literature shows that split ejaculate technique for the inseminations include oligozoospermia, hypervolemia, and poor motility as indications for the split technique. The insemination of whole ejaculate or otherwise collected semen is recommended in the case of retrograde ejaculation, hypospadia, hyperspermia and

displacement of the cervix. All these indications were used for split ejaculate insemination as well as a group that is considered to be "no reason infertility". In this group of "no reason" infertile couples, no abnormalities are found in the complete evaluations of the female and the male.

It certainly goes without saying that if there are other female reasons for infertility, these should be corrected prior to attempting split ejaculate insemination techniques. If there are reasons that can be determined for the decreased fertility potential in the male, correction of the reasons should be done prior to utilization of the split ejaculate technique.

8. REVIEW OF THE LITERATURE

Results of studies range from no improvement in fertility with the split ejaculate technique all the way to a 40% success rate using split ejaculate techniques (Table 1). Fetal wastage was increased in some studies and non-existent in others.

9. CONCLUDING REMARKS

The fertility potential of a couple is based upon many variables. One of the important variables is proper sperm density presented to the appropriately prepared cervical mucus. It appears that the use of the cup for insemination using a split ejaculate semen specimen can in some instances allow a better sperm density to be applied to the cervical mucus. Further, the cup use allows other manipulations such as the addition of surface tension lowering agents to improve the chances of preg-

Table 1. Results reported with split ejaculate insemination.

Author	No. of patients	% of pregnancy
Whitlow*	87	13
Nunley	53	21
Dmowski**	27	15
Coucke	143	27
Taymor	57	30
Moghissi	62	24
Stahl***	50	36

*   Using self-capping
**   Polyzoospermia
*** Author's ongoing series

nancy. There seems to be little doubt that the male with hypervolemia can have his fertility potential improved by the use of split ejaculate techniques. There is some controversy about those patients with oligozoospermia or decreased motility, but it is believed there is little doubt that a better sperm density can be achieved using split ejaculate techniques in many of these patients.

It has been suggested that many times this does not improve the overall fertility rate, but perhaps only decreases the time necessary for the achieving of conception in some patients, especially those with "no reason infertility". It is not believed that there is any evidence that this technique, except on rare occasions, may cause a worsening effect of the fertility potential. There may be some patients in whom artificially attempting conception may be so psychologically traumatic that pregnancy does not occur. These patients should be identified and eliminated from this technique.

The end result for the couple who does achieve pregnancy is the same whether the split ejaculate technique or normal coitus is used — that is, a couple who desires a child can achieve that end. This is after all the purpose in the practice of infertility.

REFERENCES

Coucke W, Steeno O (1979) Pregnancy rate after homologous insemination. Arch Androl 2: 73.

Dmowski WP, Gaynor L, Lawrence M, Ramaa R, Scommegna A (1979) Artifical insemination homologous with oligospermic semen separated on albumin columns. Fertil Steril 31: 58.

MacLeod J, Hotchkiss RS (1942) The distribution of spermatozoa and of certain chemical constituents in human ejaculate. J Urol 48: 225.

Moghissi KS, Gruber JS, Evans S, Yanes J (1977) Homologous artificial insemination: a reappraisal. Am J Obstet gynecol 129: 909.

Nunley WC Jr, Kitchin JA, Thiagarajah S (1978) Homologous insemination. Fertil Steril 30: 150.

Stahl NL: Unpublished data.

Steinman RP, Taymor ML (1977) Artificial insemination homologous and its role in the management of infertility. Fertil Steril 28: 146.

Whitlow JS (1979) The cervical cup self-applied in the treatment of severe oligospermia. Fertil Steril 31: 86.

Author's address:
Dr N.L. Stahl
Department of Obstetrics and Gynecology University of Tennessee
Center for the Health Sciences;
Clinical Education Center;
Chattanooga, TN 37403, USA

22. IMPROVED FERTILITY RESULTS WITH SPLIT EJACULATE INSEMINATION AND IMPROVED CERVICAL MUCUS

J.H. Check

Infertility problems have been conveniently divided into male factor, ovulatory factor, cervical factor, and tubal factor. However, frequently the problem in conception involves a combination of several of these factors. Furthermore, occasionally the correction of one factor leads to worsening of another factor.

The split ejaculate insemination is one method of improving the male factor. A count of 20×10^6 with 65% motility achieved via the split ejaculate may be considered normal. However, if there is inadequate sperm survival in the mucus, then either the semen must be improved further or the mucus must be enhanced.

This chapter will describe methods to improve the success of split ejaculate inseminations by emphasizing the interrelationships of the male, cervical, and ovulatory factors. Evidence will be provided for a new technique aimed at accomplishing these goals by treating ovulatory defects in normoprolactinemic women with bromocryptine in conjunction with split ejaculate insemination. In contrast to clomiphene citrate, bromocryptine improves ovulation without adversely affecting cervical mucus. This results in improved fertility when inseminating borderline quality sperm achieved by split ejaculate insemination.

1. THE SPLIT EJACULATE

Splitting the ejaculate into two portions (approximately 1/3 of the total in the first portion and 2/3 in the second) is a common fertility technique. In the majority of samples evaluated the first portion is significantly improved compared to the entire specimen (Amelar et al., 1965). In a minority of cases the portions are equal or the second portion is superior to the first. Improved fertility results have been

suggested by a withdrawal intercourse technique (Amelar et al., 1975). However, there are many advantages to inseminating the better portion.

The main advantage of insemination is that the semen is guaranteed in reaching the cervical os. In contrast, because of the lowered volume, sperm–cervix contact may not occur with the withdrawal technique. Another advantage is that direct insemination bypasses the hostile vaginal environment. This may be especially important for already weakened sperm.

2. OTHER METHODS OF IMPROVING THE SEMEN

If splitting the ejaculate does not result in an adequate spermogram, then other therapies may be tried in conjunction with the split. A varicocele should be sought and if present, varicocelectomy can be performed (Charney, 1962; Dubin et al., 1976; Tulloch, 1955). Alternatively, the varicocele-associated oligospermia may be treated medically with clomiphene citrate (Check, 1980).

Idiopathic oligospermia and asthenospermia has been treated with several drugs with varying success, including: clomiphene citrate (Check et al., 1977; Epstein, 1977; Paulson et al., 1976), various androgens (Brown, 1975; Check et al., 1977a; Giarola, 1974; Urry et al., 1976), human chorionic gonadotropins (Amelar et al., 1973), cyproheptadine (Segal et al., 1975), human menopausal gonadotropins (Davies, 1965; Lytton and Kase, 1966; MacLeod, 1970; Martin, 1967), testosterone rebound (Charny et al., 1978), and bromocryptine (Check, 1980a; Masala et al., 1979; Montanari et al., 1978; Nencioni et al., 1978; Saidi et al., 1977; Segal et al., 1979). There have also been attempts to improve the motility of the sperm prior to insemi-

Hafez ESE & Semm K (Eds) Instrumental insemination.
© *1982 Martinus Nijhoff Publishers, The Hague/Boston/London. ISBN 90-247-2530-5. Printed in the Netherlands.*

nation by treating with caffeine (Bunge, 1973; Haesungcharern and Chulavatnatol, 1973; Schoenfeld et al., 1975), or kallikrein (Schill, 1975). Some success in reducing an immunological factor with high doses of methylprednisolone has also been reported (Schulman et al., 1978).

3. IMPROVING THE CERVICAL MUCUS

Following AIH with the split ejaculate, the wife is asked to return two hours following the insemination to have the cervical mucus withdrawn to check sperm survival.

If a minimum of 3–5 sperm per high powered field with good linear progressive motion is not seen then attempts at improving the mucus are made even if the appearance appears adequate. Cervical mucus quality is judged by quantity, cellularity, clarity, spinnbarkeit, and ferning. The cervical factor has been nicely reviewed by Blasco (1977) and treatment includes low dose estrogen (Blasco, 1977), antibiotics (Blasco, 1977), cryosurgery (Blasco, 1977), baking soda douche (Blasco, 1977), donor cervical mucus (Check et al., 1977b), and high dose estrogens combined with human menopausal gonodatropins (Check, 1980b). Occasionally, condom therapy (Ansbacher et al., 1973) or high doses of glucocorticoids for a possible immunologic problem (Schulman et al., 1978a) can be employed.

Thus treatment of the cervical factor may be required only because of subfertile sperm in that normal semen might survive adequately. If semen is considered low normal and if everything has been done that is possible for the mucus, then therapy should be changed for the male to get the sperm to an even better quality.

4. OVULATION AND CERVICAL MUCUS

4.1. Anovulation itself as a cause of poor mucus

In some anovulatory states, e.g. polycystic ovarian disease, cervical mucus may be of good quality the entire cycle. However, in certain other anovulatory situations the cervical mucus is poor from one menses to the next. In this circumstance, the poor mucus is secondary to an altered hypothalamic–pituitary–ovarian axis resulting in inadequate cervical mucus. Simply correcting the anovulatory state results in good periovulatory mucus without any specific therapy aimed at correcting the mucus.

4.2. Clomiphene citrate and poor mucus

The frustrations of infertility related to a male factor problem may result in an anovulatory state in the wife (Check, 1978). Thus, it is very common to find in an infertile couple both a male factor problem and an ovulation defect. The most frequently employed drug for anovulation is clomiphene citrate. Unfortunately one of the side effects of this drug is a hostile cervical mucus secondary to the anti-estrogen nature of this drug. (Greenblatt et al., 1975). Frequently, this can be corrected by the addition of estrogen beginning the day after the clomiphene citrate is stopped up to the time of ovulation. However, when dealing with borderline semen quality, often times the addition of estrogen is insufficient to allow adequate sperm survival. This is even despite the intracervical insemination of the better portion of the split ejaculate.

If the mucus cannot be corrected then less potent ovulatory measures may be employed such as human chorionic gonadotropin (Bergman, 1958), glucorcorticoids (Greenblatt et al., 1956), or decreasing the clomiphene dose and adding glucocorticoids (Check et al., 1977c), or trying luteal phase support only with progesterone or 17-hydroxyprogesterone (Tho et al., 1979; Andrews, 1979). If these techniques are insufficient to induce ovulation, then the next conventional step would be the use of human menopausal gonadotropins (HMG) (Vande Wiele et al., 1965). Unfortunately, in view of its expense and potential risk of multiple births, HMG would not be available to the majority of patients.

4.3. Use of bromocryptine if hyperprolactinemia exists

Another way of overcoming the hostile mucus induced by clomiphene citrate would be by the use of bromocryptine which has no adverse effect on the cervical mucus. Conventionally, this treatment modality would only be employed if the serum prolactin was elevated (Del Pozo et al., 1972). Unfortunately, only a minority of anovulatory but menstruating women have elevated serum prolactins.

4.4. *Bromocryptine in normoprolactinemic women*

There have been a few case reports of ovulation induction with bromocryptine in women with normal serum prolactins (Seppala et al., 1976; Tolis and Naftolin, 1976; Van der Steeg et al., 1977) and even a couple pregnancies (Nencioni et al., 1978). However, this was challenged in a study by Croisignani et al., (1975) as being nothing more than a placebo. However, we now have accumulated 21 cases of pregnancies in normoprolactinemic women treated with bromocryptine who failed to conceive on other ovulation regimes because of the inability of the sperm to survive in the cervical mucus.

Bromocryptine and split ejaculate insemination. Of the 21 pregnancies achieved with bromocryptine treatment of the wives, there were nine pregnancies with associated male factor where part of the treatment of the husband required split ejaculate insemination. The patients selected all had an infertility duration greater than one year. In all cases clomiphene citrate was employed without success in achieving a pregnancy. Clomiphene was used for over five months in each case with two exceptions. Many patients had concomitant problems with endometriosis and tubal factor. They were started on 2.5 mg bromocryptine daily. If ovulation was not judged as adequate after two months treatment the dose was increased to 5 mg. If the endometrial biopsy or serum progesterone level were still too low, but yet indicative of probably ovulation, luteal phase support with 50 mg/day of progesterone suppositories was used. The nine pregnancies have occurred in a total of 22 couples tried on that treatment modality. The importance of these nine pregnancies is that these patients all represented couples who had many prior failures with other treatment modalities and conceived quickly on bromocryptine. In these cases the failures were related to hostile cervical mucus as a complication of clomiphene citrate. The other less potent ovulation therapies which allowed adequate

mucus were unable to successfully induce the appropriate ovulation response. A summary of the results on the nine pregnancy cases is seen in Table 1.

5. CASE REPORTS ILLUSTRATING CONCOMITANT TREATMENT OF MALE FACTOR AND CERVICAL FACTOR AND BROMOCRYPTINE TREATMENT OF OVULATION FACTOR

5.1. *Case I*

The couple had been trying to conceive for 6 years. Their infertility problem was secondary to an inadequate corpus luteum and oligospermia and asthenospermia. The mid-luteal phase serum progesterone was 7.9 ng/ml with an 11 day rise on the basal body temperature chart, and the endometrial biopsy taken three days prior to the menses dated day 19 of a 28 day cycle. The husband previously had an unsuccessful varicocelectomy. His baseline spermogram even with a split ejaculate showed a count of only 16×10^6, 45% motility grade 2 out of 10 in the better first portion. He was treated with clomiphene citrate 25 mg daily. His spermograms improved to an average of 30×10^6, 75% motility grade 8 after three months of treatment. One count increased to 72×10^6. The count remained increased for 20 months but no pregnancy was achieved. A summary of the ovulation and mucus treatments is seen in Table 2. The couple stopped all treatments and tried on their own for 9 cycles. The first portion of the ejaculate was now 12×10^6, 65% motility, grade 7. This time he did not respond to clomiphene. His semen did improve to 28×10^6, 75% motility, grade 8 in the first portion of the split ejaculate after 2 months on bromocryptine

Table 1. Fertility statistics on nine pregnancy cases with bromocryptine ovulation therapy and split ejaculate insemination.

1. Average infertility duration prior to therapy: 3.7 years
2. 5 cases anovulation; 4 cases inadequate corpus luteum
   a. based on endometrial biopsy dating at least 3 days early and/or serum progesterone in midluteal phase under 7
3. Average of 11.2 treatment cycles in our office before switching to bromocryptine.*
4. Average of 2.3 treatment cycles with bromocryptine before pregnancy achieved.
5. Average serum prolactin level was 11.0 ng/ml (2 patients had levels of 20.6 and 20.3 and two had levels of 4.3 and 6.8)
6. Average prolactin level when pregnancy achieved: 8.8 ng/ml
7. In 6 cases 2.5 mg bromocryptine used; 3 cases dose was 5 mg daily.

*The treatments during the unsuccessful cycles included clomiphene citrate with and without supplemental estrogen, low dose estrogen, tetracycline, baking soda douche, progesterone support of the luteal phase, HCG at mid-cycle, and human menopausal gonadotropins.

2.5 mg daily. The wife was started on bromocryptine 2.5 mg daily. Her baseline serum prolactin was 20.6 ng/ml. Her level dropped to 12.6 ng/ml after 6 weeks of treatment. A mid-luteal phase progesterone level on the second treatment cycle was 17.5. An endometrial biopsy taken four days prior to her menses on the third treatment cycle dated appropriately. A pregnancy was achieved on the fourth cycle.

5.2. Case II

The couple had been trying to conceive for 6 years. The etiology of their problem was related to oligospermia and asthenospermia, hostile cervical mucus, and anovulation. The husband's poor spermogram was not improved following varicocelectomy. However, treatment with clomiphene citrate 25 mg daily improved the count in the first portion of a split ejaculate to an average of 35 million/cm^3 with 70% having good linear progressive motion. The wife was first treated with DES 0.1 mg day 5 to 15, then 0.2 mg DES but there was no sperm survival two hours after the insemination of the first portion of the split ejaculate. The addition of tetracycline did allow good sperm survival but the serum progesterone level was only 5.4 ng/ml one week prior to her menses. Supplementation with progesterone suppositories 50 mg/day and HCG still failed to achieve a pregnancy. This was stopped after 6 cycles. The wife was now placed on clomiphene citrate 50 mg days 5 and 6 and 100 mg days 7–9 of her cycle with supplemental conjugated estrogens 2.5 mg daily until ovulation. The sperm survival was good but there was still evidence of an inadequate corpus luteum (luteal phase

only 10 days long; serum progesterone 6 days prior to menses 7.2 ng/ml). For the next six cycles progesterone suppositories 50 mg per day was used to supplement the luteal phase following clomiphene and premarin. Since no pregnancy occurred after six cycles the patient was switched to human menopausal gonadotropins. There was still evidence of inadequate luteal phases by duration of rise on temperature charts and serum progesterone levels. A serum prolactin level was 20.6 ng/ml. The patient was started on bromocryptine 2.5 mg daily. Repeat prolactin 2 months later was 9.6 ng/ml. The luteal phase now increased to 15 days with a mid-luteal progesterone level of 16.4 ng/ml. The patient conceived on her third treatment cycle with bromocryptine. She had 20 previous unsuccessful treatment cycles before switching.

6. CONCLUDING REMARKS

The importance in evaluating the male factor in reference to its survival in the cervical mucus has been stressed. In approximately 20% of the cases, splitting the ejaculate enables the first portion of the semen to attain a borderline semen quality of $20 \times 10^6/cm^3$ with at least 60% with good linear progressive motion. At least an additional 30% of the subfertile specimens may be improved to borderline quality through various other therapies including varicocelectomy, clomiphene citrate, bromocryptine and human chorionic gonadotropin.

Once at least a borderline specimen is obtained, sperm survival two hours following insemination of the first portion of the ejaculate is determined. If there is at least 3–5 sperm per high powered field then no additional treatment is given. If there is less than this amount, then treatment is directed at the male factor if the spermogram was only borderline and/or the cervical mucus if the semen quality is very good. This is especially applicable if there is evidence of some mucus problem as indicated by decrease in quantity, increased cellularity, or poor spinnbarkeit and ferning. Thus it is not so important that the sperm would survive in most women's cervical mucus, or the mucus would support most normal sperm. Of paramount importance is the survival of the husband's sperm in his own wife's mucus.

A common situation leading to suboptimal mucus is the treatment of concomitant ovulatory defects with clomiphene citrate. Even despite supplemental estrogen, frequently survival in cervical

Table 2. Treatment of ovulation and mucus defects.

Treatment	No. of cycles	Reason for failure
1. DES 0.1 mg.	1	Poor sperm survival. Inadequate corpus luteum.
2. DES 0.2 mg and tetracycline 250 mg 4 × /day for 1 week prior to ovulation.	1	Inadequate corpus luteum
3. As in no. 2 plus progesterone suppositories 50 mg daily from 3rd day of temperature rise	3	Probable inadequate ovulation.
4. As in no. 3 plus 10000 units HCG at midcyle	3	Probable inadequate ovulation.
5. Clomiphene citrate up to 100 mg for 5 days with and without supplemental conjugated estrogens up to 5 mg daily	6	Poor ovulation with low dose clomiphene and poor mucus with high dose clomiphene.
6. HMG	5	Unknown

mucus is inadequate. This is especially true when the quality of the sperm inseminated is just borderline.

Evidence was presented demonstrating that improved fertility can be achieved by treating these ovulation defects with bromocryptine even in the majority of the wives who had normal prolactins. Because of the nature of the clinical setting, a true double blind investigation was not possible. Nevertheless, the data provide much better evidence for the efficacy of bromocryptine as a drug capable of improving ovulation and improving fertility even in women with normal prolactins than the previous anecdotal reports. Not only are many more cases of success presented, but details are provided of extensive prior unsuccessful treatments with other drugs, whereas quick success was achieved with bromocryptine. Crosignani et al. (1975) suggested that bromocryptine worked by a placebo effect in normoprolactinemic women. However, the details of these cases and the illustrating case reports show that these patients had multiple prior potential placebo therapies with regimes that would not interfere with their fertility if they were not helping. Furthermore, there were enough non-treatment cycles during prior therapies to suggest that a

clomiphene rebound effect was not the mechanism behind the successful enhancement of fertility in the normoprolactinemic wives.

Without a true double blind study, one cannot completely disprove Crosignani's placebo claim. However, the quick success in achieving a pregnancy with bromocryptine even despite only borderline sperm, certainly strongly suggests that this therapy deserves further careful study for use in anovulatory normoprolactinemic women. The drug is particularly useful in conjunction with split ejaculate insemination used as a mode of improving the spermogram. It provides a much more favorable mucus environment and consequently superior sperm survival as compared to clomiphene citrate.

The mechanism of action is not known. It is possible that it works by reducing the prolactin level which was normal for the statistically average female but not for these patients. However, since in some patients the baseline prolactin levels were in the low normal range, the possibility exists that bromocryptine may induce ovulation via direct stimulation of dopaminergic receptors of the gonad (Dickey et al., 1976) or the pituitary (Tolis and Naftolin, 1976).

REFERENCES

Amelar RD, Hotchkiss RS (1965) The split ejaculate—its use in the management of male infertility. Fertil Steril 16: 46.

Amelar RD, Dubin L (1973) Male infertility—current diagnosis and treatment. Urology 1: 1.

Amelar RD, Dubin L (1975) A coital technique for promotion of fertility. Urology 5: 228.

Andrews WC (1979) Luteal phase defects. Fertil Steril 32: 501.

Ansbacher R, Keung-Yeung K, Behrman SJ (1973) Clinical significance of sperm antibodies in infertile couples. Fertil Steril 24: 305.

Bergman P (1958) The clinical treatment of anovulation. Int J Fertil 3: 27.

Blasco L (1977) Clinical approach to the evaluation of sperm-cervical mucus interactions. Fertil Steril 28: 1133.

Brown JS (1975) The effect of orally administered androgens on sperm motility. Fertil Steril 26: 305.

Bunge RG (1973) Caffeine stimulation of ejaculated human spermatozoa. Urology 1: 371.

Charny CW (1962) Effect of varicocele on fertility: results of varicocelectomy. Fertil Steril 13: 47.

Charny CW, Gordon JA (1978) Testosterone rebound therapy: a neglected modality. Fertil Steril 29: 64.

Check JH, Rakoff AE (1977) Improved fertility in oligospermic males treated with clomiphene citrate. Fertil Steril 28: 746.

Check JH, Rakoff AE (1977a) Androgen therapy of a varicocele. J Urol 118: 494.

Check JH, Rakoff AE (1977b) Treatment of cervical factor by donor mucus insemination. Fertil Steril 28: 113.

Check JH, Rakoff AE, Roy BK (1977c) Induction of ovulation with combined glucocorticoid and clomiphene citrate therapy in a minimally hirsute woman. J Reprod Med 19: 159.

Check JH (1978) Emotional aspects of menstrual dysfunction. Psychosomatics 19: 178.

Check JH (1980) Improved semen quality in subfertile males with varicocele-associated oligospermia following treatment with clomiphene citrate. Fertil Steril 33: 423.

Check JH (1980a) Improved spermatogenesis following treatment with bromocryptine in men with low normal serum prolactins. Infertility 3 (1): 91.

Check JH (1980b) Treatment of cervical factor with combined high-dose estrogen and human menopausal gonadotropins. Fertil Steril 33: 562.

Croisignani PG, Reschini E, Lombroso GC, Arosio M, Perracchi M (1975) Comparison of placebo and bromocryptine in the treatment of patients with normoprolactinemic amenorrhea. Br J Obstet Gynaec 85: 773.

Davies AG (1965) Eunuchoidism treated with gonadotropins. Proc R Soc Med 58: 580.

Del Pozo E, Brun Del Re, R, Varga L, Friesen (1972) Inhibition of prolactin secretion in man by CB-154. J Clin Endocrin Metab 35.

Dickey RP, Stone SC (1976) Effect of bromocryptine on serum hPRL, hLH, hFSH, and estradiol-17-B in women with galactorrhea-amenorrhea. Obstet Gynecol 48: 84.

162

Dubin L, Amelar RD (1976) Varicocelectomy as therapy in male infertility: a study of 504 cases. J Urol 113: 640.

Epstein J (1977) Clomiphene treatment in oligospermic infertile males. Fertil Steril 28: 741.

Giarola A (1974) Effect of mesterolone on the spermatogenesis of infertile patients. In Mancini RE, Martini L, eds. Male fertility and sterility, p 479. New York: Academic Press.

Greenblatt RB, Barfield WE, Lampros CP (1956) Cortisone in the treatment of infertility. Fertil Steril 7: 203.

Greenblatt RB, Zarete AT, Mahech VB (1975) Other ovulating-inducing agents: clomiphene and other regimens. In: Gold JJ, ed. Gynecologic endocrinology, 2nd edn, p 391. Harper and Row.

Haesungcharern A, Chulavatnatol M (1973) Stimulation of human spermatozoal motility by caffeine. Fertil Steril 24: 662.

Lytton B, Kase N (1966) Effects of human menopausal gonadotrophin on a eunuchoidal male. N Engl J med 274: 1061.

MacLeod J (1970) The effects of urinary gonadotropins following hypophysectomy and in hypogonadotropic eunuchoidism. In Rosenberg E, Paulsen CA, eds. Conference on human testis, Poitano, Italy. New York: Plenum Press.

Martin FIR (1967) The stimulation and prolonged maintenance of spermatogenesis by human pituitary gonadotropins in a patient with hypogonadotropin hypogonadism. J Endocrin 38: 431.

Masala A, Delitala G, Alagna S, Devilla L, Rovasio PP, Lotti G (1979) Dynamic evaluation of prolactin secretion in patients with oligospermia: effects of treatment with metergoline. Fertil Steril 31: 63.

Montanari GD, Volpe (1978) Bromocryptine treatment for oligospermia and asthenospermia with normal prolactin. Lancet 1: 160.

Nencioni T, Miragoli A, Dorato F, Polvani F (1978) Bromocryptine-induced pregnancy in two cases of euprolactinemic hypothalamic amenorrhea. J Endocrinol Invest 1: 65.

Paulson D, Wacksman J (1976) Clomiphene citrate in the management of male infertility. J Urol 115: 73.

Saidi K, Wenn RV, Sharid F (1977) Bromocryptine for male infertility. Lancet 1: 250.

Schill WB (1975) Improvement of sperm motility in patients with asthenozoospermia by kallikrein treatment. Int J Fertil 20: 61.

Schoenfeld C, Amelar RD, Dubin L (1975) Stimulation of ejaculated human spermatozoa by caffeine. Fertil Steril 26: 158.

Segal S, Sadovsky E, Palti Z, Pfeifer Y, Polishuk WZ (1975) Serotonin in 5-hydroxyindoleacetic acid in fertile and subfertile men. Fertil Steril 26: 314.

Segal S, Yaffe H, Laufer N, Ben-David M (1979) Male hyperprolactinemia: effects on fertility. Fertil Steril 32: 556.

Seppala M, Hirvonen E, Renta T (1976) Bromocryptine treatment of secondary amenorrhea. Lancet i 1154.

Shulman S, Harlin B, Davis P (1978) New method of treatment of immune infertility. Urology 12: 582.

Shulman S, Harlin B, Davis P, Reynick JV (1978) Immune infertility and new approaches to treatment. Fertil Steril 29: 309.

Tho PT, Byrd JR, McDonough PG (1979) Etiologies and subsequent reproductive performance of 100 couples with recurrent abortion. Fertil Steril 32: 389.

Tolis G, Naftolin F (1976) Induction of menstruation with bromocryptine in patients with euprolactinemic amenorrhea. Am J Obstet Gynecol 126: 426.

Tulloch WS (1955) Varicocele in subfertility: results of treatment. Br Med J 2: 356.

Urry RL, Cockett ATK (1976) Treating the subfertile male patient: improvement in semen characteristics after low dose androgen therapy. J Urol 116: 54.

Van der Steeg HJ, Coelingh Bennink HJT (1977) Bromocryptine for induction of ovulation in normoprolactinemic post-pill anovulation. Lancet i 502.

Vande Wiele RL, Turksoy RN (1965) Treatment of amenorrhea and anovulation with human menopausal and chorionic gonadotropins. J Clin Endocrin 25: 369.

Author's address:
Dr J.H. Check, M.D.
1015 Chestnut Street
Suite 1020
Philadelphia, PA 19107, USA

23. AIH WITH THE HOME INSEMINATION CAP

K. Semm

Donor or heterologous insemination (AID) is illegal in Germany. Only semen of high quality is used for AIH. Instruments are limited to a simple insemination cap or a glass tube for application of semen into the posterior fornix of the vagina. The plastic cap, placed in front of the cervix, pervents

the contact of semen with the sperm-hostile vagina (pH 4 to 4.5). Any vaginal contamination reduces the servival time of spermatozoa.

Several prerequisites are emphasized in men and women participating in AIH.

The endocrine profile is measured to predict ovulation time (Fig. 1; also see Chapter 17). Psychological stress of the couple should by avoided. Damaged tubes are identified by hysterosalpingography, and diagnostic pelviscopy. The penetrability of spermatozoa in cervical mucus is tested in a post coital test and *in vitro* penetration test. It is often difficult to obtain ejaculates from certain husbands by masturbation because of physical stress and psychosomatic factors. Thus instruments were developed for home insemination (Fig. 2). After ovulation prediction (Fig. 1), the insemina-

Prerequisites of men	Prerequisites of women
1. Spermiocytogram	1. Estimation of ovulation time
2. Proof e.g. exclusion of sperm auto-antibodies	2. Hormonal parameters (e.g. prolactin)
3. Bacteriological examination (including tests for anaerobic bacteria, mycoplasma etc.)	3. Patency of the Fallopian tube checked by pelviscopy
	4. Sanitation of vaginal flora
	5. Proof e.g. exclusion of sperm allo-antibodies
	6. Proof of the sperm penetration capacity for cervical mucus (sperm penetration test)

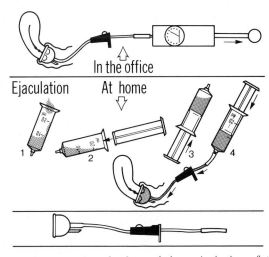

Figure 2. Home insemination technique. Aspiration of the insemination cap (SEMM) onto the cervix with the vacuum pump in the consultation room. The following is performed at home: 1. Semen is collected into a 20 ml syringe; 2b. Five minutes are allowed for semen liquefaction; 3. The syringe is fixed; 4. Liquefied semen is deposited in cervix cap after opening the roll clamp.

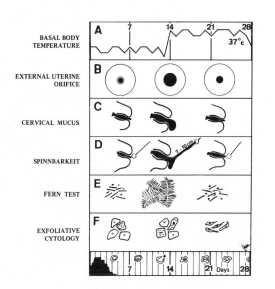

Figure 1. Method used to predict ovulation.

Hafez ESE & Semm K (Eds) Instrumental insemination.
© *1982 Martinus Nijhoff Publishers, The Hague/Boston/London. ISBN 90-247-2530-5. Printed in the Netherlands.*

164

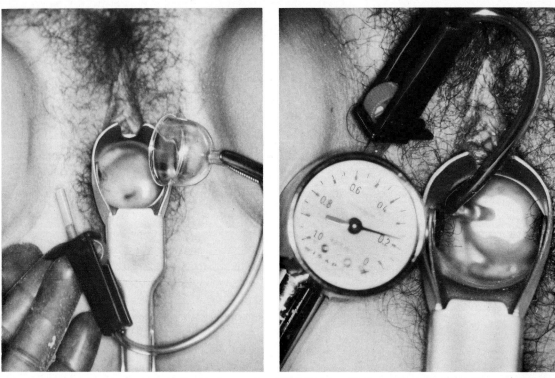

Figure 3. (a) Presentation of the portio vaginalis with the speculum (SEMM) and application of the vaginal cap with grasping forceps. (b) Aspiration of the insemination cap with a vacuum pump up to 0.2 bar.

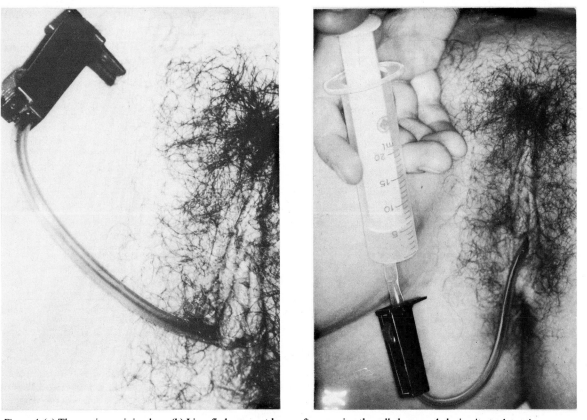

Figure 4. (a) The cervix cap is in place. (b) Liquefied semen at home after opening the roll clamp and closing it at a later time.

tion cap (Fig. 3) is placed on the cervix with a negative pressure of 0.2 (Fig. 3b). Suction with a 20 ml syringe creates a vacuum which results in hematomas and bleedings of the cervix and reduces the success of insemination. Thus a vacuum pump with manometer is recommended. After adapting the cervix cap onto the cervix, a plastic tube with a roll clamp hangs out from the vagina (Fig. 4a). The patient returns home with it, where semen is collected into a 20 ml syringe or into a small cap. After opening the roll clamp the liquefied semen is instilled by the patient herself. Then she remains lying, on her back for 6 to 8 hours. During this time, the plastic tube remains in its place (Fig. 4b). During one year 96 women were inseminated over a period of 20 months during 156 cycles (286 inseminations). Eleven women became pregnant and of these 10 had a normal delivery. There was one abortion. The spermeograms included three cases of normozoospermia, three cases of oligozoospermia, one case of asthenozoospermia, one case of impotentia coeundi, and four cases of normozoospermia with multiple negative post coital test (PCT).

24. AID USING FRESH DONOR SEMEN AND CERVICAL CAP

J.A. Rock, C.A. Bergquist and G.S. Jones

The instrumental insemination of fresh donor semen for management of infertility as a result of a male factor appears to be gaining increasing acceptance by the general public as a solution to childlessness. Although still unacceptable by certain religious groups, increasing numbers of infertile couples are relieved to find a cause of infertility which can be treated with good expectation of success. Approximately 10 million couples in the United States are infertile (Menning, 1980) and 2 or 3 million of them have a significant male factor (20–30%). It is estimated that 6000 to 10000 children are born yearly in the United States as a result of artificial insemination by donor (AID) (Curie-Cohen, 1979). This suggests that only a fraction of couples who have a significant male factor choose AID. Slightly higher pregnancy rates are obtained if only fresh donor semen than if frozen semen is used (Richardson, 1975; Ansbacher, 1978).

Those who utilize frozen semen cite advantages of the 'sperm bank' as ready accessibility, availability of specimens from the same donor for repeated inseminations in a given cycle, and for subsequent pregnancies. Pre-testing for gonorrhea may be completed and there is evidence to suggest that a lower miscarriage rate occurs with frozen semen. However, the pregnancy rate is less. A conception rate of 40% required one-third more inseminations with frozen semen than if fresh donor semen was used (Jackson, 1977). Another study reported a 72–75% conception rate in $4\frac{1}{2}$ months with fresh donor semen and 52–60% conception rate in the same length of time with frozen donor semen (Behrman, 1979). Thus, it appears that fresh donor semen offers a better pregnancy rate. The ready availability of cooperative donors at the Johns Hopkins Medical Institution has provided for an adequate number of specimens for AID and our experience has been limited to the use of fresh donor semen.

1. PATIENT SELECTION

The evaluation of a couple requesting AID should include a detailed history and physical examination of the wife, carefully eliciting details of previous gynecological conditions or surgical procedures which could be associated with an infertility factor in the female. Semen analysis should be performed on at least two occasions and urological evaluation of the male is strongly recommended. In some instances, correction of varicocele or other urological disorder may result in improvement of semen quality and subsequent pregnancy. Furthermore, a urological consultation may assist in reassuring the infertile male that a low sperm count is not a rare condition and also that his masculinity and virility need not be in jeopardy, nor is his general health at fault.

A frequency distribution of male categories is listed in Table 1, where oligospermia and azoospermia are the largest groups. The use of AID for couples in whom the male is oligospermic has been criticized because of pregnancies that have occurred, where counts as low as 1 million/cm^3 have been documented (Behrman, 1961). It has been suggested that these couples should have attempted pregnancy for at

Table 1. Categories of male factor in 278 couples undergoing artificial insemination.

Parameters	Number of patients
Azoospermia	103
*Oligospermia	124
Vasectomy	27
Genetic disorder	1
Other	11
Not known	12
Total	278

* Oligospermia is defined as having a count of 20 million sperm/cm^3 or less.

Hafez ESE & Semm K (Eds) Instrumental insemination.
© *1982 Martinus Nijhoff Publishers, The Hague/Boston/London. ISBN 90-247-2530-5. Printed in the Netherlands.*

least 5 years before AID is considered. However, such an arbitrary time limit is difficult for patients to accept and a couple may request AID sooner because of advancing age of the female or because of unwillingness to wait.

Vasectomy is the third largest category. Most of these individuals have previously fathered children, are remarried and wish to have a child by their new spouse. Only a small number of these men attempted reversal of vasectomy, presumably because of limited chances of success. Genetic disease is an infrequent indication for AID. Diabetes mellitus, cystic fibrosis, Rh factor incompatibility, Huntington's disease, Tay-Sachs disease and sickle cell disease are some of the inherited conditions which may be avoided in the offspring by AID. Other reasons may include impotence, exposure of husband to environmental mutagens, or immunological incompatibility.

2. PSYCHOLOGICAL ASPECTS

Evaluation of the couple should also include an assessment of psychological factors, of their adjustment to the knowledge of male infertility, and the process whereby a decision was made to attempt to have a child by AID. A diagnosis of male sterility may result in impotence and withdrawal in the male and hostility and guilt in the wife (Berger, 1980). Usually a number of months or years have passed from the time the diagnosis of male infertility was

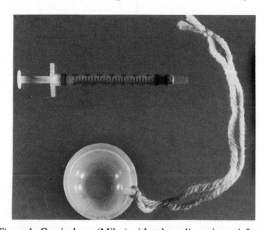

Figure 1. Cervical cap (Milex) with tuberculin syringe. A.I. procedure: 0.2 ml of semen is placed at the external cervical os, the remainder of the semen is placed in the cervical cap which is applied to the cervix. The cap is removed by the patient 4 hours later.

first made until the couple reached a decision to request AID. Often there has been a trial of therapy of the male deficiency with poor results before AID becomes an acceptable option.

Some of the psychological problems of a couple undergoing AID involve secrecy about male infertility and AID, fantasies about the donor and, when pregnancy occurs, development of appropriate family relationships. The couples who request AID are usually highly motivated and mature, and have dealt with many of these problems. The divorce rate among AID couples has been reported to be much less than that of the general population, possibly indicating a greater degree of maturity and stability in their relationships (Banks, 1968).

3. THE AID PROGRAM

In our AID program, a nurse is employed to coordinate the AID program. She is often the first telephone contact of couples inquiring about AID and she participates in the initial visit by providing information and establishing a relationship with the couple. She discusses donor selection and timing of procedures, including instruction in recording basal body temperature, if necessary. The nurse coordinator performs the artificial insemination using the cervical cap technique (Fig. 1) under the supervision of a physician. An individual approach is taken to each patient and if the day of ovulation is not exactly predictable, the patient may come in to have a cervical mucus evaluation performed by the nurse. Sometimes 2 or 3 such visits may be necessary before the mucus is judged to be pre-ovulatory based on characteristics such as the amount, spinnbarkeit and ferning. In these instances, the nurse coordinator has arranged with the donor to be on 'standby' and if the time is deemed appropriate, he is then contacted and a semen specimen is obtained for artificial insemination on that day. Using this approach we have eliminated the need for agents such as clomiphene citrate to regulate the cycle except for patients with oligo-ovulation or anovulatory cycles. It also allows early detection of a cervical factor which can then be treated immediately.

At the time of each insemination, the nurse coordinator usually spends a considerable length of time with the patient, providing information and reassurance. The husband is also invited to be present at the time of insemination and for many couples this has provided the feeling of sharing the experience rather than something that is "done to" the wife alone. When conception occurs the couple is encouraged to attend childbirth education classes which enables the husband to be an active participant during labor and delivery.

An infertility evaluation of the wife is not performed prior to the initiation of AID unless indicated by a positive finding in the history or physical exam, such as a history of pelvic infection, previous abdominal surgery, or findings suggestive of endometriosis.

4. DONOR SELECTION

Donors of semen are selected from volunteer medical students and resident physicians who are carefully screened by a thorough evaluation, including past medical history and family history with careful inquiry regarding birth defects and mental retardation or any inherited illness. A laboratory evaluation includes semen analysis, serological test for syphilis, and urethral culture for *N. gonorrhea* with additional testing for Tay-Sachs disease and sickle cell trait where indicated. Additionally, each semen specimen used for insemination is cultured for *N. gonorrhaea*. It has not been our practice to abtain karyotypes on donors. In a survey of physicians performing AID only 12.5% stated that they routinely obtained a karyotype (Curie-Cohen, 1979).

Matching of donors is based on race, height, weight, hair and eye color of the husband; A, B, O and Rh blood groups are considered if the wife is Rh negative or if there is an obstetrical history of blood group incompatibility. The couple is encouraged to express personal preferences regarding physical

characteristics of the donor if precise matching is not available. At all times, anonymity of the donor and recipient is maintained. Records are kept of the identity of the donor during the cycles where conception occurred, in code, in a separate locked office.

5. LEGAL ASPECTS

In a number of states, laws have been passed to clarify the legal status of AID. The legal questions to be addressed are 1) the status of the physician performing the AID, 2) the legitimacy of the offspring and its relationship to the couple, and 3) the protection of the anonymity of the donor. The State of Maryland passed a law in 1976 which states, "A child conceived by artificial insemination of a married woman with the consent of her husband is the legitimate child of both of them for all purposes. Consent of the husband is presumed." The wife and husband are required to sign a consent form in the presence of a witness prior to the initiation of AID.

6. SUCCESS RATES

The reported pregnancy rate of AID varies from 22% to 78% (Schoysman, 1976; Behrman, 1979). A recent survey of doctors who perform AID in the United States calculated an average national success rate of 57% and an average treatment time to conception of 3.7 months (Curie-Cohen, 1978). The same study states that AID was discontinued if pregnancy had not occurred after 6.7 months of treatment.

At the Johns Hopkins Hospital a study was made of 278 couples undergoing AID for 1 to 14 months. There were 163 pregnancies for a crude conception rate of 58.6%. The median length of time to conception was 4.9 months (Fig. 2). It is evident that most pregnancies occurred by 6 months. However, the application of the life table method of analysis to the data shows that for patients who continue to undergo AID beyond 6 months, the chances of conception are similar to those who conceived in the first 6 months. The cumulative pregnancy rate for those who underwent 6 months of AID is 67% if adjustment is made for those who dropped out of the program prior to conception (Table 2). By 12 months, 85% of patients who continued with AID

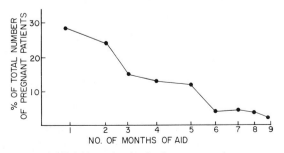

Figure 2. Artificial insemination by donor conception rate.

had conceived, and by 14 months, 90% had conceived. These figures are similar to the pregnancy rates for fertile couples engaging in normal coitus without contraception.

A cumulative pregnancy curve may be summarized in terms of a small number of clinically meaningful parameters. A model was developed (Guzick and Rock, 1980) for the estimation of pregnancy following infertility therapy in which cumulative pregnancy was expressed as a function of two parameters: the "cure" rate (i.e., the percentage of patients who after therapy have the potential for conception) and the probability of pregnancy among those cured. The points of the observed cumulative pregnancy rate lie close to the predicted curve (Fig. 3a). The estimated cure rate in this group of patients was 97% which was not significantly different from 100%.

The fecundability rate and the cumulative pregnancy rate demonstrate a continuation of chances for conception for those patients who persist with AID beyond 6 months. This is contrary to current practice where patients are often discouraged from further attempts to conceive with AID if pregnancy does not occur by 6 months. These findings support the concept that the conception rate and the fecundability rate in women undergoing AID is comparable to that of women conceiving by normal coitus (Jackson and Richardson, 1977) and that for each

month of AID the percentage of remaining women who conceive is constant (Schoysman, 1976).

6.1. Effect of age

In normal fertile couples practicing regular coitus the fecundability rate has been shown to be a maximum at age 24 years and begins a slow decline thereafter (Behrman, 1975, Sheps, 1965). Similarly, the fecundability rate in patients undergoing AID was maximal in the age group less than or equal to 24 years (17%) (Table 3). For the age group 25–30 years it was 15%, and for those women over 30 years of age, fecundability dropped to 11%. These differences were all statistically significant at $p < 0.05$.

6.2. Effect of parity

Parity was seen to have a beneficial effect on ease of conception. There were 186 nulliparous patients of whom 101 (54%) conceived and fecundability rate was 13%. A fecundability rate of 18% was found in 91 women with one or more previous pregnancies of whom 62 conceived (67%) (Table 3). Another parous sub-group, couples who had a previously successful AID and returned for a second pregnancy, demonstrated even greater ease of conception. In this group of 49 patients, 39 conceived for a pregnancy rate of 80% and fecundability rate of 24%. The monthly

Table 2. Life table analysis of the occurrence of pregnancy in 278 couples undergoing AID.

Interval starting time	No. entering interval	No. withdrawn during interval	No. of pregnancies occurring	Cumulative pregnancy rate	Fecundability rate
1	278	15	50	0.19	20%
2	213	20	28	0.30	15%
3	165	15	18	0.38	12%
4	132	18	26	0.51	24%
5	88	15	20	0.63	28%
6	53	7	5	0.67	11%
7	41	11	3	0.70	9%
8	27	4	3	0.73	13%
9	20	1	3	0.77	17%
10	16	1	5	0.85	38%
11	10	4	0	0.85	0%
12	6	0	0	0.85	0%
13	6	1	2	0.90	44%
14	3	0	0	0.90	0%

* Fecundability rates reported in this column are calculated according to the life-table method and represent the "hazard rate" of survival analysis. These rates do not correspond exactly to those calculated according to the formula "conception divided by months of exposure" since the method of computation is different. From Bergquist et al. (1980).

probability of pregnancy for this sub-group was significantly higher than that of the whole group (Fig. 3b).

7. INFERTILITY EVALUATION OF THE WIFE

Even as wives of infertile males undergoing AID would be expected to have the same fecundability rate as women of similar age and parity whose husbands are fertile, so also one should expect to find additional factors contributing to infertility in 10–15% of women undergoing AID. An infertility evaluation was performed in 38 women who had failed to conceive after 3 to 6 months. In 10 patients no treatment was given, but further AID was performed; 5 subsequently conceived (50%). For the remaining 28 women who were treated, the diagnosis

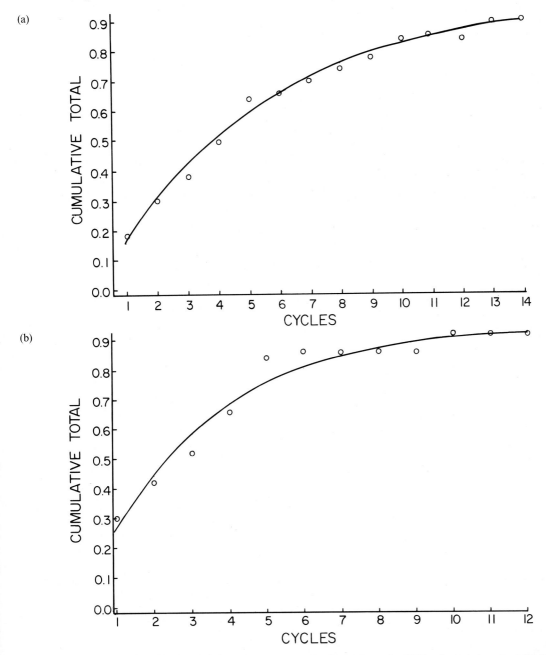

Figure 3. (a) Observed and predicted cumulative pregnancy curves for the total sample of 278 patients undergoing AID. (b) Observed and predicted cumulative pregnancy curves for 49 patients with a previously successful AID.

Table 3. Effect of age and parity on outcome of AID.

Parameters	No. of patients	Percentage pregnant by AID	No. of cycles treated	Fecunda- bility rate*
Age				
≤24	53	68%	211	17%
25–30	157	59%	608	15%
>30	68	50%	300	11%
Parity				
0	186	54%	773	13%
1 or more	92	67%	346	18%

* Differences in fecundability rates significant at the 0.05 level.

and the number who conceived are listed in Table 4. Of these 28 women, 18 conceived (64%). The fecundability rates were 11% and 13%, respectively, for the untreated and treated groups. The number of patients in each diagnostic category is small, but it appears that chances of conception approach that of women with fertile husbands and similar infertility factors. When the other factors have been recognized and treated, the patient should be encouraged to persist with AID for one

similar to that expected in a normal fertile population with a spontaneous abortion rate of 14%. An equal number of boys and girls were born as a result of AID in this series. This occurrence has also been reported elsewhere (Jackson and Richardson, 1977); however, other studies have noted slight increases in male infants (Richardson, 1975). Incidence of congenital anomalies noted at birth was less than 2%.

9. CONCLUDING REMARKS

AID is increasingly sought after by couples with infertility due to a male factor. A pregnancy rate similar to that of a normal fertile population should be anticipated if AID is well-timed and if it is continued for a reasonable length of time. Infertility evaluation of the female partner should be undertaken if there are positive findings in the clinical or physical examination, or if conception fails to occur after one year.

Table 4. Occurrence of pregnancy in 28 women undergoing AID who were treated for additional infertility factors of whom 18 conceived (64%)*.

	Ovulatory factors	Endometriosis	Tubal factor	Uterine factor	Multiple factors
Number of patients	20	13	3	3	6
Number of pregnancies	8	8	1	1	2

* Fecundability rate 13%

year or more to permit optimal chances of conception.

8. OUTCOME OF PREGNANCY

The outcome of pregnancy as shown in Table 5 is

Table 5. Pregnancy outcome following conception with AID.

	Percent
Full term delivery	84
Premature delivery	2
Spontaneous abortion	14
Ectopic	0
Total	100

REFERENCES

Ansbacher R (1978) Artificial insemination with frozen semen. Fertil Steril 29: 375.
Banks AL (1968) Aspects of adoption and artificial insemination. In Behrman SJ, Kistner RW, eds. Progress in infertility, 1st edn, chap 31. Boston: Little, Brown.

Berger DM (1980) Couples reactions to male infertility and donor insemination. Am J Psychiat 137: 9.
Bergquist CA, Rock JA, Miller J, Guzick DS, Wentz AC, Jones GS: Artifical insemination with fresh donor semen using cervical cap technique: a review of 278 cases. Submitted for publication.
Behrman SJ (1961) Artificial insemination. Int J Fertil 6: 291.
Behrman SJ, Kistner RW (1975) A rational approach to the

evaluation of infertility. In Progress in infertility, chap 1, p 1 Boston: Little, Brown.

Behrman SJ (1979) Artificial insemination. Clin Obstet gynecol 22: 245.

Curie-Cohen M, Luttrell L, Shapiro S (1979) Current practice of artificial insemination by donor in the United States. N Engl J Med 300: 585.

Guzick DS, Rock JA: Estimation of a model of cumulative pregnancy following infertility therapy. Submitted for publication.

Jackson McN, Richardson DW (1977) The use of fresh and frozen semen in human artificial insemination. J Biosoc Sci 9: 251.

Matthews CD, Broom TJ Crenshaw KM, Hopkins RE, Kern JFP, Srugos JM (1979) The influence of insemination timing and semen characteristics on the efficiency of a donor insemination program. Fertil Steril 31: 45.

Menning BE (1980) The emotional needs of infertile couples. Fertil Steril 34: 4.

Richardson DW (1975) Artificial insemination in the human. Modern Trends Human Genet p 404.

Schoysman R, Schoysman-Deboeck A (1976) Results of donor insemination with frozen semen. Prog Reprod Biol 1: 252. Basel: Karger.

Sheps MC (1965) An analysis of reproductive patterns in an American isolate. Popul Stud 21: 65.

Author's address:
Dr J.A. Rock
Division of Reproductive Endocrinology,
Department of Gynecology and Obstetrics,
The Johns Hopkins Hospital,
Baltimore, MD 21205, USA

25. RESULTS OF ARTIFICIAL INSEMINATION BY DONORS

A. Campana, U. Gigon, F. Maire, M. Litschgi, P.F. Tauber and M. Balerna

The purpose of this chapter is to evaluate the results of artificial insemination by donor (AID), with emphasis on the main factors influencing the success of the treatment. This will be done by presenting the results of five Centers belonging to the Swiss-German Society for Human Artificial Insemination, as compared with the results of other authors.

1. EVALUATION OF AID DATA

Medical literature abounds with papers on the results of AID. Most of these, however, give only incomplete information, which renders a correct evaluation and comparison of the given data with those of other authors difficult. This problem was realized by Potter, who in 1958 published the paper "Artificial insemination by donors. Analysis of seven series" (Potter, 1958). Potter concluded his own analysis suggesting that any AID report should include the following items of information:

'1. the number of months of insemination preceding each pregnancy or dropout of a patient
2. description of the nature and timing of all physical examinations administered to the patients, and the standards governing the patient's acceptance for insemination
3. description of the scheduling and number of inseminations per menstrual cycle
4. description of the technique and site of the semen deposit
5. average age of the semen specimens at the time of office arrival, together with a description of their handling prior to this time
6. duration of the 'cooling off' periods between first office visit and first insemination, together with a description of any special provisions for emotional tension, including advice given about

persisting despite several months of failure
7. providing valuable supplementary information e.g. a) the patient's miscarriage rate, b) the patient's age and c) any data pertaining to rates of anovulatory cycles before or during months of insemination.'

All the indices which consider the total number of pregnancies without taking into account the number of treatment cycles are entirely without comparative value, since the number of cycles depends upon the multiple non-explicit factors for which the frequency varies for each study (Schwartz and Mayaux, 1980). The per cycle and actuarial rates calculated on the basis of the entire population, and not only on pregnant women, avoid this problem and permit valid comparison.

Table 1. Results of AID of 5 centers (Basel, Bern, Essen, Liestal, Locarno).

| Cycle no. | No. of patients | Rates per cycle (%) | | No. of dropouts | Dropout rate |
		No. of successes	Success rate		
1	1348	352	26	61	6
2	935	215	23	58	8
3	662	148	22	48	9
4	466	76	16	24	6
5	366	75	21	36	12
6	255	43	17	25	12
7	187	33	18	15	10
8	139	19	14	15	13
9	105	17	16.2	12	14
10	76	9	12	6	9
11	61	6	10	7	13
12	48	2	4.2	3	7
13	43	4	9.3	4	10
14	35	8	23	1	4
15	26	5	19	3	14
16	18	4	22	2	14
17	12	0	0	1	8
18	11	4	36	1	14
19	6	2	33	1	25
20	3	2	67	0	0

Hafez ESE & Semm K (Eds) Instrumental insemination.

According to Schwartz, the following rates have to be taken into account:

A. *Rates per cycle*
   — lost to follow-up rate
   — success rate
   — dropout rate
   — open cases rate

B. *Cumulative rates*
   — theoretical cumulative success rate
   — effective cumulative success rate
   — cumulative dropout rates.

2. THE SUCCESS AND DROPOUT RATES PER CYCLE

The results of five AID centers (Basel, Bern, Essen, Liestal and Locarno) are summarized in Table 1. In four of these centers the AID was being practiced with a Finkentscher-Semm cervical cap, by giving 0.5 to 1.0 ml semen per insemination. In Essen the AID was practiced intracervically. The average number of inseminations per cycle was three, with one insemination every 24–28 hours. The use of fresh or frozen semen varied from one centre to another, divided up as follows: Basel and Essen using fresh semen only, Bern 90% fresh, Liestal 20% and Locarno 50% fresh and 50% frozen sperm.

Between 1974 and 1978 treatment was started in a total number of 1348 cases; 53% of these cases were from Bern, 23% from Locarno, 16% from

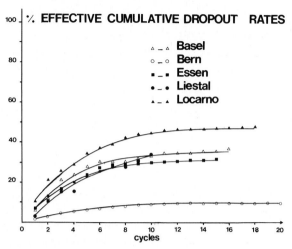

Figure 2. Effective cumulative dropout rates of five AID Centers (Basel, Bern, Essen, Liestal, Locarno).

Essen, 5% from Basel, and 3% from Liestal. A total of 81% of the artificial inseminations were performed with fresh and 19% with frozen semen. The success and dropout rates were calculated according to the statistical evaluation proposed by Schwartz. For that purpose we used a written BASIC program, run on a HP-85 table-top computer. The success rate in the first insemination cycle was 26.1%. This figure was strongly influenced by the results achieved in Bern, which presented a success rate of 30.9% in the first cycle, while the success rate of the other four centers varied between 17.9% and 24.4%. In the first ten insemination cycles the success rate per cycle remained above 10%. Between the 10th and 15th insemination cycle the success rate was still relatively high. This proves the indication to persist in the practice of the AID even after many unsuccessful cycles. The dropout rate per cycle varied in the first twelve cycles from 6.1 to 13.6%. We will see later that, again, this low rate was strongly influenced by the results achieved in Bern.

3. THE THEORETICAL CUMULATIVE SUCCESS RATE

The theoretical cumulative success rate estimates the probability of success without taking into account the dropouts. Figure 1 shows that Bern had the highest theoretical cumulative success rate, followed by the results of Essen. The figures of

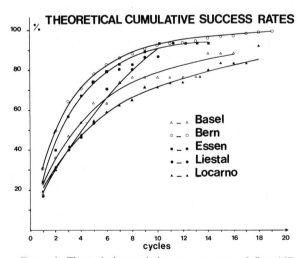

Figure 1. Theoretical cumulative success rates of five AID Centers (Basel, Bern, Essen, Liestal, Locarno).

Basel and Liestal have little indicative value because of the reduced number of cases. The results of Locarno show the lowest theoretical cumulative success rate. This can be explained by the fact that in 50% of the cases in Locarno frozen semen was employed, whereas at Bern and Essen AID was performed using 90% and 100% fresh semen respectively.

4. THE EFFECTIVE CUMULATIVE DROPOUT RATE

The effective cumulative dropout rate assesses the probability of dropout after x insemination cycles. Figure 2 shows the marked difference between Locarno, with an elevated dropout rate, and Bern, with a very low one. In a previous report (Lucciarini et al., 1978) it was concluded that the most important causes of an early dropout were: 1. insufficient conviction of the couple for AID; 2. insufficient information on the part of the physician about the many insemination cycles which will probably be necessary to obtain a positive result; 3. economic problems; 4. anonymity problems; and 5. acceptance of a request for adoption.

5. EFFECTIVE CUMULATIVE SUCCESS RATE

The effective cumulative success rate estimates the probability of success, taking into account the

Table 2. Comparison of conceptions following inseminations with fresh or frozen semen.

	No. of insemination cycles	No. of successes	Success rate (%)
Fresh and frozen semen	993	114	12
Fresh semen	250	35	14
Frozen semen	199	14	7

dropouts. A patient beginning the AID in Locarno had an effective chance of success of 52.4%, while this probability was 68.9% in Essen, and 90.2% in Bern (Fig. 3). The figures of Locarno and Essen are within the range which can be found in the literature. The results of Essen are better than those of Locarno, and this is in part due to the use of fresh or frozen semen, and in part due to the lower dropout rate of Essen. The results of Bern are exceptionally good, due to a high success rate per cycle and, above all, due to a very low dropout rate.

6. COMPARISON OF THE RESULTS OF AID WITH FRESH VS FROZEN SPERM

When using frozen sperm the overall success rate of AID is lower than when using fresh sperm. What is the reason for this difference? Steinberger et al. (1980) found no significant difference in the overall success rate between two groups of patients, inseminated with either fresh or frozen sperm: 76% success with fresh, and 64% with frozen sperm. However, the number of AID cycles necessary to obtain pregnancy was significantly different: 2.8 $\pm$ 0.3 for fresh sperm, 6.3 $\pm$ 0.6 for frozen sperm. This confirms the results of a previous study performed by the same author (Steinberger and Smith, 1973). In this study it is particularly interesting to find that the success rate in the first cycle was 12.5% with fresh sperm, and 7% with frozen sperm. Our own results showed a success rate per cycle of 14% and 7% using fresh or frozen sperm respectively; the difference between the two groups is significant (Table 2) (Campana et al., 1980).

The decisive factor is the dropout rate during the first few insemination cycles. If we compare, for example, the results of Friedman with those of Steinberger we note that Friedman has an overall

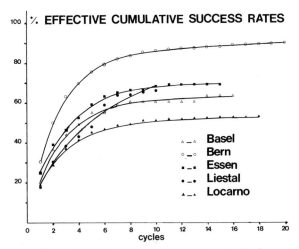

Figure 3. Effective cumulative success rates of five AID Centers (Basel, Bern, Essen, Liestal, Locarno).

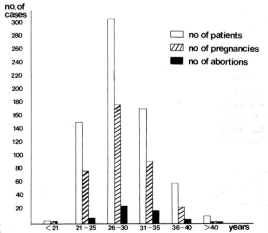

Figure 4. Age of the patients and results of the AID of four Centers (Basel, Essen, Liestal, Locarno).

success rate of 40%, Steinberger of 61%, both using frozen sperm exclusively. Friedman has a mean dropout rate per cycle of 13% in the first six cycles, Steinberger 6% (Friedman, 1977; Steinberger and Smith, 1973). Friedman's high dropout rate compared to Steinberger's is the most important factor in explaining the difference in the overall success rate because the use of frozen sperm determines a lower success rate per cycle, and thus a delay in obtaining a pregnancy.

7. AGE OF THE PATIENTS AND RESULTS OF THE AID

Figure 4 shows the AID results of four centers (Basel, Essen, Liestal and Locarno) in relation to the age of the patients. Most of the women, that is 43% were 26 to 30 years old, 24% 31 to 35, and 21% 21 to 25 years old. The overall success varied from 52 to 58% in the groups between 21 and 35 years, and dropped to 40% in the 36 to 40 year age group. It is interesting to note how the abortion rate increased with the age of the patients, starting with 10% in the 21 to 25 year age group, and going up progressively to 25% in the age group between 36 to 40 years.

Regarding women above the age of 40, in 2 out of 17 cases pregnancy occurred, resulting, however, in spontaneous abortions. In the study of David with a large number of cases, using only frozen semen, the patients were divided into four age groups: under 26, 26 to 30, 31 to 35, and over 35. The probability of success decreased progressively with age, the mean success rates being 13.8, 10.6, 8.7 and 6.3% respectively, and the theoretical cumulative success rates at twelve months being 90.0, 70.3, 62.6 and 51.3% respectively (David et al., 1980).

8. CONCLUDING REMARKS

The analysis of the results of five AID Centers operating in Switzerland and in Germany, compared with those of other authors, allows several conclusions: The use of either fresh or frozen sperm is one of the most important factors regarding the success rate of the AID; In comparing the results of the centers using mostly or exclusively fresh sperm, we notice that the dropout rate is a determinant for the success of the AID; Women older than 35 show a lower success and a higher abortion rate.

REFERENCES

Campana A, Kaplan E, Balerna M Il tasso di concepimento dopo IAD e fattori che lo condizionano. In: Atti del seminario internazionale sulla inseminazione artificiale umana Bari: Cofese 1980. In press.

David G, Czyglik F, Mayaux MJ, Martin-Boyce A, Schwartz D (1980) Artificial insemination with frozen sperm: protocol, method of analysis and results for 1188 women. Br J Obstet Gynaecol 87: 1022.

Friedman S (1977) Artificial donor insemination with frozen human sperm. Fertil Steril 28: 1230.

Lucciarini G, Sommadossi L, Campana A (1978) Tecnica e risultati della IAD Quaderni di sessuologia 3: 11.

Potter RG (1958) Artificial insemination by donors. Analysis of seven series. Fertil Steril 9: 37.

Schwartz D, Mayaux MJ (1980) Mode of evaluation of results in artificial insemination. In David G, Price WS, eds. Human artificial insemination and semen preservation, pp 197–210. New York: Plenum Press.

Steinberger E, Smith KD (1973) Artificial insemination with fresh or frozen semen: a comparative study. J Am Med Assoc 223: 778.

Steinberger E, Rodriguez-Rigau, LJ, Smith KD (1980) Comparison of results of AID with fresh and frozen semen. In David G, Price WS, eds. Human artificial insemination and semen preservation, pp 283–294. New York: Plenum Press.

Author's address:
Dr A. Campana
Servizio di Endocrinologica Ginecologica
Ospedale La Carità;
6600 Locarno, Switzerland.

26. INSEMINATION WITH CRYO-PRESERVED SEMEN

S. LETO and J.D. PAULSON

INTRODUCTION

The concept of cryopreservation of germinal cells is attributed to Spallanzani; Mantegazza was the first to suggest the use of frozen semen banks (Sherman, 1973). The results of attempted cryopreservation of semen have been quite variable and related to the development of the field of cryobiology. The discovery of the superior cryoprotective properties of glycerol (Polge et al., 1949), a polyhydric alcohol, launched the establishment and widespread use of cryopreservation of sperm as we know it today. Some of the earliest reports as to effects of freezing spermatozoa involved human sperm; however, as the establishment of human cryo-banks lagged behind the rapid development in the field of animal husbandry efforts in human sperm cryopreservation and banking proceeded slowly. The introduction of a liquid nitrogen vapor freezing technique caused a rapid expansion in the successful clinical application of frozen human semen (Sherman, 1963).

The explanation of the salt buffering capacity of glycerol and other cryoprotective agents (Farrant, 1969), and more theoretical considerations in the freezing of living cells (Mazur, 1970) have been milestones in the field of cryobiology. However, since the introduction of the nitrogen vapor method (Sherman, 1963) little improvement has been made in the field related to sperm cryo survival. Advances in methodology and the equipment have been reported (Sherman, 1977) and despite no significant breakthroughs in improved cryo survival, the establishment of cryobanks for clinical use of frozen semen have flourished worldwide.

2. FACTORS IN ARTIFICIAL INSEMINATION

The general considerations in the use of AIH or AID revolve around male and/or female factors, or both (Fig. 1).

2.1. Male factors for AIH

AIH can be considered in cases of varicocele, hypospadias, impotence, retrograde ejaculation, high or low semen volume, high viscosity, oligospermia, or asthenospermia. In addition, there are cases where male parameters are all normal, but the timing of intercourse leaves insufficient exposure.

2.2. Female factors

1) *Cervical factors:* Physiological or immunological

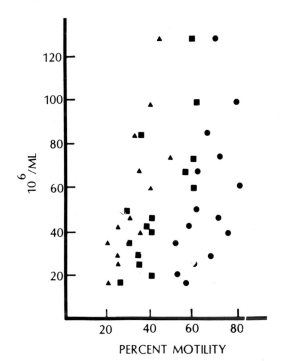

Figure 1. Freeze recovery with straw [▲] and pellet [■] methods compared to initial motility [●].

Hafez ESE & Semm K (Eds) Instrumental insemination.

in nature which prevent proper penetration and activation of the sperm.

2) *Ovulatory factors:* Cases where some form of therapy, hormonal or drug, is required to regulate ovulation with the concomitant necessity for the delivery of semen, properly timed, to enhance the probability of fertilization.

3) *Vaginismus:* Cases where the ejaculate cannot be naturally introduced into the vagina.

2.3. Male factors for AID

The use of AID to circumvent some of the above listed male factors, is not always as clear as in the case where the male is functionally azoospermic (Ansbacher, 1978). The exceptions to this would be in a case of Rh incompatibility where the wife is Rh negative and highly sensitized to the Rh positive fetus. Any unfavorable hereditary factors such as Tay-Sachs, sickle cell anemia, and other deleterious transmitted genetic factors involving the husband is, also, an indication.

2.4. Cryo-banking for AID

The American Association of Tissue Banks (AATB) reproductive council has outlined proposed guidelines in the procurement, screening and processing for storage of donor semen. Careful adherence to the guidelines should ensure the availability of a donor with an excellent background to meet the requirements of the requesting couple. The couple undergoing therapeutic donor insemination does so at great financial and emotional cost (Menning, 1980); therefore, the physician should ensure that certain minimal information is transmitted to, and understood by, the requesting couple. At least one interview is essential with the couple so that all aspects of the donor procurement, screening and insemination technique of AID are fully understood. The confidentiality, both for donor and recipient, must be stressed. Likewise, risk factors and conception rates expected with the procedure, regardless of whether fresh or frozen semen is used, must be fully understood by the couple. It is assumed that regardless of the husband's fertility status, the recipient wife has been thoroughly screened and found ready to accept donor insemination. Legal, ethical, religious

and emotional factors must be discussed (Beck, 1976; Menning, 1980; Kraft et al., 1980). It is important to dispel any fears the couple may have surrounding the procedures and confidentiality. Time taken at this point to discuss the subject freely will be well spent in the future management of the couple. The recipient's background for possible genetic interaction should be discussed, since it is fixed, while the donor can be selected or rejected depending on his genetic background.

2.5. Cryo-banking for AIH

Whatever semen qualities the husband has, is what must be dealt with, and obviously, a relaxation of standards in storing the husbands' semen is made as opposed to that of a donor. The storage for AIH may involve one or several reasons applicable to the patient:

a) Storage pre-vasectomy

This procedure prompted a rapid proliferation of commercial sperm banks in the early 70s to store sperm prior to vasectomy. This expectation did not materialize (Sherman, 1973, 1977) but unexpected interest in using cryogenic techniques in the treatment of infertility developed as a result of the publicity given these commercial ventures.

b) Retrograde ejaculation

The use of cryo-storage of semen from retrograde ejaculators has been applied with limited success. Washing with saline and other additives has improved some of the motility recovery, but the freeze–thaw loss and post-thaw survival generally has been disappointing.

c) Oligospermia

Generally, with oligospermia, other parameters considered important to a semen analysis are also compromised, i.e., motility, morphology and survival. Sperm from oligospermic males generally has poor or borderline cryo-survival characteristics (Leto, 1980; Sherman, 1973; Singer, et al. 1979; Dmowski, 1979). At least one or two attempts should be made at freezing spermatozoa in couples before considering AID. Combinations of techniques in selected cases may prove fruitful — the use of various concentration techniques such as centrifugation, filtration and split-ejaculate can be used to enhance the oligospermic specimens.

Careful concentration and resuspension, if centrifugation and filtration techniques are used, is important. Likewise, the proper collection of a split-ejaculate will give freeze recovery that generally is superior to the total specimen, especially the forward progression.

d) Storage prior to therapy that may lead to azoospermia

Individuals faced with the prospect of sterility as a result of radiotherapy or chemotherapy, surgical procedures for certain neoplasms or other reasons, may seek out cryo-banking facilities, hoping for a chance to father children at some future time. In order to store sufficient semen to make attempts at homologous insemination worthwhile requires a reasonable amount of time prior to treatment, generally two or three weeks.

3. PROCESSING FOR CRYO-STORAGE FOR AIH OR AID

It is generally found that the initial qualities of semen will determine the final success in freeze-recovery, an unfortunate situation in general for oligospermic men (Leto, 1980; Sherman, 1964b, 1973; Singer et al, 1979). The success of cryo-preservation has been previously measured in terms of motility recovered on the post-thaw. Others (Behrman, 1971) have reported that post-thaw motility of human semen was not an index or a determinant of that specimen's subsequent fertility; that is, pregnancies achieved from donors do not necessarily relate to specimens that have outstanding qualities.

In terms of the ease of evaluation of the specimen, motility measurement is the easiest parameter to determine. When correlated to other factors, they may be predictive of an improved index of subsequent fertility. While complete sperm immobilization must be considered as sterility (Amelar et al., 1980), any motility in the specimen allows the possibility of fertilization.

3.1. Semen collection and pre-freeze treatment

Straight collection of the total specimen which can be processed for freezing once a complete analysis has been performed. This sample can also be treated in one of several ways to "clean" and concentrate

the sperm quality and quantity to enhance freeze recovery. Variations in length of abstinence and method of cellection (i.e., masturbation vs coitus interruptus) can influence the quantity and quality of the ejaculate.

3.2. Split-ejaculate

In animal species studied as well as in man, sperm cell distribution is not uniform throughout the ejaculatory process (Eliasson and Lindholmer, 1972; Amelar and Hotchkiss, 1965; Amelar et al., 1980; Marmar et al., 1979). Evaluation of split-ejaculates into two fractions reveals increased concentration, better motility and morphology in the first portion in almost 90% of the ejaculates.

4. OTHER SEPARATION OR CONCENTRATION TECHNIQUES

Centrifugation, filtration through Milipore filters or glass wool columns (Paulson and Polakowski, 1977; Paulson et al., 1979) to reduce viscosity and remove debris have been utilized. The use of suitable physiological resuspension media can be important in cases where seminal plasma contains immobilizing or agglutinating factors (Shulman, 1978), and in cases of retrograde ejaculation where rapid removal of possible solid and soluble toxic contents from the isolated sperm is important.

Methods developed to "clean" and "free" sperm from poor sperm and other cells and seminal debris, and separate X and Y spermatozoa by utilizing a serum albumin column, have met with limited succes (Ericcson, 1973, 1977; Dmowski, 1979).

5. CHEMICAL TREATMENT

Current in vitro treatment to enhance sperm motility recovery involves the use of methylxanthines (caffeine, a phosphodiasterase inhibitor) and pancreatic kallikrein, a kinin-liberating proteinase (Schill, 1975, 1979; Makler et al., 1980). These and other studies (Johnsen et al., 1974; Harrison, 1978; Harrison, 1980; Barkay et al., 1977) have shown that addition of caffeine to human semen increased motility of cryo-preserved sperm when added either prior to freeze down, or during the thaw process (Table 1). Other additives (Makler et al., 1980) including L-arginine (Keller and Polakowski, 1975) have also been shown to stimulate sperm motility pre-or post-freeze.

6.1. Basic considerations

The biophysical principles underlying freeze preservation of living cells ultimately involve factors affecting the speed and character of intracellular ice crystal formation, extent of dehydration, salt buffering and salt concentrations (Mazur, 1970; Farrant, 1969; Sherman, 1964a; Behrman, 1971; Mullhaupt, 1978). There are great variations in preliminary requirements and additives which help maximize freeze recoveries of sperm from various mammalian species (Graham, 1978; Sherman, 1964a; Berndtson and Pickett, 1978); however, in man these factors seem to be of minor importance. In man, as many as 15% of a sperm population can survive freeze—thaw if the raw semen is frozen. However, the use of glycerol enhances this recovery markedly. Glycerol in final concentrations of 5–10% has been the most successful (Sherman, 1977). Different aditives such as egg yolk-citrate and variation in freezing containers and rates have yielded very little improvement in recovery rates (Sherman, 1977; Behrman, 1971; Leto, 1980).

The storage time of viable specimens seems to be related to the final temperature reached; variations are seen in recovered motility at temperatures of −79°C and above. Little or no changes have been reported at −196°C for as long as 15 years (Sherman, 1977). Reduced motility of samples stored over three years in liquid nitrogen (Smith and Steinberger, 1973) has been attributed to possible improper handlong and monitoring (Sherman, 1977) especially relative to temperature rises and light exposure.

Successful cryo-preservation seems to be compatible with a broad range of conditions in freeze and thaw rates (Sherman, 1977; Behrman, 1971; Graham and Crabo, 1978; Leto, 1980). This is not the case in other mammals or other classes (Sherman, 1964a; Graham, 1978, Graham and Crabo, 1978; Jones, 1979, Berndtson and Pickett, 1978). However, this does not imply that an optimal set of conditions does not exist, but rather than clinical applications demand a certain amount of process stability.

6.2. Methodology and instrumentation of current technology

Instruments

It has been found that sperm can be frozen successfully at temperatures below −30°C; however, sperm survival at temperatures between −100°C and −50°C was linearly related to storage temperature (Behrman, 1971). Other reports (Sherman, 1977) have pointed to a loss of motility and vital staining during storage at dry ice temperatures (−75°C to −79°C) but little or no loss at liquid nitrogen temperature (−196°C). Freezing at dry ice temperature and transfer to liquid nitrogen for final storage can be utilized and is one method in current use, utilizing either a mechanical refrigerated system which can be static or programmed to slow cool and freeze specimens. When the specimen temperature reaches −80°C to −100°C, it is transferred to liquid nitrogen. In earlier studies, a variety of coolants were used to freeze human sperm such as alcohol baths, dry ice slabs, liquid

le 1. Effect of caffeine on sperm activity*

Caffeine	£ Change over control Semen form	Motility Progression	Progression	Reference
6 mM	Fresh ejaculate	+100[1]	0	Harrison (1980)
6 mM	Fresh ejaculate	+100[1]	−30	Harrison (1980)
10 mM	Fresh ejaculate	+36[2]	−10	Makler (1980)
5 mM	Fresh ejaculate	+104[1]	+100	Schill (1979)
5 mM	Fresh ejaculate	+81[1]	+110	Schill (1979)

* Calculated from indicated references
[1] Incubated 1 h
[2] Incubated 30 min

nitrogen and liquid helium. With the exception of dry ice, only liquid nitrogen has proven practical. Liquid nitrogen, because of its superior maintenance qualities in addition to relative safety and convenience in handling in office or field conditions, is the cryo-refrigerant of choice.

Several refrigerators for longterm storage as well as field use have been developed. These include Dewar Flasks, wooden and styrofoam boxes for use with dry ice and, the more practical liquid refrigerant containers of insulated aluminum or stainless steel. A modification of such equipment was also developed for freezing human semen in pellet form (Barkay et al., 1974; Barkay and Zuckerman, 1978).

7. METHODOLOGY

7.1. Introduction

Cryopreservation of human sperm, as currently practiced, involves one or a combination of several methods. Freezing in air that is cooled by a mechanical refrigerator, dry ice or liquid nitrogen vapor is employed and then the specimen is transferred into liquid nitrogen for final storage. Factors that introduce variations include insulation characteristics of the container, air or vapor circulation (forced or otherwise) and control capability exerted on the container. One of the simplest methods is the nitrogen vapor freezing technique introduced in 1963 (Sherman, 1963). This method suffers from variations in vapor temperature and, therefore, freezing rates; but because of satisfactory survival of human sperm over a broad range of freezing rates, this method is simple, practical and compares favourably with the newer more precisely controlled methods.

7.2. Current freezing methods

Semen, prepared as to collection method, additives, extenders and freezing equipment, is frozen in one of three ways. The earliest method utilizing glass ampules currently has limited application. The paillette or plastic straw system developed by the French, is currently the most popular. The freezing of semen in the form of pellets has had application

in animal studies (Nagase and Niwa, 1964; Graham, 1978) but because of possible problems in labeling, packaging, handling and contamination, this method has had limited application for human use (Barkay et al., 1974; Nakamura and Ramos, 1975).

Reports have suggested that different freezing rates (Behrman, 1971; Graham 1978; Graham and Crabo, 1978) affect recovery of human sperm, while others report the differences to be inconsequential (Sherman, 1963, 1977). Furthermore, processing raw semen (Sherman, 1963) or with extenders (Behrman, 1971), does not seem to affect cryo-survival differently to any appreciable extent (Friberg, 1971; Leto, 1980). Sherman (1977) suggests that the egg yolk-citrate method (Behrman, 1966) may improve cryo-survival. However, others (Friberg, 1971; Leto, 1980) demonstrate no difference between use of glycerol alone or with egg yolk-citrate although electron microscope studies (Friberg, 1971) demonstrate less damage to sperm frozen by the egg yolk-citrate method as compared to addition of glycerol. Reports have appeared favouring different physical arrangement in the freezing vessels in addition to the packaging meth-

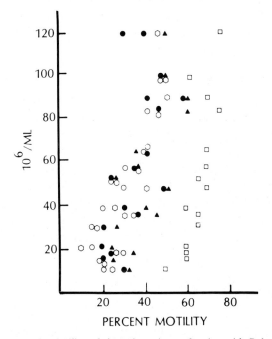

Figure 2. Motility of thawed specimens freezing with Baker's solution and egg yolk-citrate solution with pellet and straw methods compared to initial motility (pellet method with Baker's solution [○]; pellet method with egg yolk-citrate [●]; straw method with Baker's solution [○]; straw method with egg yolk-citrate [▲]; initial motility [□]).

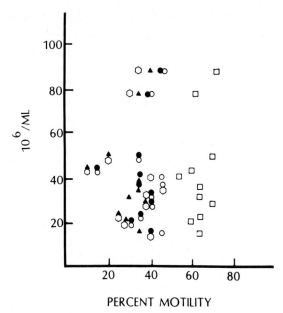

10⁶/ML (y-axis label: 10^6/ML)

PERCENT MOTILITY

Figure 3. The addition of human serum albumin added to a final concentration of 1% (pellet method [○]; pellet method with HSA [▲]; straw method [○]; straw method with HSA [●]; initial motility [□]).

od (Sherman, 1977). Some prefer freezing straws placed horizontally in nitrogen vapor (Emperaire and Riviere, 1974; Ulstein, 1973), while others prefer the pellet (Barkay and Zuckerman, 1978; Nakamura and Ramos, 1975).

7.3. Results

Modern cryo-biology has made possible the storage of various cells, tissues and organs (American association of Tissue Banks). The use of frozen in comparison to fresh semen has been reported to be associated with a lower incidence of pregnancy rates (Ansbacher, 1978; Smith and Steinberger, 1973; Steinberger and Smith, 1973; Friedman, 1977). However, recent work has found that pregnancy rates of fresh and frozen semen are similar,

Table 2. Motility and % live with Baker's buffer versus HSA buffer, pH 7.4

	Straw % motility	Live/dead	Pellet %motility	Live/dead
Initial	63	65	63	65
Buffer	26	31	30	33
Buffer and HSA	32	30	37	32

Number = 20

Table 3. The effect of freezing on morphology in straws with LN vapor versus pellet freezing on LN surface.

Group	Normal oval	Amorphous	Spermid	Tapered	Other
Initial	60	28	7	4	1
Post-thaw straw	52	35	7	2	4
Post-thaw pellet	57	30	6	2	5

Number = 18

but it requires more cycles to achieve pregnancies with frozen semen (Rodriguez-Rigau, personal communication). For practical reasons, the use of frozen semen has numerous advantages, not only in animal husbandry but for human use as well, despite reported lower pregnancy rates. Conditions applicable to freezing and storage of non-human semen may be quite different (Graham, 1978 ; Graham and Crabo, 1978; Jones and Stewart, 1979; Sherman, 1964a; Berndtson and Pickett, 1978), therefore results from such research is of limited value in furthering human efforts. Regardless of the procedure, additives, and other manipulations, the ultimate procedure is that method or combination which yields the greatest and safest number of pregnancies. The criteria of all methods described for successful cryo-preservation is based on recovered post-thaw motility. However, good correlation between post-thaw motility and fertility has not been observed (Behrman, 1971; Ansbacher, 1978).

The authors have found no difference in freeze recovery in liquid nitrogen with horizontal or vertical straw orientation. Freezing from room temperature or slow cooling to 5° C and freezing at different rates revealed no appreciable difference in post-thaw recover. Pellet formation at −79° C was performed on slabs of dry ice with depressions formed on the surface. The results were comparable to or better than any of the other procedures.

Cryo-preservation of pellets has been described at higher temperatures but it has been pointed out (Sherman, 1977) that ultra-rapid rates of freezing are lethal to most sperm cells. However, the authors observed a consistent and high motility recovery with pellets formed on the surface of liquid nitrogen with raw semen, split-ejaculates or specimens with additives.

The better the initial qualities of the specimen prior to freezing, the better the qualities after recovery. In addition very little loss in progressive motility or quality of forward movement is observed. This is not a consistent observation with standard freezing procedures using ampules or straws. Freezing from room temperature (22–24° C) is accomplished directly onto liquid nitrogen. Freeze recovery is also seen to vary directly with sperm concentration; therefore, this is still a problem for oligospermic individuals (Fig. 1); however, the pellet method gave consistently higher recoveries than the straws (Fig. 1). Certainly in cases where freeze recovery is at best marginal with the straw, the pellet may offer these cases a new option, despite some drawbacks associated with packaging, labeling and possible contamination. When a phosphate buffer (Bakers' solution) is compared to egg yolk-citrate (Fig. 2), no major difference is noted in motility recovery. The Baker's buffer compared to the same buffer to which human serum albumin is added to a final concentration of 1% (Fig. 3, Table 2) demonstrates that the pellet freeze recovery of motility and forward progression are superior to the straw. The addition of 1% human serum albumin further increases the recovery. Morphology evaluation using the MacLeod classification (MacLeod, 1964) (Table 3.) revealed a closer agreement between the initial morphology and that of the post-thaw pellets than with the straws.

Currently there is no known in vitro method which correlates cryo-survival and fertility, but there are some promising test which may resolve this dilemma in the near future. Among these tests currently being evaluated are the Humster system (Fujita et al., 1980; Binor et al., 1980), the repeat freeze–thaw technique (Ansari, 1980) and the use of flow cytometry to detect changes in resistance to in situ denaturation of spermatozoal DNA in post–thaw sperm.

8. POST-THAW OBSERVATIONS

Loss of sperm motility and forward progression, regardless of the process and method of storage (straw, ampule, pellet), is well documented. In addition to loss of motility, changes are seen in ultrastructure (Sherman, 1977; Jones and Stewart, 1979; Pederson and Lebeck, 1971; Friberg, 1971). Freezing with a cryo-protective agent results in mid-piece damage with swollen and sometimes ruptured mitochondria. The acrosome is also ruptured or wrinkled (Friberg, 1971); similar observations are noted in bull semen (Jones and Stewart, 1979). Freezing human sperm with protective agents protects and allows retention of most mitochondrial morphology, while the additional presence of egg yolk-citrate is more protective to the acrosome than glycerol alone (Friberg, 1971). By combining scanning (SEM) and transmission (TEM) electron microscopy, it is observed that freeze–thaw may cause membrane distortion and some loss of acrosomal material (Sherman, 1977). There appears to be less pro-acrosin in frozen thawed sperm than in fresh samples (Zaneveld, personal communication). Acrosin is a spermatozoal serine proteinase that is involved in various processes leading up to, and including, sperm penetration of the ovum (Anderson et al., 1980; Morton, 1977). The release of other enzymes from sperm on freeze-thaw has also been measured in an attempt to correlate cryo-injury to changes in fertilizing capacity (Graham and Crabo, 1978).

9. CONCLUDING REMARKS

Although the use of frozen semen in pellets has several drawbacks, investigators (Barkay and Zuckerman, 1978; Nakamura and Ramos, 1975) have used the method successfully. The finding by others (Graham and Crabo, 1978) and confirmed by us that of all treatment groups, ultra-rapid freezing in pellets produces the best recovery, allows the consideration that this process has great merit for special applications. Excellent retention of forward progression is also noted. Although cervical mucus penetration depth is not as good with frozen-thawed sperm as with fresh spermatozoa (Fjallbrant and Ackerman, 1969; Friberg, 1971; Ulstein, 1973), it is demonstrated (Ulstein, 1972) that a loss of forward progression, as well as motility, is seen on the thaw; if forward progression drops below certain critical levels it is associated with low fertility. The motile sperm count is positively correlated to pregnancy rates (Marmar et al., 1979) and, when the motile count is below 18 million, no pregnancies are seen. Some (David, 1979) consider motility and morphology prime factors to successful cervical mucus penetration; however, Mathews et al. (1980) presents a caveat. Cervical mucus penetration is related to obtaining mucus at the proper time, which can be variable for a given patient from month to month. Even if the study with the mucus penetration is successful, it is felt that equating satisfactory mucus penetration with fertilization potential is incorrect. The use of bovine mucus or egg white as controls may prove to be successful in evaluation of cervical mucus penetration studies (Gaddum-Rosse et al., 1980; Hansen and Hjort, 1979; Marmar et al., 1980).

Motility recovery, especially forward progression, is excellent, consistent and at least as good as other methods when spermatozoa are frozen on the surface of liquid nitrogen. Furthermore, Stranzinger et al. (1971), demonstrated no significant difference between fresh and pellet frozen semen on dry ice with regard to pregnancy rates and number of young rabbits born; however, ampules, straws or tubing used to freeze sperm produced significantly fewer young. There is no evidence at this time that sperm in pellets frozen at ultra high rates on the surface of liquid nitrogen will fertilize. These studies are currently under investigation.

REFERENCES

Alexander NJ (1977) Surface structure of spermatozoa frozen for artifical insemination. Andrologia 9: 155.

Amelar RD, Dubin L, Schoenfeld C (1980) Sperm motility. Fertil Steril 34: 197.

Amelar RD, Hotchkiss RS (1965) The split ejaculate: its use in the management of male infertility. Fertil Steril 16: 46.

Anderson RA, Oswald A, Leto S, Zanneveld LJ (1980) Inhibition of human acrosin by fructose and other monosaccharides. Biol Reprod 22: 1079.

Ansari AH (1980) Repeated freeze-thawing for assessment of semen freezability. In Emerpaire JC, Audebert A, Hafez ESE, eds. homologous artificial insemination, p 177–182. The Hague: Martinus Nijhoff.

Ansbacher R (1978) Artificial insemination with frozen spermatozoa. Fertil Steril 29: 375.

Barkay J, Zuckerman H, Heiman M (1974) A new practical method of freezing and storing human sperm and a preliminary report on its use. Fertil Steril 25: 399.

Barkay J, Zuckerman H, Sklan D, Gordon S (1977) Effect of caffeine on increasing the motility of frozen human sperm. Fertil Steril 28: 175.

Barkay J, Zuckerman H (1978) Further developed device for human sperm freezing by the twenty-minute method. Fertil Steril 29: 304.

Barkay J, Zuckerman H (1979); 1st pan american congress of andrology. Caracas, Venezuela, March 13–16, 1978.

Beck WW Jr (1976) A critical look at the legal, ethical, and technical aspects of artificial insemination. Fertil Steril 27: 1.

Behrman SJ (1971) Preservation of human sperm by liquid nitrogen vapor freezing. In Ingelman-Sundberg A, Lunnell N, eds. Current problems in fertility, pp 10–16. New York: Plenum Press.

Berndtson WE, Pickett BW (1978) Techniques for the preservation and field handling of bovine spermatozoa. In: The integrity of frozen spermatozoa, pp 53–77. Proc Nat Acad Sci, Washington DC.

Binor Ž, Sokoloski JE, Wolf DP (1980) Penetration of the zona-free hamster egg by human sperm. Fertil Steril 33: 321.

Dmowski WP, Gaynor L, Lawrence M, Rao R, Scommenga A (1979) AIH with oligospermic semen separated on albumin columns. Fertil Steril 31: 58.

Eliasson R, Lindholmer CHR (1972) Distribution and properties of spermatozoa in different fraction of split ejaculates. Fertil Steril 23: 252.

Emperaire JC, Riviere J (1974) La congélation du sperme human normal. J Gyn Obstet Biol Reprod 3: 215.

Ericcson RJ, Langevin CN, Nishiro M (1973) Isolation of fractions rich in human sperm. Nature 246: 421.

Ericcson RJ (1977) Isolation and storage of progressively motile human sperm. Andrologia 9: 111.

Evenson DP, Darzynkiewicz Z, Melamed MR (1980) Relation of mammalian sperm chromatin heterogeneity to fertility. Science 210: 1131.

Farrant J (1969) Is there a common mechanism of protection of living cells by polycinylpyrcolidone and glycerol during freezing? Nature 222: 1175.

Fjallbrant B, Ackerman DR (1969) Cervical mucus penetration in vitro by fresh and frozen-preserved human semen specimens. J Reprod Fertil 20: 515.

Fribert J, Nilsson O (1971) Motility and morphology of human sperms after freezing in liquid nitrogen. In Ingelman-Dundberg A, Lunnel N, eds. Current problems in fertility, pp 17–22. New York: Plenum Press.

Friedman S (1977) Artificial donor insemination with frozen human sperm. Fertil Steril 28: 1230.

Fujita JS, Van Campen H, Rogers BJ (1980) The effect of freezing on fertilizing capacity of human sperm assayed using zona-free hamster eggs. (Abstr) J Androl 1: 77.

Gaddum-Rosse P, Blandau RJ, Lee WI (1980) Sperm penetration into cervical mucus in vitro — II. Human spermatozoa in bovine mucus. Fertil Steril 33: 644.

Graham EF (1978a) Fundamentals of the preservation of spermatozoa. In: The integrity of frozen spermatozoa, pp 4–44. Proc Nat Acad Sci, Washington DC.

Graham EF, Crabo BG 1978b Some methods of freezing and evaluating human spermatozoa. In: The integrity of human spermatozoa, pp 274–304. Nat Proc Acad Sci, Washington DC.

Hansen KB, Hjort T (1979) The penetration of antibody covered spermatozoa into cervical mucus and egg white. Arch Androl 3: 245.

Harrison RF (1978) Insemination of husbands' semen with or without addition of caffeine. Fertil Steril 29: 532.

Harrison RF, Sheppard BL, Kaliszer M (1980) Observations on the motility, ultrastructure and elemental composition of human spermatozoa incubated with caffeine. Andrology 12: 34.

Johnsen O, Eliasson R, Abdel-Kader MM (1974) Effects of caffeine on the motility and metabolism of human spermatozoa. Andrology 6: 53.

Jones RC, Stewart DL (1979) The effects of cooling to 5° C and freezing and thawing on the ultrastructure of bull spermatozoa. J Reprod Fert 56: 233–238.

Keller DW, Polakowski KL (1975) L-arginine stimulation of human sperm motility in vitro. Biol Reprod 13: 154.

Kihlma BA (1977) Caffeine and chromosomes. Amsterdam: Elsevier.

Kraft AD, Palombo J, Mitchell D, Dean C, Meyers S, Schmidt AW (1980) The psychological dimensions of infertility. Am J Orthopsychiat 50: 618.

Leto S (1980) Human semen cryopreservation — a re-evaluation. Presented at the American Association of Tissue Banks, Washington, DC, May 12–14.

Leto S et al. (1981a) A re-evaluation of current techniques of human semen cryopreservation. 2nd Pan American Congress of andrology, Mexico City, Jan 26–30, 1981.

Leto S et al. (1981b) A prospective study of semen qualities of donors selected for AID. 2nd Pan American Congress of Andrology, Mexico City, Jan 26–30, 1981.

Makler A, Makler E, Itzkovitz J, Brandes JM (1980) Factors affecting sperm motility — IV. Incubation of human semen with caffeine, kallikrein, and other metabolically active compounds. Fertil Steril 33: 624.

Marmar JL, Praiss DE, DeBenedictis TJ (1979) An estimate of the fertility potential of the fractions of the split ejaculate in terms of the motile sperm count. Fertil Steril 32: 202.

Marmar JL, Praiss DE, DeBenedictis TJ (1980) Functional role of sperm agglutinating antibodies in men. Fertil Steril 34: 365.

Mathews CD, Makin AE, Cox LW (1980) Experience with in vitro sperm penetration testing in infertile and fertile couples. Fertil Steril 33: 187.

Mazur P (1970) Cryobiology: the freezing of biological systems. Science 168: 939.

MacLeod J (1964) Human seminal cytology as a sensitive indicator of the germinal epithelium. Int. Fert 9: 281.

Menning BE (1980) The emotional needs of infertile couples. Fertil Steril 34: 313.

Morton DB (1977) The occurence and function of proteolytic enzymes in the reproductive tract of mammals. In Barrett AJ, ed. Proteinases in mammalian cells and tissues, pp 445–500. Amsterdam: North Holland.

Mullhaupt JT (1978) Molecular factors affecting gametic integrity during storage at low temperatures. In: The integrity of frozen spermatozoa pp. 126–143. Nat Acad Sci, Washington DC.

Nagase H, Niwa T (1964) Deep freezing bull semen in concentrated pellet form. 5th Int Congr on Animal Reproduction and Artificial Insemination, Trento vol 4, p410,

Nakamura MS, Ramos RM (1975) Frozen human semen: a new simplied technique of cryopreservation. In Campos da Paz A, Drill VA, Hayashi M, Rodriquez W, Schelly AN, eds. Recent advances in human reproduction, pp 66–69. Amsterdam: Excerpta Medica.

Paulson JD, Polakowski KL (1977) A glass wool column procedure for recovering extraneous material from the human ejaculate. Fertil Steril 28: 178.

Paulson JD Polakowski KL, Leto S (1979) Further characterization of glass wool column filtration of human semen. Fertil Steril 32: 125.

Pederson H, Lebeck PE (1971) Ultrastructural changes in the human spermatozoa after freezing for artificial insemination. Fertil Steril 22: 125.

Polge C, Smith AV, Parker AS (1969) Revival of spermatozoa after vitrification and dehydration at low temperatures. Nature 164–666.

Rogers BJ, VanCampen H, Ueno M, Lambert H, Bronson R, Hale R (1979) Analysis of human spermatozoal fertilizing ability using zona-free ova. Fertil Steril 32: 664.

Schill WB (1975) Caffeine and kallikrein induced stimulation human sperm motility: a comparative study. Andrologia 7: 229.

Schill WB, Pritsch W, Preissler G (1979) Effect of caffeine and kallikrein on cryopreserved human spermatozoa. Int J Fertil 24: 27.

Schoenfeld CY, Amelar RD, Dubin L (1975) Stimulation of ejaculated human spermatozoa by caffeine. Fertil Steril 26: 158.

Sherman JK (1963) Improved methods of preservation of human spermatozoa by freezing and freeze-drying. Fertil Steril 14:49.

Sherman JK (1964a) Low temperature research on spermatozoa and eggs. Cryobiology 1: 103.

Sherman JK (1964b) Research on frozen human semen; past, present and future. Fertil Steril 15: 485.

Sherman JK (1973)Synopsis of the use of frozen human semen since 1964: state of the art of human semen banking. Fertil Steril 24: 397.

Sherman JK (1977) Synopsis of the use of frozen human semen since 1964: state of the art of human semen banking. Fertil Steril 24: 397.

Sherman JK (1977) Cryopreservation of human semen. In Hafez ESE, ed. Techniques of human andrology, p. 399. North Holland Biomedical Press: Elsevier.

Shulamn S, Harlin B, Davis P, Reyniak JV (1978) Immune infertility and new approaches to treatment. Fertil Steril 29: 309.

Singer R, Barnet M, Allalouf D, Chowers I (1979) Sensitivity of human spermatozoa to various isolation procedures: differences in relation to sperm counts. Int J Fertil 24: 33.

Smith KD, Steinberger E (1973) Survival of spermatozoa in a human sperm bank: effects of long-term storage in liquid nitrogen. JAMA 223: 774.

Steinberger E, Smith KD (1973) Artificial insemination with fresh and frozen semen. JAMA 223: 778.

Stranzinger GF, Maurer R, Paufler SK (1971) Fertility of frozen rabbit semen. J Reprod Fertil 24: 111.

Tyler E (1973) The clinical use of frozen semen banks. Fertil Steril 24: 413–416.

Ulstein M (1973) Fertility, motility and penetration in cervical mucus of freeze-preserved human spermatozoa. Acta Obstet Gynecol Scand 52: 205.

Ulstein M (1972) Sperm penetration of cervical mucus: a criterion of male fertility. Acta Obstet Gynecol Scand 51: 335.

Author's address:
Dr. S. Leto
Washington Fertility Study Center
2600 Virginia Avenue, N.W.
Washington, DC 20037, USA

27. ORGANIZATION OF THE FRENCH SPERM BANKS — C.E.C.O.S.

M. SERVOZ GAVIN

In France, artificial insemination with donor semen (AID) has encountered difficulties in the past for religious and moral reasons. Consequently, the technique had to be practiced in a clandestine manner. AID was performed by only a few private gynecologists using fresh semen obtained from donors. This practice provided only a scant number of donors with limited guarantees regarding the quality of semen and the protection of anonymity.

All of these factors, combined with the development of cryobanking techniques, catalyzed the creation in Paris in 1973 of the first two sperm banks (David and Lansac, 1980). This was the beginning of C.E.C.O.S. (Centre d'Etude et de Conservation du Sperme). Since then, AID has become accepted as a service in the public hospitals and is recognized officially by government authorities. The success and efficiency of these initial two sperm banks has resulted in the creation of official sperm banks all over France, following a homogenous geographic distribution. Presently, there are 14 C.E.C.O.S. Centers (Fig. 1).

Since its start, the functions and a strict number of principles concerning the rules and regulations of all C.E.C.O.S. Centers were defined in order to ensure medical, biological and moral guarantees in the practice of AID. The Centers maintain a close relationship with one another through regular meetings of their directors which has resulted in a close cooperation and exchange of ideas. The Centers recently formed the French Federation of C.E.C.O.S. in order to increase their common efforts in facilitating AID and to coordinate their activities in fundamental research. There is, however, no formal central organization or director and the centers are independent of each other.

1. STRUCTURE OF C.E.C.O.S.

The C.E.C.O.S. Centers are generally located within University Hospital Centers (C.H.U.) and are usually associated with a service of reproductive biology. They are independent of the hospital administration and have their own budget. They are managed by an administrative board which includes representatives from the Ministry of Health, the hospital administration, social security, and different interested medical specialists. The budget of C.E.C.O.S. is independent of the Hospital and is derived mainly from income arising from charges for frozen semen, for AID and services such as spermiograms and semen auto-cryopreservation. The principle exists of a non-profit policy.

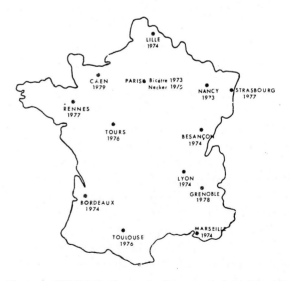

Figure 1. C.E.C.O.S. Centers in France and their dates of opening.

Hafez ESE & Semm K (Eds) Instrumental insemination.

The Ministry of Health provides financial support for the equipment and the development of fundamental research (25% of the total budget).

The budgetary and managerial autonomy of the C.E.C.O.S. has allowed the centers to respond to the needs of both hospitals and private physicians.

2. FUNCTIONS OF C.E.C.O.S.

The following functions of the C.E.C.O.S. Centers are performed: 1) semen preservation for AID, 2) semen autopreservation, and 3) development of fundamental research of cryopreservation of semen and on problems related to sterility and fertility.

2.1. C.E.C.O.S. and AID

AID as a method of controlled conception involves four protagonists: the donor, the couple requesting AID, the medical team (gynecologist, biologist) which performs AID, and the society which has to take responsibility for AID with respect to legal, ethical and religious aspects.

2.1.1. Semen donation. The following three principles govern the C.E.C.O.S. policies:

First, semen donation has to be benevolent and no payment is ever provided as in the case of organ donations. Sperm banking allows the donor to come to the center at his convenience and anonymity is preserved.

Secondly, the donation is made by a couple. Only married men less than 50 years of age having one or more normal children may donate. The agreement of their spouses is also required. This point has important moral and psychological benefits: the notion of 'the donor' is replaced by 'the donor couple' and 'woman recipient' by that of 'recipient couple'.

Thirdly, only five or six ejaculates, equivalent to approximately 100 doses, are obtained from a given donor. The number of pregnancies obtained with one donor is limited to five in order to limit risks of consanguinity.

Donors can be accepted by fulfilling a certain number of conditions based on personal and family medical history, physical examination, karyotype and semen quality (>50 million/ml, $>40\%$ motility after freezing, $>50\%$ normal forms).

2.1.2. Indications and contraindications for AID. The couple requesting AID is either sent to the C.E.C.O.S. Center by a referring physician or consults the Center directly. During the first interview, the director of the Center or his assistant provides information on the procedure of AID and discusses the medical, biological and psychological problems. Necessary information is also obtained to establish the indication for AID.

The indications for AID are:
1. The most obvious indication is irreversible male sterility due to secretory as well as excretory azoospermia.
2. In the case of spermatozoal insufficiency (oligozoospermia, asthenozoospermia, teratozoospermia), AID requests are accepted only if all other treatments of improving fertility have failed.
3. The presence of genetic risks due to a male dominant heredity or a recessive disorder.
4. More rately, AID has been indicated for cases of Rh incompatibility with severe isoimmunization of the woman or for problems of ejaculation.

C.E.C.O.S. Centers always seek the advice of various specialists dealing in male sterility. The fertility of the woman has to be demonstrated as normal through a complete gynecological examination. Finally, each couple undergoes an interview with a psychiatrist in order to provide an opportunity for deeper reflection regarding their motivation and concerns. The main contraindications for AID are unproven male sterility, female infertility, or psychological disorders. The percentage of refused couples, however, remains low (4.6%).

2.1.3. Semen freezing. The same cryopreservation technique has been adopted throughout C.E.C.O.S.: a cryoprotective medium of glycerol – citrate – egg yolk, semen packaging in 0.25 ml plastic straws, rapid (7 min) freezing and storage in liquid nitrogen (David and Czyglik, 1977).

2.1.4. Insemination procedure. The choice of donor semen for a couple requesting AID is based on the principle that one tries to avoid introducing a character which does not exist in either partner of the couple (morphotype, blood group). Inseminations are carried out by gynecologists who are required to respect the protocol established by C.E.C.O.S. A very close collaboration between gynecologists and the C.E.C.O.S. Center enhances the success of AID.

2.2. Collection and analysis of data

All information on donors, couples requesting insemination, associated gynecological treatment, occurrence and evolution of conceptions, and conditions of the child at birth are collected and codified for computer processing. The data are treated at the Statistical Research Center of INSERM; Schwartz and Mayaux (1980) proposed a method of analysis of results in artificial insemination. Following this method, results of insemination are calculated on a per cycle basis. Four groups of patients are defined at each cycle: those lost to follow-up, successes, dropouts, and open cases at the end of each cycle. Cumulative rates established on the basis of a given population are used to quantify theoretical and effective success rates. Only women seeking a first child are considered. This standardized approach has been used in other fields such as in the evaluation of survival or of the effectiveness of contraceptive methods. The per cycle and actuarial rates calculated on the basis of the entire population permit valid comparisons.

2.3. C.E.C.O.S. activity and results

The level of activity and overall results for all French C.E.C.O.S. Centers and for the Grenoble Center are given in Table 1.

The mean success rate per cycle (David et al., 1980) calculated for each cycle, from cycle one to twelve, is 9.8%. In the C.E.C.O.S. Center of Grenoble, it is somewhat lower (7.5%). The differ-

ence by comparison may be due to the relatively low number of cases especially after 6 cycles (496 cases). Nevertheless, the cumulative success rates are quite similar at 12 cycles being 55.4% and 58.6% respectively.

Using published data, David et al. (1980) were able to calculate per cycle success rates obtained by other authors of 14.7% (Lebech, 1972), 15.4% (Jondet et al., 1975), and 5.1% (Bromwich et al., 1978).

3. CONCLUSIONS

The French C.E.C.O.S. system is still in the developmental stage. AID requests and autocryopreservations are continually increasing. Based on current demand, there is an estimated need for at least one sperm bank per 2 to 4 million inhabitants: an increase of 14 to a total of about 20 centers. The creation of the French Federation of C.E.C.O.S. reinforced the link between the Centers which have maintained a stronger position in wich to confront public opinion and official authorities in their goal to facilitate AID practice. A bill concerning AID practice that has already been approved by the Senate has now been submitted to the French Government.

Table 1. Activity and results of the French C.E.C.O.S. Centers in France and Grenoble.

		France (1973–1978)	Grenoble (1978–1980)
AID requests accepted		7130	207
No. women treated		4253	135
Pregnancies		1852	48
Births	1158		21
Miscarriages	290		9
Pregnancies in progress	404		18
Donors		1324	54

REFERENCES

Bromwich P, Kilpatrick J, Newton JR (1978) Artificial insemination with frozen stored donor semen. Br J Obstet Gynaecol 85: 641.

David D, Czyglik F (1977) Tolérance à la congélation du sperme humain en fonction de la qualité initiale du sperme. J Gyn Obst Biol Repr 6: 601.

David G and Lansac J (1980) The organisation of the centers for the study and preservation of semen in France. In David G, Price W, eds. Human artificial insemination and semen preservation, pp 15–26. New York Plenum Press.

David G, Czyglik F, Mayaux MJ, Martin Boyce A, Schwartz D (1980) Artificial insemination with frozen sperm: protocol, method of analysis and results for 1188 women. Br J Obstet Gynaecol 87: 1022.

Jondet M, Millet D, Cornuau J, Picaud C, Netter A (1975) Utilisation du sperme congelé pour l'insémination humaine hétérologue. Gynécologie 26: 285.

Lebech E (1972) Banques de sperme humain. In Thibault C, ed. Fécondité et Stérilité du mâle. Acquisition récentes, pp 349–359. Paris, Masson.

Schwartz D, Mayaux MJ (1980) Mode of evaluation of results in artificial insemination. In David G, Price W, eds. Human artificial insemination and semen preservation, pp 197–210. New York: Plenum Press.

Author's address:
Maria Servoz-Gavin
C.E.C.O.S.
Laboratoir d'Histologie et Embryologie
Faculté de Médecine
38700 La Tronche
France

28. FACTORS AFFECTING PREGNANCY RATE AFTER AID

J. KREMER

Achieving pregnancy by AID depends on several factors. Factors which can be influenced are occurrence and time of ovulation, timing and technique of insemination, quality of donor semen and psychological stress of the woman. Psychological stress may inhibit sperm transport in the female genital tract. The number of spermatozoa reaching the ampulla of the tube is depressed in ewes showing signs of discomfort or fright (Mattner 1963; Thibault and Wintenberger-Torres, 1967). This inhibition may be mediated through the release of epinephrine, which in turn reduces the contractility of the myometrium to oxytocin (Bedford, 1970). The influence of psychological stress on the result of AID in women is difficult to assess. Psychological stress may, however, have a depressing influence on achieving pregnancy by AID (a pregnancy is often unexpectedly achieved when a situation of tense expectation by whatever means is relieved).

Unadjustable factors that influence pregnancy by AID are: age of the woman, fertilizability of the oocytes, transport of the gametes and of the fertilized ovum through the (patent) female genital tract beyond the uterine cervix, nidation capacity of the blastocyst, and the presence of antispermatozoal antibodies in the woman.

1. AID OUTCOME AND NUMBER OF INSEMINATION CYCLES

Between 1973 and 1979, achieving the first pregnancy by AID was attempted in a group of 305 women. In 106 couples, the husband was azoospermic; while in 199 couples, the husband's semen contained spermatozoa but the total number of progressively moving spermatozoa in the ejaculate was less than 20 million. The fertility investigations in the women in the latter group did not reveal any abnormality. Since all couples could not normally achieve pregnancy for at least 4 years, semen deficiency was considered the cause of infertility. The ages of the women ranged from 22 to 40 years.

All women were inseminated 2 or 3 times per cycle with fresh donor semen containing at least 40 million progressively motile spermatozoa per ml ejaculate. The inseminations were performed with an interval of about 48 hours, by means of a combined intracervical–paracervical technique. Cervical caps or intrauterine inseminations were never used. Cycle irregularity was adjusted in 41 women by administering 50 – 100 mg. of clomid from the 5th to the 9th cycle day. The results of the investigation are indicated in Fig. 1.

The pregnancy percentage for each cycle, is calculated with the life table method which calculates the chance of achieving pregnancy in couples who are willing to continue AID treatment as long as possible (Schwartz and Mayaux, 1979). This chance tends to decrease when the number of insemination cycles increases, although the results in the 16th and 18th insemination cycle were comparable with the results during the first four insemination cycles. The life table pregnancy % after 18 cycles was 78.9. There were no pregnancies in seven women where the inseminations were continued for longer than 18 cycles. This does not, however, indicate that pregnancy by AID cannot occur after the 18th insemination cycle. In a larger group of women 12 pregnancies occurred between the 24th and 60th insemination cycle (Schoysman et al., 1979). It is not known when the chance of achieving pregnancy has been reduced to zero; however, a choice must be made. Eighteen insemination cycles are enough to offer a couple a fair opportunity for achieving pregnancy.

Hafez ESE & Semm K (Eds) Instrumental insemination.
© *1982 Martinus Nijhoff Publishers, The Hague/Boston/London. ISBN 90-247-2530-5. Printed in the Netherlands.*

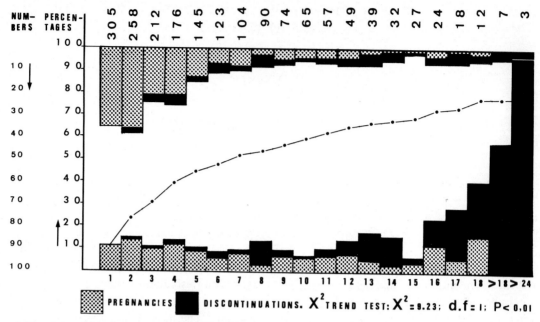

Figure 1. Chance to achieve first pregnancy by AID in 305 women where AID was performed during 1-11-73 and 10-12-79. The numbers along the lower and upper horizontal line indicate the number of the insemination cycle and the couples per insemination cycle, respectively. The upper bars represent the *number* of pregnancies and discontinuations; the lower bars represent the pregnancy- and discontinuation *percentage*. The curve represents the cumulative pregnancy percentage per cycle calculated with the life table method.

2. AID OUTCOME AND AGE OF RECIPIENT

A second investigation concerned the influence of age on the chance of achieving the first pregnancy by AID within 18 insemination cycles in a group of 209 women (Table 1).

Neither the chance of achieving pregnancy nor the mean number of insemination cycles per pregnancy differed significantly in all age groups between 25 and 39 years. The group of 7 women, aged 20–24 years, was not sufficient for statistical assessment. Similar results have been reported by Chong and Taymor (1975). In a group of 186 women treated with donor insemination, the pregnancy rate remained stable from ages 20 to 39.

Table 1. Relation between age and chance of *first* pregnancy after AID in 209 women where the treatment started between 1-11-1973 and 1-8-1978.

Number of couples, pregnancies and mean number of insemination cycles (i.c.)	Age groups				
	20–24 years	25–39 years	30–34 years	35–39 years	Total
Number of couples	7	104	75	23	209
Number of insemination cycles	23	691	547	138	1399
Number of pregnancies	6	80 (76%)	50 (66%)	17 (74%)	153 (73%)**
Number of pregnancies per 100 i.c.	26.1	11.6	9.1	12.3	10.9
Mean number of i.c. per pregnant woman	3 (1–9)	4.9 (1–18)	4.2 (1–16)	3.9 (1–16)	4.5 (1–18)
Mean number of i.c. per non pregnant woman	5	12.4 (3–24(	13.4 (3–28)	12 (8–18)	12.7
Life table pregnancy percentage after 18 cycles*		87%.SE 4.4%	72%.SE 5.9%	85%.SE 11.3%	82%.SE 3.6%

* No age effect on the chance of achieving pregnancy (log rank test: $\chi^2 = 4.98$; d.f. = 3; $P > 0.10$
** Number of abortions (<16 weeks): 12 (8%)

Table 2. Relation between the chance to achieve the *first* pregnancy after AID and the grade of subfertility of the husband's semen in 209 women where the treatment started between 1-11-1973 and 1-8-1978.

Number of couples, pregnancies and mean number of insemination cycles (i.c.)	Total number of motile spermatozoa in husband's semen				
	Azoospermia	<2 million	2–9 million	≥10 million	Total
Number of couples	80	40	39	50	209
Number of insemination cycles	512	248	234	405	1399
Number of pregnancies	66 (83%)	32 (80%)	28 (72%)	27 (54%)	153 (73%)**
Number of pregnancies per 100 i.c.	12.9	12.9	12.0	6.7	10.9
Mean number of i.c. per pregnant woman	4.9 (1–8)	4.9 (1–18)	3.2 (1–7)	4.4 (1–16)	4.5 (1–18)
Mean number of i.c. per non pregnant woman	13.4 (6–24)	11.4 (3–17)	13.1 (3–26)	12.4 (3–28)	12.7 (3–28)
Life table pregnancy percentage after 18 cycles*	92%.SE 4.5%	100%.SE 6.5%	73%.SE 7.2%	62%.SE 8.4%	82%.SE 3.6%

* Significant effect of grade of subfertility of husband's semen on the chance of achieving pregnancy (log rank trend test: $\chi^2 = 6.36$; d.f. = 1; $0.01 < P < 0.025$)
** Number of abortion (<16 weeks): 12 (8%)

3. AID OUTCOME AND QUALITIES OF HUSBAND'S SEMEN

The relation between achieving the first pregnancy after AID and the grade of subfertility of the husband's semen was also investigated in the same group of 209 women where the influence of age had been investigated (Table 2).

Pregnancy by AID within 18 cycles of treatment was about 100% in the groups where the husband's semen contained less than 2 million motile spermatozoa (column 1 and 2). The mean number of treatment cycles per pregnant woman in these two groups was 4.9. This means that, on average, 4–5 insemination cycles are required for a pregnancy to occur by AID in fertile women.

The women where the husband's semen contained at least 2 million motile spermatozoa per ejaculate (column 3 and 4), yet was considered subfertile (due to a motility percentage less than 30, slow progressive movements or more than 70% abnormal headforms), proved to have a rather low chance of achieving pregnancy within 18 insemination cycles (73% and 62% resp.). This high proportion of women who were not able to become pregnant was probably due to their own (undiagnosed) infertility. The pregnancy percentage after AID is lower in a group of women married to oligozoospermic men than in a group of women married to azoospermic men (Emperaire et al., 1980; Matthew, 1980).

4. AID OUTCOME AND RESULT OF MARITAL POST-COITAL TEST

Results of the marital Post-Coital Test (PCT) taken from 42 AID couples where the husband probably had subfertile semen, were investigated (Table 3). All 50 couples were childless and, for more than five years, had unsuccessfully achieved pregnancy by coitus (Table 2).

Achieving pregnancy by AID was significantly greater in the group of 21 women with a negative result of the PCT than in the group of 21 women where the PCT showed progressively motile spermatozoa in the endocervical mucus (Table 3). In more than 50% of the couples in the latter group, the cause of the infertility was probably due to infertility of the wife.

5. CONCLUDING REMARKS

Pregnancy by AID can be achieved by nearly 100% when fresh semen and the proper insemination technique are used, and if the woman is normally fertile. The number of insemination cycles should

Table 3. Relation between the chance to achieve the *first* pregnancy after AID and the result of the Post-Coital Test in 42 women where husband's semen contained ≥ 10 million motile spermatozoa.

	Result of Post-Coital Test (normal pre-ovulatory mucus)	
	No progressively moving spermatozoa in endocervical mucus	Progressively moving spermatozoa in endocervical mucus
Number of couples	21	21
Number of i.c.	149	198
Number of pregnancies	15 (71%)	8 (38%)
Number of pregnancies per 100 i.c.	10.1	4.0
Mean number of i.c. per pregnant woman	4.8 (1–16)	4.4 (1–10)
Mean number of i.c. per non pregnant woman	12.8 (8–18)	12.5 (4–28)
Life table pregnancy percentage after 18 cycles*	79%.SE 11%	46%.SE 13%

* Significant difference; log rank test: $\chi^2 = 3.09$; d.f. $= 1$; $P < 0.05$ (one sided)

also be at least 18. The wife can be considered as normally fertile if she is younger than 40 years, if the total number of motile spermatozoa in her husband's ejaculate is less than 2 million, and if the routine fertility investigation did not reveal any abnormality. Hysterosalpingography and laparoscopy are superfluous. If the husband's semen is subfertile but contains at least 2 million motile spermatozoa in the whole ejaculate, then in 30–40% of the cases the female partner is responsible for not being able to conceive. In more than 50% of all cases, infertility is due to the wife provided the husband's semen contains at least 10 million motile spermatozoa in the whole ejaculate (but is subfertile due to subnormal swimming velocity or subnormal sperm morphology) and progressively moving spermatozoa are found in the pre-ovulatory endocervical mucus. The cause of infertility in the female partner, however, cannot often be discovered, creating what is known as 'unexplained infertility in the woman.'

ACKNOWLEDGEMENTS

Thanks are due to Mr. V. Fidler, Dept. of Medical Physics, University of Groningen for the statistical assessments, Mrs. A. Witteveen-de Vlaming for collecting the data and Mrs. R. Mathias for the correction of the English text.

REFERENCES

Bedford JM (1970) The saga of mammalian sperm from ejaculation to syngamy. In Gibian H, Plotz EJ, eds. Mammalian reproduction. Berlin: Springer Verlag.

Chong AP, Taymor ML (1975) Sixteen years' experience with therapeutic donor insemination. Fertil Steril 26: 791.

Emperaire JC, Gauzere E, Audebert A (1980) Female fertility and donor insemination. Lancet 1: 1423.

Matthew C (1980) The technique and outcome of AID. In Wood C, ed. Artificial insemination by donor. Melbourne: Brown Prior Anderson.

Mattner PE (1963) Spermatozoa in the genital tract of the ewe — III. Role of spermatozoa motility and of uterine contractions in transport. Austr J Biol Sci 16: 473.

Schoysman R, Schoysman A, Devroey P (1980) A thousand pregnancies by AID. Text of lecture given at Dept Gyn/Obstet, Free University of Brussels.

Schwartz O, Mayaux M (1979) Mode of evaluation of results in artificial insemination, pp 197–220. In: Proc Int Symp Human Artificial Insemination and Semen Preservation, April 9–11, 1979. New York: Plenum.

Thibault C, Wintenberger-Torres S (1967) Oxytocin and sperm transport in the ewe. Int J Fertil 12: 410.

Author's address:
Prof Dr J. Kremer
Parklaan 16
9724 AN Groningen
The Netherlands

29. FAILURE IN AIH AS A METHOD OF FERTILITY INDUCTION IN MEN WITH SPERM AGGLUTINATION

ANNE M. JEQUIER, N.J. BULLIMORE and JOAN P. CRICH

The spontaneous agglutination of spermatozoa that may occur in human semen at or very soon after ejaculation is a well recognised cause of infertility in the male (Rumpke, 1968; Halim et al., 1974). This spontaneous sperm agglutination is traditionally ascribed to the presence in the semen of specific antibodies directed against the surface antigens of the spermatozoa (Hansen and Hjort, 1971). It is the polyvalency of these antibodies which are said to cause the sperm to stick together in clumps in the semen. These antibodies can be demonstrated in the serum not only in men with spontaneous spermagglutination but also in men with a wide variety of different disorders producing their infertility (Rumpke and Hellinga, 1959). For example, the Gel Agglutination Test which is a commonly used method for demonstrating sperm antibodies (Halim et al., 1974) may, if applied to different groups of infertile men, result in an incidence of between 3.3 and 14.2% positive responses (Rumpke and Hellinga, 1959; Beer and Neaves, 1978; Jequier et al., 1980; Rumpke et al., 1974). The demonstration of spermagglutination in the serum of infertile men is not a very good prognostic index as far as fertility is concerned.

Although an immune orchitis and an immune aspermatogenesis can easily be produced experimentally both in laboratory animals (Johnson, 1970) and in man (Mancini et al., 1965), the fact that no spontaneously occurring initiating factor for the development of such autantibodies has ever been satisfactorily described, makes the whole concept of sperm antibodies as a cause for infertility in man a little hard to believe. Also, that such an "autoimmune" disease is so common a cause for infertility again causes one to question the whole idea of sperm antibodies in relation to human infertility.

Spontaneous spermagglutination is always due to the presence of antisperm antibodies is a conclusion that really cannot be justified. That sperm aggluti-

nation is due to sperm autoimmunity is an assumption that is too often made in the absence of any unequivocal evidence of the presence of such antibodies. In reality, there could in fact be many other causes of sperm agglutination which have no immune basis and the steroid related beta-macroprotein described by Boettcher et al. in 1970 is such an example.

However, the general consensus supports the belief that spermagglutination is indeed antibody-induced. Thus the current methods of treatment of this problem are directed in two main ways: 1) the attempted removal of these antibodies by various washing procedures (Usherwood, 1978) and 2) the use of parenteral immuno-suppressants such as methyl prednisolone in large doses (Shulman, 1976) to decrease the production of these antibodies.

1. "ANTIBODY COATED" SPERMATOZOA

Spontaneous agglutination of sperm may involve a varying percentage of the total sperm complement in the ejaculate. However, in some patients, sperm agglutination may be very marked, and in some 10 to 15 min after ejaculation, almost all the sperm may be held together in clumps. However if this sperm agglutination is caused by a surface coating of antibody, and bearing in mind the high surface area to volume of a cell as small as a spermatozoa, then this antibody would have to be present in high concentration if it were to clump together many thousands or millions of spermatozoa. If it is present in high concentration its presence should therefore be easy to demonstrate and one of the ways that could be used to demonstrate such antibody is direct immunofluorescence.

Antigen specific immunoglobulins, in particular those of the IgG class, have affinity constants that lie

Hafez ESE & Semm K (Eds) Instrumental insemination.
© *1982 Martinus Nijhoff Publishers, The Hague/Boston/London. ISBN 90-247-2530-5. Printed in the Netherlands.*

between 10^5 and 10^{12} litres per mole (Holborow and Reeves, 1977). From the theoretical point of view, it should therefore be very difficult, due to the dilution alone, to wash off such an antibody were it specifically bound to surface antigens on spermatozoa. It should thus be impossible to wash off any antibody from the surface of the spermatozoa during their preparation for any procedure whether it be investigatory or therapeutic. During a simple washing process, any significant amounts of immunoglobulins that are removed from the surface of these sperm, cannot be specifically bound to them. conversely, as the seminal fluid normally contains immunoglobulins, in particular IgA (Friberg, 1974), the demonstration of antibodies on the surface of unwashed sperm does not prove the presence of specific antibody directed against the surface antigens of these spermatozoa.

In order to test this hypothesis, ten infertile men all with varying degrees of spontaneous sperm agglutination of rapid onset were studied. Of these ten patients, eight men had other possible causes of their infertility. Of these patients, two had reduced testicular size associated with a raised follicle stimulating hormone level in their serum, i.e. they had a primary spermatogenic failure. Two men had a unilateral varicocoele and four more had markedly retractile testes, pyospermia, hyperprolactinaemia and incomplete liquefaction respectively. Two more men had spontaneous sperm agglutination as their only diagnosable abnormality.

Spontaneous sperm agglutination in the semen of these patients was detected by microscopy within 1 hour of production. It was graded visually. The sign + signified less than half the total sperm were agglutinated, the sign + + that half or more of the sperm were agglutinated and the sign + + + denoted almost complete agglutination of all the sperm in the specimen.

Freshly produced semen specimens were obtained from each patient and were gently centrifuged for five minutes and the supernatant aspirated. The spermatozoa were then resuspended in 0,01 M phosphate buffer containing 0.18 M sodium chloride at pH 7.5 (P.B.S.) and then recentrifuged. The sperm from each patient were washed in this way three times and the resuspended spermatozoa were then smeared onto clean glass slides in the same way as a blood film is made. In no specimen examined after washing was there any evidence of reduction in the proportion of agglutinated sperm. Further aliquots from each semen specimen were also subjected to as many as 10 washes and still at no time was any disruption of the clumped sperm noted. The smears of sperm were air dried and fixed in 70% methanol for 10 min.

Florescein conjugated antisera raised against human IgG and subgroups, IgM and IgA immunoglobulin classes and obtained from Dacopatt A/S, Denmark, were used to detect the presence of immunoglobulin on the surface of the sperm. The fluorescein conjugated antisera were diluted 1 in 10 in P.B.S. A drop of the diluted conjugate was placed on the smear and left for 30 min at room temperature. The excess conjugate was then gently washed off and further excess removed by soaking the glass slide in P.B.S. for one hour with at least two changes of buffer in that hour. Excess buffer was then

Table 1. A group of ten infertile men who were studied in relation to sperm agglutination and direct sperm immunofluorescence.

Patient No.	Diagnosis		Degree of sperm agglutination	Direct immunofluorescence of sperm
1	Clumping alone		+ + +	IgA
2	Clumping alone	(a)	+ + +	Negative
		(b)	+ + +	Negative
		(c)	+ + +	Negative
3	Incomplete liquefaction		+ +	Negative
4	Hyperprolactinaemia		+	Negative
5	Pyospermia	(a)	+ + +	Negative
		(b)	+ + +	IgA × IgC
6	Retractile testes		+	Negative
7	Varicocoele		+	Negative
8	Varicocoele		+	Negative
9	Seminiferous tubular failure		+	Negative
10	Seminiferous tubular failure		+ +	Negative

removed with filter paper and the slide dried at room temperature. The stained sperm were then covered with a coverslip, sealed with varnish and viewed under a Leitz microscope using ultra violet light.

Semen from all the ten patients were treated in this way. However from one patient, two separate specimens of semen were obtained and from another, three specimens were obtained. Of the ten men studied, only two of these patients showed a positive direct immunofluorescence of their sperm and in one the immunofluorescence was not repeatable on a second specimen of semen. In both patients, the immunofluorescence was positive to IgA and in one was positive to IgG. However, the positive response to IgG was not repeatable in a second specimen. These data are summarised in Table 1.

Repeated washing of sperm with P.B.S. did not disrupt spontaneously agglutinated sperm. There was also no demonstrable relationship between sperm agglutination and positive direct immunofluroscence when conjugated antisera raised against the major classes of human immunoglobulins were applied to these clumped sperm. In all of these patients, sperm that had been repeatedly washed in phosphosaline buffer were used for AIH in the wives of each of these patients. Inseminations were performed for between 2 to 6 cycles. No pregnancy resulted in any of the women so treated.

The washing of sperm, a manoeuvre frequently described as a method of freeing clumped sperm of antibody, is not a feasible method of treatment even is such spontaneous agglutination were due to the presence of antibody on their surface. No such antibody was demonstrable. It would thus seem that agglutination of sperm is not always due to immunoglobulins binding to the surface of sperm. Nevertheless, many such reports in the literature suggest the presence of such antibody by finding positive immunofluorescence on such sperm. However, careful washing of the sperm is often not carried out and such studies may thus be reporting the presence of non-specific antibody which is adherent to, rather than specifically bound to the surface of sperm. Thus if the direct immunofluorescence is negative because the antibody is being washed off, then washing should unclump these sperm. As this was not the case, these data suggest that spontaneous sperm agglutination may have other causes which are not necessarily of an immune aetiology.

2. ISOLATION OF POSSIBLE ANTAGGLUTININ FROM SEMEN

In the search for the aetiology of sperm agglutination, it is becoming clear that such sperm clumping may far from always have an immune cause. It is possible that spontaneous sperm agglutination could be due to the presence of a non-immune substance which coats sperm causing them to clump together. However, it is equally possible that sperm agglutination could be due to the absence of a specific substance that, in normal circumstances, prevents sperm sticking together. As spontaneous agglutination may occur in normal semen on incubation, there thus existed a possibility that in normal semen there is a substance which prevents agglutination but which may be unstable. With this possibility in mind, it was decided to begin a search for a substance in semen that would act as an antagglutinin.

In 1954, Lindahl and Kihlström reported the isolation of a sperm antagglutinin from bull semen. It was therefore decided to try to identify and to isolate this substance from human semen. As whole semen from normal fertile men was difficult to obtain in large quantities, it was decided to use pooled semen from men who were routinely attending for semen analyses following vasectomy. This had the advantage that these men were all of proven fertility but had the disadvantage that the testicular and epididymal contributions to the ejaculate would be, in the main, absent. The method of extraction used was a minor modification of that described by Lindahl and Kihlström in 1954.

Using fresh pooled semen (the volume dependent on availability) the mixture was centrifuged for 5 min to remove cellular debris and any remaining sperm. The supernatant plasma was aspirated off the cells at the bottom of the tube. The seminal plasma was now gently oxidised by placing it in a small piece of platinum wire and bubbling air through it for about 20 min. Salting out of the protein content of the oxidised seminal plasma was now achieved using a saturated ammonium sulphate solution. This was acieved by the addition of 0.037 ml of a saturated solution of ammonium sulphate prepared at $4°C$ to each millilitre of seminal plasma. The pH was adjusted to 7.8 using 0.1 M sodium hydroxide. After storage for 5–10 min at $4°C$, the solution was centrifuged at 9000 *g* for a further 10 min, the supernatant aspirated and discarded. The precipitate was then redissolved in a volume of distilled water equal to that of the discarded supernatant. The salting out procedure was then repeated for a second time. The second precipitate so formed was now redissolved in distilled water to a volume equivalent to some 25% of the original seminal plasma. The pH of this solution was then readjusted to pH 8.5 using the 0.1 M sodium hydroxide.

One gram of calcium carbonate will absorb out all the antagglutinin from 60 ml of bull semen. Using an appropriate weight of calcium carbonate for the volume of seminal fluid used, a calcium carbonate sus-

pension was packed into a Pasteur pipette above a small plug of glass wool. The extracted protein was now applied to the calcium carbonate and the column washed with a sodium hydroxide solution at pH 8.5. During this process the antagglutinin is absorbed onto the calcium carbonate. The antagglutinin is now eluted off the column using a weak solution of carbonic acid. This carbonic acid is prepared simply by bubbling carbon dioxide through distilled water until the pH reaches 5.5. This acid solution was now applied to the calcium carbonate column and the eluate collected as fractions of about 2 ml. The antagglutinin is found in the first fraction and can be identified by its pattern of extinction of

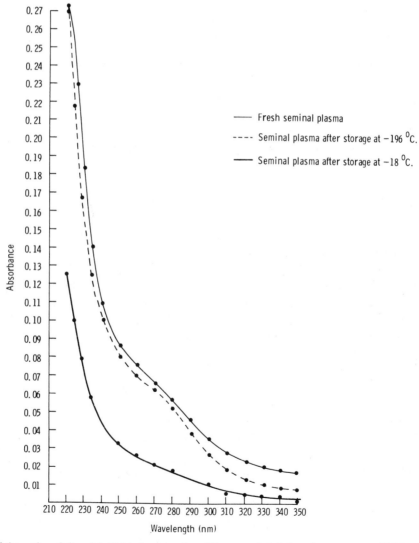

Figure 1. Profiles of absorption of ultra violet light after extraction of the antagglutinin from human semen which has been extracted a) from fresh seminal plasma b) from seminal plasma stored for 24 hours at $-196°$ C and c) from seminal plasma stored for 24 hours at $-18°$ C.

ultra violet light. The absorbance pattern of ultra violet light by the solution of antagglutinin was tested in an ultra violet spectrophotometer using wavelengths between 220 and 350 nm. Between this range absorbance is measured using light of increasing wavelength of 10 nm.

When this method was applied to pooled human seminal plasma, the first 2 ml elution fraction obtained from the calcium carbonate produced a pattern of extinction of ultra violet light identical to the described by Lindahl and Kihlström (1954a) in bull semen. The extinction pattern from an extraction of antagglutinin from 30 ml of pooled human post vasectomy semen is depicted in Fig. 1.

Another pool of fresh human post vasectomy semen was now divided into three aliquots. One aliquot was subjected to the extraction procedure while fresh. A second aliquot was stored in liquid nitrogen, i.e. at $-196°$ C, for 24 hours prior to extraction and a third aliquot was stored at $-18°$ C for 24 hours prior to extraction. The semen stored in an ordinary deep freeze at $-18°$ C provided a much lower concentration of antagglutinin than did those aliquots of semen extracted fresh or after storage in liquid nitrogen. These extinction patterns are depicted graphi-

cally in Fig. 2. This antagglutinin in unstable in semen after storage even at $-18°$ C. However after removal from semen, the antagglutinin remained stable at $-18°$ C. These data suggest that this substance may be degraded in semen and the disappearance of this substance may account for the spontaneous agglutination that occurs in normal semen on incubation.

The most important question to ask, however, is whether this substance that has been extracted from human semen, in fact acts as an antagglutinin on human spermatozoa. In order to test this possible affect, the extracted antagglutinin was applied to the semen of two more infertile men both of whom had severe ($+++$) spontaneous sperm agglutination. Equal volumes of the extracted antagglutinin were mixed with each of these two semen samples and the effects on the sperm clumps observed by microscopy. On microscopy of a wet preparation, severe agglutination is noted. After application of the antagglutinin, the clumps of sperm which were mostly of the head-to-head agglutination become markedly looser and some dispersed altogether. However, it is now possible to see that more than half of these now unagglutinated spermatozoa were grossly morpho-

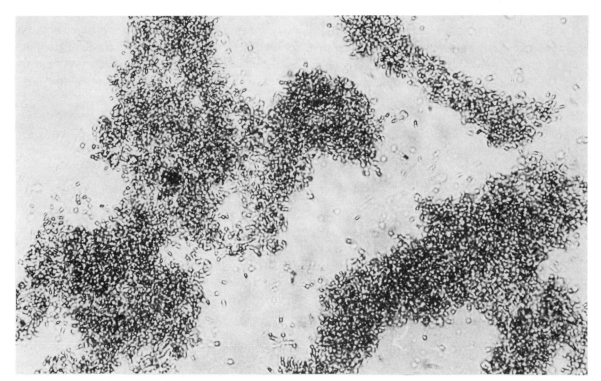

Figure 2. Photomicrograph of a wet preparation of fresh semen (-145) which shows marked spontaneous spermagglutination

logically abnormal. Some demonstrated abnormal heads while others showed distal displacement of the nucleus and absent middle pieces. These findings were confirmed on fixing and staining with haematoxylin and eosin.

The fact that this substance can be extracted from human semen in the same way as from bull semen and that the human extract has a very similar extinction pattern to ultra violet light as that from bull semen, suggests but by no means proves, that this substance is the same in both human and bull semen. That this substance can be extracted by salting out demonstrates that it is a protein but whether it is a single protein or a group of proteins remains, in the man, to be elucidated.

This substance is also unstable in semen stored at $-18°$ C but is maintained in semen stored at $-196°$ C. Enzyme activity is not halted at $-18°$ C and it may be that enzyme activity is responsible for the degradation. This phenomenon may occur in normal semen for it is quite common to see spontaneous sperm agglutination of otherwise normal fertile spermatozoa. At 6 hours after production, quite large clumps of sperm may be present in normal semen. Where this substance is produced is unclear. In the bull Lindahl and Kihlström (1956) suggest that it is part of the prostatic ejaculate. The fact that it is present in post-vasectomy human semen would indicate that it does not come from the testis or epididymis. However it must be remembered that not all the human post-vasectomy semen used in this study was completely azoospermic and so a testicular or epididymal source for this factor cannot be excluded.

What feature of this substance or substances produces the high extinction pattern of ultra violet light is not known in the human. However a tocopherol molecule has been demonstrated by Lindahl and Kihlström (1954b, 1956) to be incorporated into or bound to this factor extracted from bull semen and this is therefore likely to be the case in the human. It is of course entirely possible that it is the tocopherol molecule that is supplying the bulk of the absorption of the ultraviolet light by this anti-agglutinic factor and that the protein moiety of this molecule may, in man, differ substantially from that in the bull.

The presence of gross morphological abnormalities was noted in these agglutinated sperm after their release from the clumps by this antagglutinin. Such abnormalities were not seen when normal unclumped sperm were treated with the extracted antagglutinin and thus these changes did not seem to be produced artifactually (Bullimore, unpublished data).

Spontaneously agglutinated sperm cannot be made to unclump by simple washing and that washing these clumped sperm and their use in AIH does nothing to improve their fertility potential. No coating antibody could be demonstrated on the surface of these agglutinated sperm and thus spontaneous sperm agglutination may have other causes which may be unrelated to antisperm antibodies or, for that matter, to any other aspect of immunology. As in bull semen, there may well be an antiagglutinic factor in human semen but what role this plays in normal sperm physiology as well as in pathological sperm agglutination remains to be elucidated. The high numbers of abnormal sperm found among the clumped sperm suggest that sperm agglutination may be only a manifestation of abnormal sperm and not a cause of infertility per se. The assumption that all sperm agglutination is due to the presence of antisperm antibodies is simply not justified both on theoretical grounds as well as experimental grounds. In the meanwhile, infertility due to spontaneous sperm agglutination remains an untreatable condition.

ACKNOWLEDGEMENTS

Thanks are due to Mr. Stuart Carlton from the Department of Immunology, Queen's Medical Centre, for performing tests for immunofluorescence on the spermatozoa.

REFERENCES

Beer AE, Neaves WB (1978) Antigenic status of semen from the viewpoints of the female and male. Fertil Steril 29: 3.
Boettcher B, Hay J, Kay DJ, Baldo BA, Roberts TK (1970) Sperm agglutinating activity in some human sera. Intern J Fertil 15: 143.

Friberg J (1974) Sperm agglutinating antibodies and immunoglobulins G and A in stored human seminal fluid. Acta Obstet Gynecol Scand Suppl 36: 59.

Halim A, Antoniou D, Lane J, Blandy J (1974) The significance of antibodies to sperm in infertile men and their wives. Br J Urol 46: 65.

Hansen KB, Hjort T (1971) Immunofluoroscent studies on human spermatozoa. II. Characterisation of spermatozoal antigens and their occurrence in spermatozoa from the male partners of infertile couples. Clin Exp Immun 9: 21.

Holborow EJ, Reeves WG (1977) Immunology in medicine, chap 1, p. 11. In Holborow EJ, Reeves WC, eds. New York: Academic Press.

Jequier AM, Crich JP (1980) Gel agglutination test: its application to infertile men. Arch Androl 5: 205.

Johnson MH (1970) Changes in the blood testis barrier of the guinea pig in relation to histological damage following isoimmunisation with testis. J Reprod Fertil 22: 119.

Lindahl PE, Kihlström JE (1954a) An antiagglutinic factor in mammalian sperm plasma. Fertil Steril 5: 241.

Lindahl PE, Kihlström, JE (1954b) A constituent of male sperm antiagglutinin related to vitamin E. Nature 174: 600.

Lindahl PE, Kihlström JE, Ross S (1965) On some properties of the aromatic constituent of sperm antiagglutinin and its "active group" Acta Chem Scand 10: 1597.

Mancini RE, Andrada JA, Saraceni D, Bachmann AE Lavieri JC, Nemirovsky M (1965) Immunological and testicular response in man sensitised with human testicular homogenate. J Clin Endocrin Metab 25: 859.

Rumpke P, Hellinga G (1959) Autoantibodies against spermatozoa in sterile men. Am J Clin Pathol 32: 357.

Rumpke P (1968) Sperm agglutinating antibodies in relation to male infertility. Proc R Soc Med 61: 275.

Rumpke P, Van Amstel N, Messer EN, Bezemer PD (1974) Prognosis of fertility in men with spermagglutinins in the serum. Fertil Steril 25: 393.

Shulman S (1976) Treatment of immune male infertility with methyl prednisolone. Lancet ii: 1243.

Usherwood MM (1978) Sperm washing and artificial insemination. In Cohen J, Hendry WF, eds. Spermatozoal antibodies and infertility. London: Blackwell.

Author's address:
Dr Anne M. Jequier
Department of Obstetrics and Gynaecology
University of Nottingham
Hucknall Road
Nottingham, UK

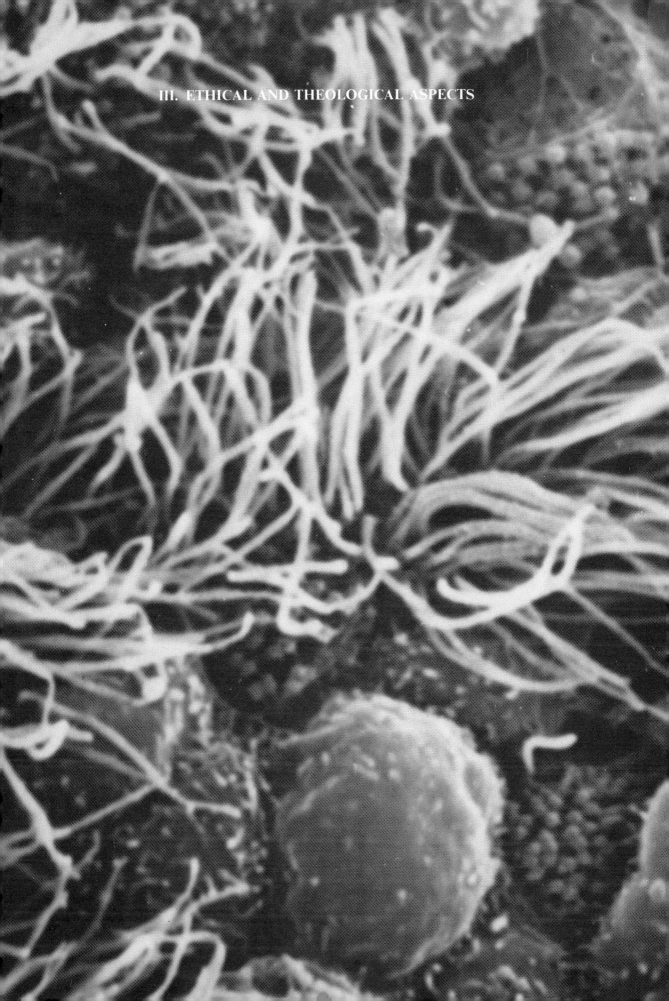

30. ETHICAL IMPLICATIONS OF AID

E.S.E. HAFEZ

In general, some 13% of all married couples have an infertility problem, directly related to the male. Overall, 15% of all married couples have an infertility problem. Therefore, there is a substantial and potential need for AID, as several thousand children are born annually in U.S.A. and Europe (Schellen, 1957; Behrman, 1975). There is also a great demand for AID primarily due to impatience for wanting a child, without extensive testing on the husband. In general, AID is performed with the husband's consent only when sterility is established. There has been some biological anxiety that the children born from AID might in some way be defective. At present there are several AID babies who have grown up, married and had children, without any apparent psychological problems attributed to AID.

The purpose of this review is to evaluate — in view of rapidly changing attitudes — the ethical and moral status of AID as affected by differences in culture, religion, social and economic conditions. Basic and clinical research should not be discontinued in view of the present population crisis, and the sharp increase in illegitimate and homeless children in some societies.

1. SELECTION OF AID DONORS

In most cases, an attempt is made to match the donor to the husband as closely as possible; whereas, in some cases, mixed semen from different donors is used so that the actual father of any given baby is never known. Thus, the andrologist exercises a certain positive eugenic selection, since he only uses donors who he believes are physically and mentally sound, with a good medical record and semen of high quality. The andrologist may also introduce value judgements as to which personality types (for example) would make the best fathers (McLaren, 1973). The effect of this selection, however, is minimal over the whole population, unless the amount of AID progeny from a given donor becomes extensive. It would inevitably appear that the selection of donor may not be satisfactory since the selector chooses what he or she believes to be good characteristics.

The recipient of AID sometimes may not be informed about the donor; however, some details concerning physical characteristics and level of education may be supplied. Choosing AID also provides the choice of selecting an improved I.Q. The improvement that could be introduced by medical, educational and cultural measures would be more effective than many centuries of intense eugenic efforts (McLaren, 1973). The physical and mental development of AID children is not inferior to controls, whereas I.Q. is strongly affected by the family environment, which then can significantly exceed the mean level (Ilizuka et al., 1968).

Several factors involving ethical problems of AID applies to the father, paternity, religious aspects, adultery, illegitimacy and adoption. In the interest of positive eugenics it is unlikely that AID will be used in the near future for the genetic improvement of the human race or to further some less reputable social or political aim. In most AID clinics, the donor either collects his semen in an excitingly decorated 'masturbation parlor', or delivers the semen at a different door from that used by AID patients. Most AID donors are either needy medical students, male nurses who receive a financial incentive, or the husbands of patients at infertility clinics. Concern has been expressed that willingness to become a donor might reflect some undesirable personality trait which would then be transmitted to a disproportionate number of progeny (McLaren, 1973). At present, most donors in

Hafez ESE & Semm K (Eds) Instrumental insemination.
© *1982 Martinus Nijhoff Publishers, The Hague/Boston/London. ISBN 90-247-2530-5. Printed in the Netherlands.*

the U.S.A. are not prepared to give their semen without some financial reward, as when they donate blood.

Paid donors have demonstrated the medical and economic inferiority of blood transfusion services in which donations are paid for. The financial reward encourages the indigent to conceal relevant facts in medical history, and so increases the supply of infected blood. By analogy, payment to those donating semen, with no evidence of genetic suitability other than unverified assurances about parenthood and medical record, implies the taking of highly unethical risks from which the patient to be inseminated, her husband and the child to be conceived might prove to be the victims (Dunstan, 1973).

An attempt is being made to match the external characteristics of the husband with those of the donor, e.g. color of skin, hair and eyes. No serious attempts have been made for some genetic compatibility as in the case of adoption agencies.

The andrologist may inquire about illnesses and diseases in the family history among uncles, aunts, brothers, cousins, parents and grandparents. It may be advisable to provide semen from a more intelligent donor to a less intelligent recipient. Pedigrees can be useful for a few obvious genetic diseases such as hemophilia, rhesus-negative and sickle cell anemia. The assessment of the donor according to the pedigree and medical history merely excludes honest donors with good memories. It is irresponsible to use a donor again if his semen produces anomalies of unknown etiology, e.g. spina bifida. It is possible that AID children conceived from the same donor, and who were therefore half-brothers and half-sisters, might unwittingly marry and have children of their own (Law and Ethics, 1973).

2. AID CONSENT

AID is performed when the husband is either infertile, azoospermic or suffers from a severe hereditary disease. Most andrologists feel than AID should not be used when the husband has either not given his consent or is fertile. It is also feasible that AID can be performed on unmarried women and lesbians who wish to conceive and raise a child.

Women over the age of 16 can validly consent in writing the performance of AID. AID should not be provided for a wife without the informed and deliberate consent of the husband (Appendix I). When AID is performed without the consent of the husband, the husband might then have grounds for divorce.

3. AID REGISTER

Registered records should be kept of each donor. Unfortunately, there is no AID national register in any country. It may be advisable to collect highly confidential information for possible subsequent use. Such records can be of great use to some psychiatric departments, clinics of venereal disease, and for administrative purposes. It is the responsibility of the andrologists to ensure that their records are carefully preserved and not misused. The AID register can be used to evaluate the fertility of the donor and to ensure the production of satisfactory progeny. The disadvantage of such a register is the potential misuse of its information.

Some andrologists do not wish that the husband be legally registered as the father of an AID child since they would consider it to be falsifying the records. From the ethical point of view, the correct method of birth registration would not record any name for the father, and so testify to the illegitimacy of the certificate (Law and Ethics, 1973). Amendments of the laws are needed with respect to legitimacy or registration of birth after AID.

4. AID CHILDREN

Some people believe that the AID child should not know the circumstances of his conception, and that the husband and wife should be advised of keeping the insemination a secret from their families. Others feel that the husband and wife may wish to inform the child at their discretion that he is the descendant of only one of them. In the U.K., AID children are generally not told about their origins. In the U.S.A., the child will eventually know of his origin because of certain judicial proceedings. Even if the secret of his origin is kept from the child for as long as possible, the child is likely to find out at adolescence, when most healthy adolescents become independent of their parents.

The secrecy involved in AID obliges the andrologist, the husband, the wife, and the donor to conspire together to deceive the child and society as to the child's true parentage — his genetic identity (Dustan, 1973). Truth is violated; credibility is undermined; and these are serious ethical matters. From the ethical viewpoint it may be in the child's best interest to be deceived as to his true parentage, at least before adolescence. An AID child is at least comparable to the adopted child. Prenatal adoption can be incorporated and considered in the husband's consent to AID (Appendix II).

5. NUMBER OF CHILDREN PER DONOR

Theoretically, one healthy donor has enough semen to produce 20000 AID children per year for some 20 years. The maximal recorded number of AID live births from a given donor is 17. If 1000 live children a year, for example, were to be born in Great Britain as a result of the successful use of AID and if each donor has produced five children, an unwitting incestuous marriage is unlikely to take place more than once in 50–100 years (Glass, 1960). Even under unfavorable conditions, the expected increase of consanguineous marriages in the future generation due to unintended half-sib matings is negligible when compared to the actual consanguinity or even incest rate.

If the number of AID children from each donor is strictly limited, not only are the risks of incestuous marriage minimized, but any demographically undesirable effects of donor selection are also minimized (McLaren, 1973). A further advantage is that there will be less risk of disproportionate spread of any harmful recessive genes that the donor may be carrying. In cattle breeding, where producing a large number of progeny from genetically superior sires is one of the main objectives of artificial insemination, the danger of wide dissemination of harmful recessive genes is considerable and carriers have to be detected through matings with their oldest daughters (cf. Hafez, 1980).

6. BANKS OF FROZEN SEMEN

The use of frozen semen for AID has become increasingly common. Frozen storage of semen is possible for men about to undergo vasectomy, thus providing some insurance against any future change of mind. Certain circumstances may offer semen from a wide range of donors of different blood groups and external physical characteristics, thereby allowing the andrologist considerable flexibility in 'matching' the donor to the husband. Human semen may also be frozen for future use as donors in the controlled production of a number of children with supposedly favorable genetic characteristics (Dunstan, 1973).

The average number of inseminations per conception is 5–7 for fresh semen and 15–19 for frozen semen, whereas the conception rate is 70–80% for fresh semen and 50% after freezing for several months. Damage to the spermatozoa and reduction of their viability and motility in the female reproductive tract are most likely the result of cold storage.

Several couples undergo AID to have two to three children by using the same donor. This may not be possible however, unless several semen samples have been initially deep-frozen. One of the disadvantages of frozen semen banks is the possibility of an error in the labeling of the specimen. The andrologist should control the freezing and storage of semen specimens, thereby having total responsibility over all specimens.

7. MIXED SEMEN

Mixing semen from two or more donors, or from husband and donor, is not recommended due to immunological incompatabilities, as well as decreasing the possibility of knowing the exact physical characteristics that are desired. Mixing semen also interferes with determining whether or not a given donor is again able to produce normal children. It is also ethically unjustifiable.

8. ETHICAL FACTORS AFFECTING PROBLEMS OF AID

The paternal and maternal genomes and the contribution of gametes from donors to offspring acquired by various techniques are summarized in

Table 1. Several factors are involved in the ethical problems of AID, as it applies to the father, paternity, religious aspects, adultery, illegitimacy and adoption.

8.1. The Father and Ethics of Paternity

The father is the joint head of a family, whether or not he is the genetic father of the child. If intercourse between the husband and wife is continued while AID is being performed it is often possible that the husband is the father of the child. The genetic father donor does not carry out the responsibilities of the social father. Parents who undergo AID may appear to be more responsible parents compared to couples having a high percentage of unplanned and unwanted pregnancies.

8.2. Legitimacy

In several Western countries, the practice of AID is legal and AID children are the legitimate children of both the wife and her husband, provided the husband has given his written consent. In other countries, AID is rejected and/or considered to be a criminal offense by both the woman and her physician.

AID may lead to forgery in the childbirth certificate, but this forgery is covered by the legal presumption of the husband's paternity. Genetic paternity, when in question, can now be determined primarily by blood tests. At present there is major discrepancy in the law with respect to the right of inheritance of property from the sperm donor and from the father by marriage of an AID child.

8.3. Adoption and AID

Presently, fewer babies are available for adoption due to the availability of various effective contraceptive methods, the increased incidence of abortion and to the attitudes of women in today's society. AID may become more popular and more accepted than it is at present. It has been advisable for adopted children to be told about their adoption as early as they can understand that they are not the biological but rather the social product of their adoptive parent. Adopted children who suffer dis-

Table 1. Paternal and maternal genome and contribution of gametes from donors to offspring acquired by various techniques.

| Patterns | | Gametes | | | | |
| | | | Initial couple | | Donor | |
		Inter-course	Egg[a]	Sperm	Egg[b,c]	Sperm
Normal conception		X	X	X		
Instrumental insemination	AIH		X	X		
	AID		X			X
	AID to surrogate			X	X[b]	
	AIM (mixed semen)	X	X?			XX
Oocyte transfer	In vivo fertilization of wife's oocytes transferred to tube		X	X		
Embryo transfer	In vitro fertilization of wife's egg		X	X		
	In vitro fertilization of donor's egg; transfer to wife			X	X	
	transfer of donor blastocyst to wife				X	X
Embryo transfer and instrumental insemination	Sperm from donor male	X				X
	Egg from donor female			X	X	
Adoption					X[c]	X

[a] Genetic mother; provides the egg
[b] Gestational (uterine) [surrogate] mother: provides uterine environment for implantation, gestation and delivery
[c] Social mother: looks after child from birth onwards

turbances do fantasize about their biological parent. The fantasies manifested by AID children are likely to be modified by the knowledge that only the father is not the true genetic father.

8.4. Religious Aspects

Most Eastern and Moslem cultures are against AID. Western culture, influenced not only by the Judeo-Christian religion but also by the Graeco-Roman tradition of philosophy and law, has emphasized the nexus between the begetting and conception of children and the shared or common life of the marriage and the family (Dustan, 1973).

In the U.K., the Feverham Committee was appointed under pressure in September 1958, to re-

Table 2. Inventory of unanswered ethical questions.

Parameters	Unanswered questions
Eugenic	1. To what extend should AID involve eugenic planning? Or should it operate at some private level?
Planning and general ethics	2. Does AID of a consenting married women without her husband's knowledge or consent constitute adultery? Would the doctor be an accessory (cf. Doll, 1970; Pisapla, 1962)?
	3. Where no AID is involved, how sure are we of paternity in how large a segment of population? (What is the percentage of true paternity in cases of extramarital relationships and premarital intercourse?)
	4. If we accept termination of pregnancy should we question the ethical aspects of AID and embryo transfer from donor?
Andrologist of AID	5. What is the extent of the obligations and responsibilities of the physician who performs AID ?
	6. Is there need to seek further sanctions outside the profession?
	7. Are there any ethical considerations of the profession if there are sufficient agreement and public acceptance?
	8. Can AID be carried out by any competent midwife, carefully supervised in hospital, or only by an andrologist/gynecologist?
	9. Should we register andrologists who perform AID to avoid problems associated with AID without consent of the husband?
	10. If the first AID does not result in pregnancy how sure can the wife be that the semen she receives later is from the same donor, since it is the andrologist who finds a suitable anonymous donor?
	11. Since the child needs in his upbringing both mother and father figures would it be unethical to give a child by AID to an unmarried woman?
	12. Is AID provided to women who have already had natural children?
The donor	13. Should the donor(s) be known? Should the andrologist insist that semen is collected in the clinic rather than delivered to the premises?
	14. What are the main responsibilities of the donor once he has given semen for AID?
	15. Should donor be paid or not?
	16. Can a fertile husband give semen for the insemination of a woman other than his wife?
	17. What are the ethical and legal aspects of AID with mixed semen?
AID records	18. Is it advisable to establish a register of AID donors as for the register of adoptions?
	19. How can accurate AID biological records be maintained?
	20. What type of records should be kept about donors of AID? Who should have access to donor records?
	21. Is it ethical to store and provide information about the child to which the parents will have access?
Semen banks	22. Who takes the responsibility if an error is made in labeling of semen samples?
	23. What should be included on the label of stored semen specimen (donor's Christian name)?
	24. Why use Christian name, especially if the semen is all mixed together?
	25. If an AID child developed a disease of unknown etiology, would those in charge of a sperm bank reveal any family history of disease?
	26. Can legitimate children be conceived post mortem (from frozen semen after the death of the father)?
	27. By whom should the records of the semen bank be kept? Who has access to them?
AID children	28. Is it advisable that AID children be told their origins, like adopted children, as early as possible?
	29. At what stage should AID parents inform their AID child of their particular method of conception?
	30. What is the status of illegitimacy of AID children?
	31. Does the AID child have a claim on the sperm donor's estate if the donor dies intestate or bequeaths money to his children?

commend the prohibition of AID as an offense (H.M.S.O., 1960). A similar recommendation was submitted by a committee on behalf of the Church of England (C.I.O., 1960). The Roman Catholic Church has pronounced authoritatively against AID for the married woman as much as for the unmarried, in statements from the Holy Office in 1897, and from Pope Pius XII, in 1949 and 1956 (C.T.S., 1960).

Using recent advances in the investigation and treatment of infertility, Catholic gynecologists investigate infertile couples without identifying the infertile partner to the couple. In cases of curable infertility, the same gynecologist will inform both partners of the problem whereas, in cases of incurable infertility, he does not identify the infertile partner to the couple.

9. INVENTORY OF UNANSWERED ETHICAL QUESTIONS

Numerous ethical questions have been raised in relation to ethical, legal and moral questions as they relate to the responsibility of the andrologist who performs AID, the selection of donors, semen banks, AID records, the recipient, and the AID child (Table 2).

REFERENCES

Behrman SJ (1975) Techniques of artificial insemination. In Behrman SJ, Kistner RW, eds. Progress in infertility; 2nd edn. Boston: Little, Brown.
CIO (1960) Artificial insemination by donor: two contributions to a Christian judgement, Church Information Office, London. (The publication contains also the personal evidence of the then Archbishop of Canterbury, who disagreed with the conclusions of the Committee which he had appointed.)
CTS (1960) Artificial insemination. Evidence on behalf of the Catholic Body in England and Wales (submitted to the Feversham Committee), Catholic Truth Society, London.
Doll PJ (1970) La discipline des greffes, de transplantations et des autres actes de disposition concernant le corps humain. Paris: Masson.
Dunstan GR (1973) Moral and social issues arising from AID. Law and ethics of AID and embryo transfer. Ciba Foundation Symposium 17 (new series). Amsterdam: Elsevier.
Glass DV (1960) Sex ratio: a statistical association with the type and time of insemination in the menstrual cycle. Int J Fertil 15: 221.
Hafez ESE (1980) Reproduction of farm animals, 4th edn. Philadelphia: Lea and Febiger.

HMSO (1960) Report of the Departmental Committee on Human Artificial Insemination; London: HM Stationery Office, Cmnd 1105.
Ilizuka R, Sawaday Y, Nishina N, Ohi M (1968) The physical and mental development of children born following artificial insemination. Int J Fertil 13: 24.
Law and Ethics (1973) of AID and embryo transfer. Ciba Foundation Symposium 17 (new series). New York: Elsevier.
McLaren A. (1973) Biological aspects of AID. Law and ethics of AID and embryo transfer. Ciba Foundation Symposium 17 (new series). Amsterdam: Elsevier.
Pisapla GD (1962) Les problèmes de droit pénal posés par l'insémination artificielle. Revue de science criminelle et de droit pénal comparé, pp 47–64.
Schellen AMCM (1957) Artificial insemination in the human. Amsterdam: Elsevier.

Author's address:
Dr. E.S.E. Hafez
Andrology Research Unit
C.S. Mott Center for Human Growth and Development and Departments of Gynecology/Obstetrics and Physiology
Wayne State University School of Medicine
Detroit, Michigan, USA

APPENDIX I: CONSENT TO PERFORM ARTIFICIAL INSEMINATION

I, ——————————————————, as a voluntary participant at the Wayne State University C.S. Mott Center for Human Growth and Development, have engaged or been assigned to Dr. ————————— to perform one or more, if necessary, artificial insemination(s) with sperm from an unidentified donor. The artificial insemination procedure has been explained to me by the above-named doctor, and involves said doctor obtaining the necessary sperm from a donor who shall not be advised of my identity, nor shall I ever be advised of the identity of the donor. Furthermore, I relinquish, waive and disclaim any privilege or right I may have to determine the donor's identity. I agree to rely upon the judgement and discretion of the above-named doctor or any other physician who may be associated with him to choose a donor whose physical and mental characteristics are compatible with my characteristics. I also agree that on occasion donor sperm may be used that has been frozen for purposes of storage over periods of weeks to months.

I fully agree and understand that Doctor ————————————, or any other physician who may be associated with him, the Wayne State University C.S. Mott Center for Human Growth and Development, and/or Wayne State University, shall not be responsible for, nor have given any guarantees of warranties of, fitness for (of?) sperm or for the physical or mental characteristics of any child or children conceived or born. This agreement is not a contract to cure, a warranty of treatment, nor a guaranty of conception. I do hereby absolve, release, indemnify, protect and hold harmless from any and all liability for the mental or physical nature or character of any child or children so conceived or born, and for their affirmative acts or acts of omission which may arise during the performance of this agreement, Doctor _____, any physician associated with him, the Wayne State University C.S. Mott Center for Human Growth and Development, and/or Wayne State University. I further agree that unavoidable infections, sometimes contagious, may result from the insemination process.

I further agree that I am assuming entire responsibility for any child or children conceived or born. I agree that I will not seek support for the child or children, or any other payment, from the donor or from Doctor _____, any physician associated with him, the Wayne State University C.S. Mott Center for Human Growth and Development and/or Wayne State University. I further agree that if the child or children should seek support or any other payment from the donor of from Doctor _____, any physician associated with him, the Wayne State University C.S. Mott Center for Human Growth and Development, and/or Wayne State University, I will indemnify and hold harmless the donor, Doctor _____, any physician associated with him, the Wayne State University C.S. Mott Center for Human Growth and Development, and/or Wayne State University.

It is further agreed that the nature of this agreement is such that it must remain confidential: therefore, I agree that a sole copy of this agreement may be retained in the above-named doctor's files and shall not be disclosed except with my express written permission, except that Doctor _____, any physician associated with him, the Wayne State University C.S. Mott Center for Human Growth and Development, and/or Wayne State University may use the agreement as necessary in connection with any legal proceeding to which it is relevant.

Dated _____, 19_____   Signature _____

_____ o'clock____m   Witness _____

I consent to the above doctor–patient relationship _____

(Doctor)

(Courtesy, The C.S. Mott Center for Human Growth and Development, 275 East Hancock Avenua, Detroit, MI 48201, U.S.A.

APPENDIX IIA: CONSENT TO PERFORM ARTIFICIAL INSEMINATION AND LEGITIMACY OF CHILD OR CHILDREN

I, _____ and my spouse _____, as husband and wife and voluntary participants at the Wayne State University C.S. Mott Center for Human Growth and Development, have engaged or been assigned to Dr. _____ to perform one or more, if necessary, artificial insemination(s) with sperm from an unidentified donor, and involves said doctor obtaining the necessary sperm from a donor who shall not be advised of the identity of husband and wife, nor as husband and wife shall we ever be advised of the identity of the donor. Furthermore, as husband and wife we relinquish, waive and disclaim any privilege or right we may have to determine the donor's identity. We agree to rely upon the judgement and discretion of the above-named doctor or any other physician who may be associated with him to choose a donor whose physical and mental characteristics are compatible with our characteristics. It is also agreed that on occasion donor sperm may be used that has been frozen for purposes of storage over periods of weeks to months.

We fully agree and understand that Doctor _____, or any other physician who may be associated with him, the Wayne State University C.S. Mott Center for Human Growth and *Development, and/or Wayne State University*, shall not be responsible for, nor have given any guarantees or warranties of, fitness for *(of?)* sperm or for the physical or mental characteristics of any child or children conceived or born. This agreement is not a contract to cure, a warranty of treatment, nor a guaranty of conception. We do hereby absolve, release, indemnify, protect and hold harmless from any and all liability for the mental or physical nature or character of any child or children so conceived or born, and for their affirmative acts or acts of omission which may arise during the performance of this agreement, *Doctor _____, any physician associated with him, the Wayne State University C.S. Mott Center for Human Growth and Development, and/or Wayne State University*. It is further agreed that unavoidable infections, sometimes contagious, may result from the insemination process.

It is further agreed that from conception, I, _____, as husband, accept the act of insemination as my own and agree:
  a. That such child or children conceived or born shall be my legitimate children and heirs of my body and
  b. That I hereby waive forever any right which I might have to disclaim or omit the child or children as my legitimate heir or heirs, and
  c. That such child or children conceived or born shall be considered to be in all respects, including descent and distribution of my property, a child or children of my body.

We further agree, jointly and severally, that we are assuming entire responsibility for any child or children conceived or born. We agree that we will not seek support for the child or children, or any other payment, from the donor or from Doctor _____ _____, and physician associated with him, the Wayne State University. We further agree that if the child or children should seek support or any other payment from the donor or from Doctor _____, any physician associated with him, the Wayne State University C.S. Mott Center for Human Growth and Development, and/or Wayne State University, we will indemnify and hold harmless the donor, Doctor _____, any physician associated with him, the Wayne State University C.S. Mott Center for Human Growth and Development, and/or Wayne State University.

It is further agreed that the nature of this agreement is such that it must remain confidential; therefore, we agree that a sole copy of this agreement may be retained in the above-named doctor's files and shall not be disclosed except with our express written permission, except that Doctor _____, any physician associated with him, the Wayne State University C.S. Mott Center for Human Growth and Development, and/or Wayne State University may use the agreement as necessary in connection with any legal proceeding to which it is relevant.

Husband _____   Wife _____

Dated _____, 19_____

_____ o'clock ____m

I consent to the above doctor–patient relationship _____

(Doctor)

(Courtsey, C.S. Mott Center for Human Growth and Development; 275 East Hancock Avenue; Detroit, MI 48201, U.S.A.)

APPENDIX IIB: CONSENT TO ARTIFICIAL INSEMINATION

We, husband and wife, having considered the alternatives of continuing to try to have children by sexual intercourse, adopting a child, use of available medical therapy, and continuing our marriage without children, have decided that we desire to have one, or more if necessary, artificial insemination, using the sperm of a stranger-donor performed.

We understand that this procedure will involve the collecting of sperm from a donor and the introduction of that sperm, by Dr. _____, or his/her designated associate, into the cervix of the wife either by means of a syringe or use of a cup placed over the cervix. We understand that even though this procedure may be repeated as many times as advised, there is no guarantee that pregnancy will occur, or that if it does it will be carried to term. We also understand that there are some potential risks associated with this procedure. It is possible, although unlikely, that infection could be introduced into the wife by the procedure. In very rare cases, if the semen is injected too rapidly, cramps can result that last for about an hour.

During pregnancy, childbirth and delivery, of course, the same types of complications can arise as with a child conceived by sexual intercourse. It is also possible that the resulting child or children could be born abnormal, possess undesirable traits or hereditary tendencies, or be possessed of any of the other problems or disabilities of children conceived by sexual intercourse. In some cases the birth of a child by this method might also produce psychological problems for either or both spouses, and for the child.

We understand and agree that the donor shall be selected by the physician in his/her sole discretion, and that neither of us shall ever be advised of the identity of the donor. The physician shall select a donor to match the characteristics of the husband insofar as he/she is able if we so desire, and may use the services of a laboratory that screens donors and processes frozen semen.

We agree never to attempt to discover the identity of the donor, waive all rights we might have under any applicable law to see or copy, either in person or through a representative, records concerning the donor that may be kept by the physician or facility supplying frozen semen, and understand that at some point all records and information concerning the donor may be destroyed to protect his identity.

We, and each of us, accept this act as our own, and acknowledge our obligation to and agree to care for, support, and otherwise treat a child born as a result of this procedure in all respects as if it were our natural born child.

SIGNED: _____ (husband)
_____ (wife)
DATE: _____

(From IDANT Laboratories)

31. ARTIFICIAL INSEMINATION, JUDEO-CHRISTIAN EVALUATION AND PHILOSOPHICAL IMPLICATIONS

BÉLA SOMFAI and A. LYNCH

The final point of reference for a religious-ethical investigation is not rational evidence in itself but the goodness of God as revealed by a rational scrutiny of certain past and present religious experiences. It is assumed that human goodness is motivated or patterned by God's goodness as construed through this analysis. The initial task for such investigation, therefore, is the critical analysis of sources through which God's goodness is communicated to us; this study is then combined with an interpretation of those human symbols through which the God-experience is communicated to different communities of believers in history.

1. JUDEO-CHRISTIAN EVALUATION

In connection with artificial fertilization technology the written sources of Judeo-Christian beliefs have no direct and immediate information. An ethical evaluation therefore has to be reconstructed in reference to and in consistency with other religiously motivated value judgements of the past and present. In addition, the evaluation has to retain certain consistency with the historically conditioned system of symbols through which these religious traditions have articulated certain tenets of their beliefs. Since Judeo-Christianity represents several historically different articulations of a basically common God experience, our investigations will not lead to one single set of normative statements. Different interpretations of God's goodness, different perceptions of human potentials and of freedom, as well as the historically changing use of religious symbols all contribute to a pluralistic judgement, only with the broad outlines of a common stance prevailing.

From the viewpoint of a general ethical evaluation there are important differences between artificial insemination and embryo transfer. The latter procedure in its present form implies the necessary loss of fertilized ova and the not yet fully discounted possibility of danger to embryo and/or mother. In vitro fertilization also avails the necessary tool for a variety of experimental or therapeutic interference with the beginnings of human life, and offers the possibility of far-reaching control and transformation of our perceptions of human fertility, development and of parenthood itself. Our investigation approaches these procedures through those common aspects which received more attention in religious literature; these are: the externalization of semen or of ovum, the separation of intercourse from fertilization and the problems connected with the use of a donor's seed or ovum. Through the evaluation of these aspects we provide a brief synopsis of Judeo-Christian judgements without an analytic study of sources, and by way of critical comparisons indicate possible base points for future consensus.

Given the Biblical demand to multiply, Seymour Siegel, Professor or the Jewish Theological Seminary of America, is convinced that there is a clear consensus in contemporary Judaism on the acceptability as a last resort of artificial insemination by the husband's seed (AIH) or of extracorporeal fertilization and subsequent implantation of the embryo in cases when the gametes of husband and wife were used (Siegel, 1978; Jakobovits, 1975). Isaac Klein is in aggreement with Rabbi Siegel and points out that this is clearly not a case of onanism. Neither can artificial insemination with the donor's seed (AID) be equated with adultery in the interpretation of Jewish law; yet many good reasons exist in his opinion why it does not and should not receive general approval (Klein, 1975).

In the light of Orthodox Jewish convictions concerning marriage it is important that not only

Hafez ESE & Semm K (Eds) Instrumental insemination.

the child be conceived by partners in marriage, but also that somehow sexual intercourse remain a means of conception. Rabbi David Bleich of Jeshiva University is of the opinion that most orthodox rabbis would insist that the husband's seed be obtained only after sexual intercourse since they have objections to masturbation. He also states that from a religious point of view it is better to use one single ovum for transfer in order to avoid "man-determined destruction of life". Similarly, Fred Rosner believes that most rabbis would accept the use of the husband's semen for analysis or insemination, but would insist that *coitus interruptus* or a condom be used for obtaining it (Cross and Postal, 1978; Rosner, 1972).

Orthodox rabbis unanimously reject the donor's use, according to Siegel, not because they equate it with adultery or because they fear the possibility of later incest, but because they see a clear contradiction between the spirit of the Torah and the introduction of a stranger's sperm (or ovum) into the wife's body. Conservative Judaism on the other hand also recognizes the importance of marital happiness and satisfaction, and the contribution to marriage and society rendered by nurturing a child. Consequently in Siegel's opinion these rabbis are evenly divided on the acceptability of AID or embryonic transfer with the use of a donor's ovum. Reformed Jews are even more permissive in these matters, but even for this group the outside limit is the framework of an existing marriage. As these observations indicate a virtually unanimous judgement exists in contemporary Judaism on the necessity of marriage for human procreation through whatever methods.

The analysis of Protestant views portrays a similar diversity of perceptions. Conservative Protestantism anchors its judgement in Biblical norms releated to monogemous marriage and sexual union of spouses; liberal theology counters this conviction with arguments drawn from beneficial consequences to parents, society and to the offspring. Helmuth Thiellicke argues that securing of the donor's seed (or of the donor's ovum) is totally separated from the I–thou relationship of the partners. More importantly, however, the child produced by such methods incarnates the fact that the one flesh unity between husband and wife has been significantly distorted. The child symbolizes the achievement of

parenthood for one partner and its non-achievement for the other; in his words: "... a third person enters into the exlusive psychophysical relationship of the marriage, even though it is only his sperm that 'represents' him" (Thiellicke, 1964).

Christian understanding, Paul Ramsey argues, postulates that the "humanum in man" include the "body of his soul no less than the soul (mind) of his body". The union between the realm of personal love and "procreativity in man-womanhood" he continues, is rooted "is the image of God's creation in the midst of his love". Artificial insemination with the donor's seed or embryonic transfer with the use of a donor's ovum "puts completely asunder what God joined together". The nature of human parenthood is such "that conjugal intercourse is a life-giving act of love-making or a love-making act of life-giving" (Ramsey, 1971).

Other authors, however, are more cautious. Harmon L. Smith, for example, after reviewing the relevant Protestant and Roman Catholic literature proposes a "provisional" judgement. For the time being, he says "the most responsible (not to say only) Christian response appears to be a qualified "yes" to AIH and a qualified "no" to AID" (Smith, 1970). In AID he perceives a rather subtle denial of "mutuality" in marriage, a refusal of the commitment to share each other's life for better or for worse. It is a manifestation not of unambiguous generosity by accepting a child, but of covetousness, which claims that the personal fulfilment of parenthood by one can be achieved without the participation of the other. In face of dangers created by population explosion, he argues, it becomes more and more obvious that the non-exercise of parenthood can offer many creative possibilities, especially when fertility is achieved at such a high human cost. Although he did not have to face the problem of embryo transfer, his judgement is applicable to the moral implications of the method.

A report prepared by a task force of the Anglican Church of Canada on artificial insemination by donor well represents the contrast between two different mentalities. As the report indicates, members of this task force remained divided on the moral acceptability and social desirability of AID. After a thorough review of all aspects of the procedure they could not find clear evidence for its moral wrongness, nor indications of damage to its users or to society in general; consequently they raised no objection against its present small scale practice.

The majority of members were convinced that AID is a "fully acceptable treatment" of a legitimate human need, which in the absence of adoptable children cannot be met in any other way. They came to this conclusion because they viewed "... children as a precious and real fulfilment of a couple's love, ... in faithfulness to the belief which Christians share with many others that children are a blessing enriching marriage and society". Five members, however have expressed reservations against AID on the basis of "Christian teachings about marriage and human nature". It is possible for married people joined together before God in mutual life to be creative in true self-giving even if the blessing of children is denied to them. In addition they believe that "the creation of new life should be by husband and wife in the personal intimacy of sexual union" (Creighton, 1977). They also insisted on the importance of accepting full responsibility for the life-creating power of a person's sperm, and consequently expressed doubts about the morality of semen donation and insisted that AID should not be given to single women.

The commission of the United Church of Canada concluded without dissent that in connection with AID objection arises from legal rather than from moral difficulties. The conclusion according to this report "... appears to be when AID is used within marriage and based on mutual knowledgeable consent it is a legitimate ethical and moral option" (The United Church of Canada, 1975). A theoretical foundation for such conclusion may be found in Joseph Fletcher's thought, in whose opinion the decisively human characteristic is rational calculation, preditability and control. "Coital reproduction is therefore less human than laboratory reproduction... with our separation of baby making from love making, both become more human, because they are matters of choice and not of chance" (Fletcher, 1978).

The well-known episcopal theologian has argued in favour of AID for almost twenty-five years, and more recently with equal vehemence he defended the beneficial achievements of the new reproductive technology. Cloning, in vitro fertilization and other future possibilities are in harmony with his view on Christian marriage. Marriage is not a physical monopoly; consequently, by mutual consent husband and wife can incorporate into their relationship the product of a donor's seed or ovum. The important element in parenthood is "... a moral relationship with children, not a material or merely physical relationship" (Fletcher, 1960).

While he admits the necessity of the marriage framework for most cases of artificial reproduction, he radically separates the sexual manifestation of married love from its reproductive potentials. This stance is in contradiction not only with basic Judeo-Christian convictions, but also with observable facts. Nurture is only possible because of the love between parents, states McCormick, and married people love their children "... because they have loved each other, and because children are the visible fruit and extension of that love" (McCormick, 1978). Parenthood includes the acts of nurture and the acts of generation, both rooted in mutual love.

As our evidence indicates, a virtually unanimous consensus exists also in Protestantism on the necessity of the loving union between husband and wife to safeguard the dignity of human reproduction. Concerning the importance of means by which fertility is achieved, a variety of opinions exist. A basic acceptance however of the importance of sexual intercourse, of exclusivity in marital relationships and of the genetic continuity between parents and children is recognizable in Protestantism, since with the sole exception of Joseph Fletcher, all authors agree that artificial methods of reproduction should only be considered as last resort, when natural methods fail. Within this general stance liberal Protestantism however finds little difficulty with accepting into the framework of a family the product of a donor's seed or ovum.

The premises of a Roman Catholic judgement are very similar to those of orthodox Judaism and of conservative Protestantism, and for this reason the problem of embryo transfer is again considered through the evaluation of the common elements with artificial insemination. Artificial insemination was condemned by the teaching office of the Roman Church as early as 1897; some dissent however continued to surface during first half of the twentieth century. To counter these views Pope Pius

XII addressed the issue repeatedly between 1949 and 1958. His position provides the parameters of the Roman Catholic stance even today.

He rejected artificial insemination outside marriage since natural and divine law equally demand, in his opinion, that new human life be the fruit of married love. The desire of the spouses to bring their love to perfect manifestation is the best protection for the dignity of new life and of the personal welfare of husband and wife. Artificial insemination by the donor's seed within marriage was equally ruled out. "Only marriage partners have natural rights over their bodies for the procreation of new life, and these rights are exclusive, non-transferable and inalienable" (Pius XII, 1949). The donor's contribution to life within marriage disrupts the symmetry of this exclusive partnership vis-à-vis the child. "Between the marriage partners, however, and child which is the fruit of the active element of a third person — even though the husband consents — there is no bond of origin, no moral or juridical bond of conjugal procreation" (Pius XII, 1950). Finally the Pope had objections even against artificial insemination by the husband's seed when the procedure was carried out apart from the natural performance of sexual intercourse. In his opinion only the sexual act naturally performed may receive medical assistance, to eliminate some possible defects, and enhance the possibility of fertilization. The arguments to support this last point are somewhat laborious and not all that convincing.

The Pope's reasoning is ultimately rooted in the conviction that an integral connection exists between the exclusive and inseparable union of spouses, the sexual expression of their love and the desire to manifest and perfect this love through the offspring. The moral evaluation of any interference with the reproductive process hinges on maintaining the vital connection between these elements. It is not the fear of adultery or the traditional condemnation of masturbation that matters primarily, but the isolation of these elements from each other. It was in this context that Pius XII dismissed 1956 the possibility of in vitro fertilization as "immoral and absolutely illicit". If the sacrament of marriage is a symbol of God's creative love, then the marriage act had to be analogous with the act of creation. As in God's creation the act and his love are inseparable,

so must the act of love-giving in marriage be unfailingly connected with life-giving, according to his thought.

Relatively little disagreement exists in current Roman Catholic thought on the basic assumptions of the Pope's stance. Artificial fertilization outside marriage and the use of donor's seed or ovum within marriage are rejected by almost all theologians. Karl Rahner, for example is convinced that "... the child is an embodiment of the abiding unity of the marriage partners which is expressed in marital union". AID, or in vitro fertilization with a donor's contribution, "fundamentally separates the marital union from the procreation of a new person as this permanent embodiment of the unity of married love; and it transfers procreation, isolated and torn from its human matrix, to an area outside man's sphere of intimacy..." (Rahner, 1972). Bernard Häring can see no justification for AID either, and at least for the time being is also opposed to in vitro fertilization even when the gametes of the spouses are used. This opposition is based "... not on the fact that it is artificial, but that it is manipulation not only of sperm but of embryo itself, with no safety..." (Häring, 1975).

On the question of AIH performed in separation from an act of intercourse, however, divergent opinions have been proposed for a long time. Today few Roman Catholic moralists would object to this procedure either for the reason that masturbation is the means of producing the semen, or that fertilization occurs in isolation from the marriage act. Current moral theology is convinced that a single human act in isolation from the life orientation of the person can not exhibit a decisive moral value (McCormick, 1973; Fuchs, 1971; Janssens, 1977). Consequently the moral value of an act of masturbation for example does not depend on its physical structure alone (orgasmic manipulation of a sexual organ), but more so on the intention, on the effects of the act, and its relationship to the life orientation of the agent. It will lose its seflish character when undertaken by husband, becomes the necessary means for securing fertility and thus contributes to the most perfect manifestation and ultimate fulfillment of married love (Van Allen, 1970; Troisfontaines, 1973). Similarly, the fact that in an otherwise infertile marriage the fertilization of the wife's ovum with her husband's seed occurs in isolation from one act of intercourse is far outweighed by the benefits achieved through the birth and nurture of a child.

Further arguments in favour of AIH and of vitro fertilization by the gametes of spouses do not seem necessary, to indicate that conservative objections to these procedures can be satisfactorily answered. More difficult is the question why Roman Catholic thought and conservative Judeo-Christianity in general is reluctant to accept the donor's use in these procedures. Before taking a look at this question we have to discuss briefly the question of life-loss connected with embryo transfer, and construct the "base line" for a Judeo-Christian consensus on the ethical evaluation of these procedures.

The fact that embryo transfer at present requires the loss of fertilized ova in significant numbers constitutes the ethically most controversial aspect of the procedure. Although the parameters of a religious judgement arise in the context previously discussed, the value attached to incipient life significantly influences the position of those opposed to abortion. This includes Roman Catholics, most orthodox Jews and conservative Protestants. Even if one tends to accept a difference in the status of a non-implanted blastocyst and a fetus, the loss of human life is a serious and not yet resolved problem which argues against embryo transfer in most circumstances. It is hoped that this objection will be met in the near future through a refinement of the procedure which would reduce the rate of life loss to a level comparable to what occurs in the process of natural fertilization.

The evidence here presented indicates that the "base line" for a Judeo-Christian consensus is found in the common belief that the divinely sanctioned institute of marriage ought to be the only context for human reproduction. Judeo-Christianity therefore insists with a unanimous voice that, as a rule, the use of reproductive technologies must be confined within the framework of functioning marriages. In addition, a religious significance is attached also to the love- and life-giving dimensions of sexual intercourse, and to the genetically, socially and psychologically balanced partnership of spouses in parenthood. Consequently, artificial insemination, embryo transfer and other future possibilities of reproductive technology are considered by almost all representatives of these traditions as a last resort; they ought to be used as therapeutic means, or experimental efforts in view of future remedy against sterility in marriage.

Although the religious significance attached to these latter factors changes in the different traditions, it is safe to say that only the most conservative groups will object to AIH and extra-corporeal fertilization with the gametes of husband and wife. Since these procedures do not change the balance of partnership in reproduction and leave the family lineage undisturbed the beneficial effects of fertility outweigh the "alienation" caused by the artificiality of the method. While insistence on marriage as a necessary prerequisite separates Judeo-Christian through from a strictly pragmatic evaluation of artificial fertilization, exclusion of a donor's seed or ovum differentiates conservative and more liberal religious opinions. The permanent disequilibrium in marital partnership and the discontinuity of family lineage cannot be balanced by the benefits of children, according to the conservative view.

Not all the supporting arguments however are open to rational analysis. The meaning and significance of marriage in the context of different religious traditions and what Karl Rahner calls a "moral faith instinct", a particular sensitivity and intuition nurtured by the value system of a given faith community, exercise great influence on this judgement, and perhaps more so on the decisive firmness with which these methods are rejected or opposed.

This non-thematic element manifests itself in all forms of ethical discourse. It not only emphasizes in our case the privileged importance of covenanted relationships, but also points to the fact that in all moral judgements there is a transcendental element which ultimately resists full conceptualization. It is through this element, rather than through the physical structure of an act, that a moral decision reaches to the absolute (Rahner, 1963, 1964; Fuchs, 1970).

In the final analysis the difference of opinions is rooted in opposing convictions concerning the symbolic and functional importance of certain human and religious elements. On one side the conservative posture is convinced that the donor's presence in life-giving and his or her genetic contribution to children cannot be reconciled with a Judeo-Christian understanding of sexuality, marriage and family life. Without categorically denying the significance of these concerns the other side emphasizes the importance of empirical evidence and argues that given the practical impossibility of adoption, children even if conceived through a donor's seed or ovum, contribute to the full achievement of marital love. Marriages with children are preferable since they are a more perfect manifestation of creative spousal love, even if there remains the inevitable asymmetry between spouses in their genetic relationship to the offspring, and the discontinuity of the family lineage. In all other aspects of their family life they can and in fact do approximate the situation of a naturally reproduced family. In its insistence on children in the family and in the suggestion that even at the cost of artificiality, parental imbalance, and discontinuity, their presence brings about the most perfect fulfillment of marriage under given circumstances, this mentality draws from the traditional theological conviction which emphasizes that the primary end of marriage does consist in fertility. Under our present day conditions, however, this assumption needs a very serious re-examination.

2. PHILOSOPHICAL IMPLICATIONS

In contrast to Judeo-Christian theologians' "commonality in pluralism", philosophical ethicists find no consensus in discussion of AID – in vitro fertilization–embryo transfer. This is not surprising since the philosopher is neither constrained to consideration of material arising within a "revelation" – "religious tradition" context, nor always comfortable with the minimal unanimity derived from a shared, if variously-interpreted, value-system.

Recent British discussion regarding availability of AID (BMJ 1979a, b, c; Case Conference, 1978) reflects the diversity of philosophical view in this area. While some query any use of AID technology on both consequential and deontological grounds, other argue these same grounds in support of AID's use within and beyond marriage. Attention to the focus of philosophical argument is thus more profitable as indicative of present and future philosophical interest here than concentration on philosophical resolution via applications of varying ethical systems.

In this vein, three aspects of the philosophical discussions of AID warrant attention: a) Preoccupation with the language of "rights". Beyond discussion of availability of AID in fulfillment of the "right" of the couple, AID is mentioned as the "right" or claim of a woman (St. John Stevas, 1964; Fried, 1973; Edwards and Sharpe, 1971); defined as treatment for infertility, AID will be considered with other "rights to health care service" (BMJ a, c 1979; Jonsen, 1978; Walters, 1979); the "rights" of the AID child are examined (Annas, 1979); the "rights" of future generations may include the genetic well-being AID could provide (Golding, 1972). b) Growing concern with empirical evidence, e.g., concern with the post-AID effect on family, child. c) Focus on the genetic implications of the procedure, e.g., eugenic possibilities of AID, genetic continuity for the child, linkage between the genetic and psycho-social component in shaping the individual (Annas, 1979, citing Curie-Cohen, 1979; Fried, 1973 citing Piatelli-Palmarini, 1973).

In addition to serving philosophers' goals, development of arguments along these lines could well enhance the position of theological consensus already described. Should Annas's suggestion (Annas, 1979) of psychological testing of AID children be implemented, for example, its results could only be useful in this context. On the other side, the challenges to the Judeo-Christian understanding of "the human and religious meaning of sexual intercourse and fertility, of marriage and parenthood" which may be presented by such philosophical considerations can be ignored only to the detriment of that consensus.

Consideration of in vitro fertilization inevitably involves pre-consideration of the "moral status of the early human embryo" (Walters, 1979). Any brief discussion of a problem so central to bioethical (Engelhardt, 1975), metaphysical and epistemological speculation is impossible. It should be emphasized, however, that all philosophers and theologians agree on the significance of the question: in large measure, its resolution determines ethical judgement regarding in vitro fertilization, whether that procedure is accompanied by embryo transfer or not (Kass, 1979).

When in vitro fertilization is denoted as an extension of acceptable AID practice, i.e., when accompanied by embryo transfer, two problems have engaged philosophers' attention:

a) The procedure is perceived as proper to the more general areas of health care resource-allocation. In developing and providing it, a just social rationalization of costs and benefits must be divised (Hellegers and McCormick, 1978). The task is not simple given infrequency of use, ambiguity in the identification of in vitro fertilization–embryo transfer as "therapeutic", procedural expenses (Marsh and Self, 1980; Kass, 1978).

b) The physical, psychological, moral status of the child is a concern. Louise's well-being has offset much potential negative argument in this regard although long-range physical and psychological effects are yet to be measured (Callahan, 1978). Further, given parental or individual "rights", and the possibility of pre-natal diagnosis and abortion, will the child be seen as means satisfying adults' desires or as an end in itself (Lappe, 1972, 1978)? Finally, the possibility of in vitro fertilization–embryo transfer practice with ovum/sperm donors, surrogate mothers, raises in extreme form the genetic lineage psychosocial bonding question already noted. Who has continuing parental responsibility for the "cells-child" when gametes are artificially-derived, when conception is externally manipulated, when gestation is "hosted" in the cause of prenatal adoption? Who is one's kid or kin?

To propose laboratory in vitro fertilization without embryo transfer is to argue the beneficent research imperative as practiced on donated gametes routinely destined for destruction after use. While research using some individual gametes seems unproblematically beneficent, research using early human embryos may not (Mastroianni, 1978; Kass, 1978). Ethical assessment of the moral status of the early human embryo is one critical factor in this determination, for that judgement may render it impossible to perform this research beneficently or in an ethical fashion (McCormick, 1978). If the embryo has moral claims, then consent is a second critical factor: is the locus of that consent the individual gamete donor? For those who do not view the early human embryo as worthy of any special respect, the ends of the research will justify the means. Particularly problematic is the "cut-off" point: are there limits to types of permissible experiment vis-a-vis certain gestational age? When will "human person" be, and how will that be defined for laboratory purposes?

To many, laboratory in vitro fertilization is the inevitable culmination-initiation of an era in development of reproductive technology. AID, prenatal and carrier screening which prepared the way for laboratory in vitro fertilization and embryo transfer, now give way to parthenogenesis, cloning, hybridization, chimera-production, embryo culture in vitro. Given the success of current in vitro fertilization procedures, these potential research projects just named point towards new clinical applications in reproductive and other technologies. Does this continuing trend bode well or ill for mankind?

In summarizing the initiatives of philosophical-ethicists' in the AID – in vitro fertilization–embryo transfer area, two fundamental value issues could be identified (Veatch, 1974). In the attempt to resolve individual ethical problems, philosophical activity implicitly examines:

a) The tension between individual and social good;
b) The limit to be set to human manipulative ability.

Any single AID – in vitro fertilization–embryo transfer decision is necessarily social; any social policy first affects individuals in their group. The "right" of the child is accommodated in the "right" of adults; the cost of all beneficent research is borne by each citizen. The future of mankind rests on the steady incremental effect of continuing individual choices and actions. What constructive balance is to be established between the good of the one and the good of the many?

Ought man to apply technological skill to his own shaping? Is the "Judeo-Christian philosophical premise that man's role in the world is to dominate and subdue nature with his intellectual and technical skills" valid (Veatch, 1974 paraphrasing White, 1967)? Or is it better in these areas to let Nature take its course... "where unpredictability seems more favourable to human welfare than predictability, it is surely the former and not the latter that is truly human in this situation" (Crotty, 1972 as quoted in Veatch, 1974).

Differences in perception, in moral sensitivities and in basic assumptions with regard to these questions will remain with us in the foreseeable future. They are indications of huw Judeo-Christianity interprets human partnership with God's creative activity, of philosophical reflection on human responsibilities in the use of technology. On the level of communicable arguments, however, we would come to a better theological and philosophical understanding if further attention were given to several important and not yet fully considered questions: what is the short- and long-term significance of the "genetic make-up", i.e., of the fact that in the case when a donor is used half of the inherited characteristics in a person originate outside the family? What is the accurate extent of partnership in marriage, and what are the creative possibilities of accepting the "cross of infertility" as a mutual condition which has equal effects on both partners? Given the problems associated with overpopulation and the financial and social costs of making artificial reproductive technologies available, are we not guilty of a fertility bias when we suggest that couples should have the option for a child at whatever cost? What is the weight of the social benefit goal in justifying experimentation using the early human embryo?

Given the fact that the possibilities of today tend to become the realities of tomorrow, the common message of Judeo-Christianity is increasingly important: the child must never become the product of a choice motivated by calculation or desire, but rather her or his existence ought to be a gift bestowed upon parents by their sincere and unrestrained love to each other. As A. Hellegers and R. McCormick have cautioned (Hellegers, 1978), increase in choice and possibilities introduces the danger of "consumerism", even in the field of procreation. The more we lose the spontaneity and intimacy of marital relationships, the closer we come to the danger of reducing human reproduction to the 'processes of a biological laboratory'.

As philosophers continue to defend opposing views about human reproduction, the Judeo-Christian message may well provide the single focus on which all can agree. Indeed, there can be no less than universal concern for the child's well-being.

ACKNOWLEDGEMENTS

The preparation and presentation of Section 1 of this paper was made possible by a grant of the Social Sciences and Humanities Research Council of Canada, grant no. 461–80 0268.

REFERENCES

Van Allen R (1970) Artificial insemination (AIH): a contemporary re-analysis. The homiletic and pastoral rev pp 363.
Annas GJ (1979) Artificial insemination: beyond the best interests of the donor. Hastings Center Report 9; 4: pp 14–15; 43.
BMJ (1979a) Artificial insemination for all? (Editorial) 6188; 2: p 458.
BMJ (1979b) AID for lesbians (Letters). 6188; 2: p 495.
BMJ (1979c) AID for lesbians (Letters). 6191; 2: p 669.
Callahan D (1978) In vitro fertilization: four commentaries. Hastings center report 8; 5: p 7.
Case conference: Lesbian couples: should help extend to AID? J Med Ethics 1978; 4: 91.
Creighton PG (1977) Artificial insemination by donor, pp 61–62.
Cross D, Postal B (1978) Test-tube babies. Jewish Digest: Dec p 69.
Crotty N (1972) The technological imperative: reflections on reflections. Theol Stud 33: 440.
Curie-Cohen M, Luttrell L, Shapiro S (1979) Current practice of artificial insemination by donor in the US. NEJM 300: p 785.
Edwards RG, Sharpe DJ (1971) Social values and research in human embryology. Nature 231: 87.
Engelhardt HT (1975) Bioethics and the process of embodiment. Persp Biol Med summer: pp 486.
Fletcher J (1960) Morals and medicine, p 139.
Fletcher J (1978) Humanhood: essays in biomedical ethics, p 88.

Fried C (1973) Ethical issues in existing and emerging techniques for improving human fertility. Law and Ethics of AID and Embryo Transfer. pp 40–44.
Fuchs J (1970) Basic freedom and morality. Human Values and Christian Morality, pp 178–203.
Fuchs J (1971) The absoluteness of moral terms. Gregorianum pp 415–457.
Golding MP (1972) Obligations to future generations. Monist 56: 85.
Häring B (1975) Ethics of manipulation. p 200.
Hellegers A, McCormick R (1978) Unanswered questions on test-tube life. America 18 Aug, pp 74–78.
Jakobovits I (1975) Jew Med Ethics pp 272–273.
Janssens L (1977) Norms and priorities in a love ethics. Louvain Studies pp 207–238.
Jonsen A (1978) Health care III: right to health-care services. Encycl of Bioethics pp 623–629.
Kass L (1979) A conversation with L Kass: the ethical dimensions of in vitro fertilization. Washington.
Kass L (1979) Making babies revisited. The Public Interest Winter, 54: 32–60.
Klein I (1975) Responsa and Halakhic Studies Ktaw pp 167–168.
Lappe M (1978) Ethics at the center of life: protecting vulnerable subjects. Hastings Center Report 8; 5: 11.
Lappe M (1972) Risk-taking for the unborn. Hastings Center Report 2: p 1.
McCormick R (1973) The ambiguity of moral choice.
McCormick R (1978) Reproductive technologies. Encyclopedia of Bioethics col 1458.

Marsh FH, Self DJ In vitro fertilization: moving from theory to therapy, Hastings Center Report, 10; 3: 5.

Mastroianni L (1978) Reproductive technologies: in vitro fertilization. Encyclopedia of Bioethics pp 1448–1451.

Piatteli-Palmarini M (1973) Biological roots of the human individual . Law and Ethics of AID and Embryo Transfer pp 19–25.

Pius XII (1949) Acta Apostolicae Sedis pp 577 ff.

Pius XII (1950) Acta Apostolicae Sedis p 252.

Pius XII (1951) Acta Apostolicae Sedis p 850.

Pius XII (1956) Acta Apostolicae Sedis pp 470–471.

Rahner K (1963) On the question of formal existential ethics. Theol Investig, Vol II, pp 217–234.

Rahner K (1964) The dynamic element in the church.

Rahner K (1972) The problem of genetic manipulation, Theol Investig, Vol IX, p 246.

Ramsey P (1971) Fabricated Man pp 47–48; 87.

Rosner F (1972) Modern medicine and Jewish law. Studies in Torah Judaism 13, p 105.

Siegel S (1978) Test tube propagation. The Jewish Spectator, Winter, p 24.

Smith HL (1970) Ethics and the New Medicine p 83.

Steinfels MO (1979) In vitro fertilization: ethically acceptable research. Hastings Center Rep 9–3:5.

St John-Stevas N (1964) Artificial human insemination. Life, Death and the Law, pp 116–159.

Thiellicke H (1964) Ethics of Sex, pp 252–254 esp p 259.

Troisfontaines R (1973) L'insémination artificielle Nouvel Rev Theol pp 764–778.

The United Church of Canada (1975) Report of the Commission on Ethics and Genetics p 7.

Veatch RM (1974) Ethical issues in genetics. Progr Med Genet X: 223.

White L (1967) The historical roots of our ecologic crisis Science 155: 1203.

Author's address:
Dr Béla Somfoi
Regis College
Toronto School of Theology, Canada

APPENDIX

Strasbourg, 5 March 1979

DRAFT RECOMMENDATION
ON ARTIFICIAL INSEMINATION OF HUMAN BEINGS
AND EXPLANATORY REPORT*

(prepared by a Committee of experts of the Council of Europe and adopted by the European Committee on Legal Cooperation (CDCJ)

RULES

ARTICLE 1. These rules apply only to artificial insemination of a woman with semen of an anonymous donor.

ARTICLE 2.

a) Artificial insemination can be administered only when appropriate conditions exist for insuring the welfare of the future child.

b) Artificial insemination shall be administered only on the responsibility of a physician.

ARTICLE 3.

a) No person's semen may be utilized for artificial insemination without his consent.

b) The consent of the woman and, if she is married, of her husband, is necessary to administer artificial insemination.

c) The physician responsible for administering artificial insemination shall see that the consent is given in an explicit manner.

ARTICLE 4. A physician or medical establishment receiving semen for artificial insemination must make appropriate medical inquiries and examinations in order to prevent the transmission from the donor of an hereditary condition or contagious disease, or other factor which may present a danger to the health of the woman or the future child. In addition, the physician administering artificial insemination must take all appropriate measures in order to avoid danger to the health of the woman and that of the future child.

ARTICLE 5. The physician and the staff of a medical establishment receiving the donation of semen as well as those administering artificial insemination must keep secret the identity of the donor and, subject to the requirements of law in legal proceedings, the identity of the woman and, if she is married, of her husband, as well as the fact of artificial insemination. The physician shall not administer artificial insemination if the conditions make the preservation of secrecy unlikely.

ARTICLE 6.

a) No payment shall be made for donation of semen. However, the loss of earnings as well as travelling and other expenses directly caused by the donation may be refunded to the donor.

b) A person or a public or private body which offers semen for the purpose of artificial insemination shall not do it for profit.

ARTICLE 7.

a) When artificial insemination has been administered with the consent of the husband the child shall be considered as the legitimate child of the woman and husband and nobody may contest the legitimacy on the sole ground of artificial insemination.

b) No relationship of affiliation may be established between the donor and the child conceived as a result of artificial insemination. No proceedings for the latter's maintenance may be brought against the donor or by the donor against the child.

B. DRAFT EXPLANATORY REPORT

1. *Introduction*

1. Resolution (78) 29 on the harmonization of the legislation of member States relating to removal, grafting and transplantation of human substances, which was adopted by the Committee of Ministers on 11 May 1978, in its paragraph 2 of Article 1 of the annexed rules, excludes from its field of application 'the transfer of embryos, the removal and transplantation of testicles and ovaries and the utilization of ova and sperm'. In fact, due to the particular nature of the problems created by these operations, it was agreed that special rules should be elaborated because of the serious legal and moral consequences particularly those concerning filiation.

2. This Recommendation deals only with one of the subjects not covered by Resolution (78) 29 as it limits itself to the utilization of semen for artificial insemination. In fact, it was thought that this was the most urgent problem to be studied at present.

3. Artificial insemination of human beings is at present practiced in several member States as a remedy for childlessness due to male infertility or any hereditary conditions existing in the couple which would make it undesirable for them to procreate because of the

Hafez ESE & Semm K (Eds) Instrumental insemination.
© *1982 Martinus Nijhoff Publishers, The Hague/Boston/London. ISBN 90-247-2530-5. Printed in the Netherlands.*

possibility of the conditions being transferred to the child or his descendants. Since the number of childless couples is substantial, recourse to artificial insemination has become more frequent in certain member states in recent years as a result of difficulties in adoption and of changing social attitudes and technical developments. This practice, although it resolves a family problem, raises also a number of moral, legal and medical issues, which range from the gratuitous character of the semen donation to the legal status of a child conceived as a result of this operation.

4. Very few member States possess legal provisions on the subject, and those which exist deal only with the problem of affiliation. It is evident that, in the near future, a number of member States, especially those in whose territory artificial insemination is frequently practiced, will introduce specific legislation in this field in order to rectify injustices which may result from the application of the general legislation on affiliation and to curb any abuses of this practice.

As the aim of the Council of Europe is to achieve a greater unity between its members, in particular through harmonizing their legislation on matters of common interest, the Committee of Ministers by this Recommendation recommends the governments of member States, if they introduce legislation on artificial insemination of human beings and related matters, to do so in conformity with the rules annexed to this Recommendation, so as to achieve a harmonized regulation of the problem in Europe.

5. This Recommendation contains rules which constitute a minimum solution to the problem of artificial insemination. The States may thus adopt additional rules, particularly as to penal sanctions for violations of the rules annexed to the Recommendation. In this context, the Recommendation does not deal with the problems raised by artificial insemination administered against the system laid down by the rules. This problem is left to national legislation which may adopt specific rules in this field on the condition that the fundamental principles on which the Recommendation is based are respected.

6. The present Recommendation has been drafted by a joint Committee of Experts under the authority of the European Committee on Legal Co-operation (CDCJ) and of the European Public Health Committee (CDSP) which gave to it as terms of reference, the harmonization of legislations in the field of removal, grafting and transplantation of human substances.

II. *Rules*

ARTICLE 1

7. Article 1 defines the field of application of the rules.

They apply only to artificial insemination of a human being with the semen of an anonymous donor.

It follows from this provision that excluded from the field of application of the rules are artificial insemination with the semen of the husband, living or deceased, and, in the case of an unmarried couple, artificial insemination with the semen of the partner.

Artificial insemination of a woman with the semen of her husband or of the partner, when certain medical conditions render natural insemination impossible or difficult, does not raise the same problems which artificial insemination with the semen of a third party donor creates and consequently it was not considered useful to deal with it in this resolution.

ARTICLE 2

8. Under normal conditions, a married couple or a single woman is the sole judge as to whether to have a child by natural means or not to have one. Whatever the health, social and economic situation of the future mother and father may be, they may have a child if they so wish and no one outside the couple may interfere with their decision. A married couple or unmarried woman may be advised by a physician or family counsellor against having a child, but this advice is by no means binding. Naturally the couple or the unmarried woman are also solely responsible for the consequences of having the child.

9. The situation is somewhat different in the case of artificial insemination. The physician administering artificial insemination is also to some extent responsible for the conception of the child. As a result it is logical that the physician should have the duty to refuse to carry out such an operation when he considers that the appropriate conditions do not exist for ensuring the welfare of the future child. These 'appropriate conditions' are, in particular, that the couple or the unmarried woman shall be in good health and sufficiently well-balanced emotionally and psychologically to raise a child properly.

10. However, it should be noted that paragraph 1 of Article 2 does not define 'appropriate conditions' and does not indicate the person or the body which is to judge whether they exist. These matters are therefore left to national legislation.

In particular it is for national legislation, if any, to define by a general rule or to give the physician the task of judging case by case, whether the 'appropriate conditions' exist when the insemination is requested by an unmarried women. This legislation can also provide for additional rules in order to specify the conditions of artificial insemination in such a case.

11. Paragraph 2 requires for the benefit of the parties, that artificial insemination must be administered by a physician or under his control and on his responsibility.

ARTICLE 3

12. This article concerns the consent which is necessary in order to perform artificial insemination.

Three consents are required: That of the donor, that of the woman and that of her husband if she is married. This provision stems from the necessity that all those who are concerned in such a delicate and important operation for society, the conception of a human being, are fully aware of the consequences and agree to them.

13. Paragraph 1 prohibits the utilization of a man's semen without his consent. As semen may be received by medical establishments for other reasons than as a donation for artificial insemination, e.g. for medical analysis, this semen should not be utilized for artificial insemination without the consent of that man.

14. Paragraph 2 requires the consent of the woman as well as her husband, if she is married. It is evident that the first requirement for artificial insemination is the consent of the woman to whom it will be administered. In all member States any practice of artificial

insemination without the consent of the woman would constitute a criminal offense, no matter whether her husband consented to it or not.

15. In addition to the woman's consent the article also requires the consent of her husband if she is married. Therefore, should the husband refuse, the physician or the medical center must not administer artificial insemination, even if the woman should insist. Although the case where artificial insemination is administered to a woman following the refusal of her husband does not constitute a criminal offense in all member States, it would constitute grounds for divorce and for repudiating the legitimacy of the child in most member States. In order to avoid such a situation, which would shake or even destroy the family unit, and risk harm to the child's future, this article forbids the practice of artificial insemination without the consent of the husband.

16. As for the validity and form of the consent required by this article, these matters are left to national legislation. However, the article requires that such consent must be given in an explicit manner, the intended meaning of 'explicit manner' here being some manner of expressing a wish which would not given rise to any doubt or differing interpretation.

The purpose of putting on the physician the obligation of seeing that consent is given in an explicit manner is to draw the attention of practitioners especially to the importance of consent.

ARTICLE 4

17. This article requires any physician or medical establishment receiving semen for artificial insemination, to make appropriate medical inquiries and examinations in order to prevent the transmission from the donor of a hereditary condition or contagious disease or other factor which may present a danger to the health of the recipient woman or the future child.

18. By 'hereditary conditions', the article refers primarily to dominant hereditary conditions but also includes other gentic factors which may be of equal relevance; by 'contagious diseases' it refers to those which may be transmitted by semen (e.g. gonorrhoea) and 'other factors' refers to such factors as for example Rhesus factors of the blood. But, of course, all these are given merely as examples and if a physician or medical center discovers any trace of another hereditary condition or contagious disease, or other factor which would create a danger to the health of the mother or future child, artificial insemination with the semen of that donor must not be administered.

In addition, although the problem is one that can hardly ever arise in practice, it may be necessary to take precautions not only against consanguinity of the donor and the recipient but also against producing a large number of consanguineous children. To this end physicians should, so far as possible, avoid using the semen of a particular donor for a great many artificial inseminations in one center.

19. The rules do not contain a provision on the question of whether the physician should satisfy any wishes of the couple or the unmarried women on particular physical characteristics of the donor. It is left to the physician, in conformity with paragraph 1 of Article 2, to see whether in such case the 'appropriate conditions' exist to administer artificial insemination.

20. The second sentence of the article relates to all other measures and examinations necessary to perform the operation. Therefore, if an examination of a woman reveals that artificial insemination would create undue danger to her health the physician must not administer artificial insemination.

ARTICLE 5

21. Secrecy is a matter of the utmost importance in the administration of artificial insemination in the interest of the donor, of the couple and of the child. The article requires that all precautions should be taken to keep secret the identity of the donor, of the recipient woman and of her husband, if she is married, as well as the fact that artificial insemination was used. Therefore a physician or center receiving donations of semen or administering artificial insemination is required to keep secret the names and nay other information which could lead to the identification of the donor, the recipient woman and her husband, and moreover they must equally keep secret the fact that any particular birth results from artificial insemination.

22. The article however allows exceptions to the rules of secrecy in the case of proceedings before a court, for instance when an action is brought to contest the legitimacy of the child.

In this case the physician is authorized to reveal the existence of the artificial insemination, identity of the woman and her husband and the existence of their consent. The identity of the donor must never be revealed; a rule to the contrary might have the effect of discouraging donations of semen. The secrecy of the identity of the donor is therefore an absolute rule to which there are no exceptions.

23. The article also requires the physician to refuse to administer artificial insemination when the circumstances in which it is carried out would put at risk the maintenance of the secret. For example in certain cases family or other links between the donor and the woman or her husband might emerge, for example, from the sudden and undesirable discovery that the real father is a close relative or friend of the family..

ARTICLE 6

24. Paragraph 1 of this article is on the same lines as Article 9 of the rules annexed to Resolution (78) 29 on harmonization of the legislation of member States relating to the removal, grafting and transplantation of human substances, and which is based on the legal principle existing in most member States which treats human substances as *res extra commercium*. Semen being a human substance, the donor can receive no material consideration for his donation. However, on the same principle as in Article 9 of the annexed rules to the above-mentioned Resolution, the loss of earnings and travelling and other expenses incurred as a direct restult of the donation may be refunded to the donor.

25. Paragraph 2 prohibits the transfer of semen for profit by those who receive, conserve and treat it. It is worthwhile, however, pointing out that only profit is prohibited; the cost of production may be recovered.

ARTICLE 7

26. Where a State law has accepted that artificial insemination is a permissible medical practice, it would be illogical for it to give anyone the right to dispute the legitimacy of a child conceived by artificial insemination with the consent of the husband merely on that account. This article therefore provides that in such a case the child shall be considered as the legitimate child of the woman and her husband and that no-one may dispute the child's legitimacy on the sole ground of artificial insemination. This article covering only the case where birth results from artificial insemination, is not intended to lead to any other change in the legal provisions in force in member States which give the husband, or other interested persons, the right to dispute the child's legitimacy on grounds other than that of artificial insemination.

27. Paragraph 2 of this article prohibits the establishment of a link of affiliation between the donor and the child on the ground of artificial insemination. This is quite logical because the donor does not intend to have a child of his own, but simply to make artificial insemination possible. If the child, the mother or any other interested person had the right to bring proceedings to establish his paternity against the donor, despite the promised secrecy, very few men would feel inclined to donate their semen. As the establishment of any link of affiliation between the donor and the child is prohibited, the rules also forbid maintenance proceedings between the two.

* Reprinted with permission from David G and Price WS (1980) (eds.) Human Artificial Insemination and Semen Preservation; New York and London: Plenum Press.

SUBJECT INDEX